PRINCIPLES OF CANCER RECONSTRUCTIVE SURGERY

PRINCIPLES OF CANCER RECONSTRUCTIVE SURGERY

Edited by

Charles E. Butler, MD, FACS
The University of Texas M. D. Anderson Cancer Center
Houston, Texas, USA

Neil A. Fine, MD, FACS
Northwestern University Feinberg School of Medicine
Chicago, Illinois, USA

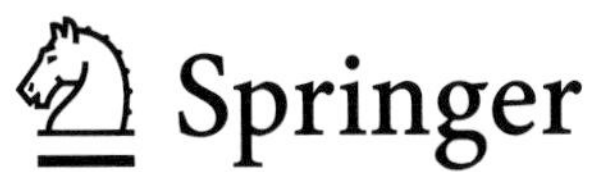

Editors
Charles E. Butler, MD, FACS
Department of Plastic Surgery
Division of Surgery
The University of Texas M. D. Anderson Cancer Center
Houston, TX 77230, USA

Neil A. Fine, MD, FACS
Division of Plastic Surgery
Department of Surgery
Northwestern University Feinberg School of Medicine
Chicago, IL 60611, USA

ISBN: 978-0-387-49502-6 e-ISBN: 978-0-387-49504-0
DOI: 10.1007/978-0-387-49504-0

Library of Congress Control Number: 2006939124

Printed on acid-free paper

9 8 7 6 5 4 3 2 1

springer.com

To Angel, Sophie, and Sadie for their eternal support and inspiration.

—CEB

To my parents, Glen and Cynthia, for getting me started on this path. To my children, Neil and Peter, for the joy that they have brought to my life. And to my wife Karen, for her 25 years of patience and support.

—NAF

Preface

Principles of Cancer Reconstructive Surgery is a reference text for medical and surgical oncologists, radiation oncologists, family practice physicians and dermatologists, providing an overview of reconstructive procedures. Interested residents, medical students, and health care professionals will find this an important resource designed to educate those involved with the management of cancer patients.

The disease-specific format facilitates quick reference for focusing on a single body area or disease. The most commonly occurring cancers, breast, melanoma, and head and neck, are covered in an overview chapter and in greater detail individually, with 300 color illustrations in a format that provides excellent detail and clarity.

Charles E. Butler, MD, FACS
Neil A. Fine, MD, FACS

Contents

Contributors

S. Baumeister, MD
Division of Plastic and Reconstructive Surgery, Duke University Medical Center, Durham, NC 27710, USA

Elisabeth K. Beahm, MD
Department of Plastic Surgery, Division of Surgery, The University of Texas M. D. Anderson Cancer Center, Houston, TX 77230-1402, USA

Gary C. Burget, MD
Department of Surgery, University of Chicago Medical Center, Chicago, IL 60657, USA

Charles E. Butler, MD, FACS
Department of Plastic Surgery, Division of Surgery, The University of Texas M. D. Anderson Cancer Center, Houston, TX 77230, USA

Joseph J. Disa, MD
Plastic and Reconstructive Surgery Service, Department of Surgery, Memorial Sloan-Kettering Cancer Center, New York, NY 10021, USA

Gregory A. Dumanian, MD
Division of Plastic Surgery, Department of Surgery, Northwestern University Feinberg School of Medicine, Chicago, IL 60611, USA

Neil A. Fine, MD, FACS
Division of Plastic Surgery, Department of Surgery, Northwestern University Feinberg School of Medicine, Chicago, IL 60611, USA

Ida K. Fox, MD
Washington University School of Medicine, St. Louis, MO 63139, USA

Margo Herron, MD
Department of Surgery, Southern Illinois University School of Medicine, Springfield, IL 62794-9653, USA

John Y.S. Kim, MD
Division of Plastic Surgery, Department of Surgery, Northwestern University Feinberg School of Medicine, Chicago, IL 60611, USA

Steven J. Kronowitz, MD
Department of Plastic Surgery, Division of Surgery, The University of Texas M. D. Anderson Cancer Center, Houston, TX 77230-1402, USA

Howard N. Langstein, MD
Division of Plastic Surgery, University of Rochester School of Medicine, Rochester, NY 14642, USA

L. Scott Levin, MD
Division of Plastic and Reconstructive Surgery, Duke University Medical Center, Durham, NC 27710, USA

H. Levinson, MD
Division of Plastic and Reconstructive Surgery, Duke University Medical Center, Durham, NC 27710, USA

Joan E. Lipa, MD
University of Toronto, Division of Plastic Surgery, Department of Surgery and Department of Surgical Oncology, Toronto General Hospital, University Health Network, Toronto, Ontario, Canada M5G 2C4

Colleen M. McCarthy, MD
Plastic and Reconstructive Surgery Service, Department of Surgery, Memorial Sloan-Kettering Cancer Center, New York, NY 10021, USA

Michael J. Miller, MD
Division of Plastic Surgery, The Ohio State University, Columbus, OH 43210, USA

Peter C. Neligan, MD
Division of Plastic Surgery, University of Washington Medical Center, Seattle, WA 98195, USA

Michael W. Neumeister, MD
Department of Surgery, Southern Illinois University School of Medicine, Springfield, IL 62794-9653, USA

Geoffrey L. Robb, MD
Department of Plastic Surgery, Division of Surgery, The University of Texas M. D. Anderson Cancer Center, Houston, TX 77230-1402, USA

Joseph M. Serletti, MD
Plastic and Reconstructive Surgery, Department of Surgery, University of Pennsylvania, Philadelphia, PA 19104, USA

Jeremy Waldman, MD
Division of Plastic Surgery, University of Rochester School of Medicine, Rochester, NY 14642, USA

Robert L. Walton, MD
Plastic Surgery Chicago, LLC, Chicago, IL 60611, USA

M. Zenn, MD
Division of Plastic and Reconstructive Surgery, Duke University Medical Center, Durham, NC 27710, USA

1

Plastic Surgery

A Component in the Comprehensive Care of Cancer Patients

Neil A. Fine and Charles E. Butler

Comprehensive cancer centers in the United States interweave subspecialty care from multiple disciplines. These centers' very existence is testimony to the broad interdisciplinary approach to cancer care today. Plastic surgery, with its ability to restore form and function, represents a small but critical component of the comprehensive care of patients with cancer. Plastic surgical reconstruction extends the capabilities of surgery and radiation therapy for patients with cancer. Without plastic surgery, many extirpative cancer surgeries could not be performed or would result in mutilating deformities. In addition, reconstructive surgery can facilitate the delivery of adjuvant radiotherapy and/or reconstruct tissue damaged by its effects. Cancer and complications of cancer treatment can involve virtually any area of the body; therefore, plastic surgeons may be called upon to address reconstructive challenges in any area of the body, from head to toe. A multi-disciplinary team approach is the optimal method of cancer treatment, and plastic surgical reconstruction, with its ability to restore form and function to the involved areas, is a critical component of that treatment. This book provides an overview of the role of plastic surgery in the multi-disciplinary approach to cancer treatment.

General Role of Plastic Surgery

Plastic surgery's primary role in cancer care is extending the ability of other surgeons and specialists to more radically or effectively treat cancer, thus offering the patient the best opportunity for cure. The contributions of plastic surgeons have enabled many advances in the treatment of breast cancer, head and neck cancers, sarcoma, and other cancers. Surgical oncology is not the only discipline that has been impacted by plastic surgery. Radiation therapy options are extended when well-vascularized tissue covers the planned area of treatment. For example, the use of soft tissue flaps enables the insertion of brachytherapy catheters for delivery of post-operative brachytherapy to large surface area wounds, which would not be possible without overlying vascularized tissue.

Plastic surgeons also interact with and advance the care given by medical oncologists in two ways. First, plastic surgery can provide well-vascularized tissue coverage to resection defects, allowing the medical oncologist to begin chemotherapy earlier after surgery by reducing the risk of infections and wound-healing complications that might delay chemotherapy. Second, plastic surgeons can aid in the treatment of infiltrates of chemotherapeutic agents and other medications into subcutaneous tissues. Prompt injection of diluting and dispersing agents can limit skin loss, and proper treatment of open wounds, with moist dressings and extremity elevation, can hasten healing. A plastic surgeon can provide advice on these treatments and perform flap or skin graft closure of wounds when necessary *(1–6)*.

Plastic surgical reconstruction can also help patients recover from the psychological impact of oncologic surgery. Although the most substantial data documenting improved psychosocial well being in cancer patients exist for breast reconstruction after mastectomy, it is reasonable to assume that most cancer patients who undergo major reconstruction to minimize deformity caused by cancer therapy feel some overall improvement in quality of life.

In major cancer centers, plastic surgeons deal with a large variety of defects in all areas of the body. Some of the most common referrals for reconstruction include those for breast, head and neck, and sarcoma.

Breast Cancer

Women who choose not to have reconstruction can adjust well psychologically to their new body image; but for women who desire reconstruction, the reconstruction offers significant psychological benefits *(7–9)*. For women who choose reconstruction, the decision of which type of breast reconstruction to use, and the timing of the reconstruction, should be individualized for each breast cancer patient *(10–12)*. It is crucial to have open and accurate communication with not only the patient but also the breast surgeon, medical oncologist, and radiation oncologist, whose treatment plan will influence the potential reconstructive options and the procedure ultimately selected.

The need for post-mastectomy radiation is frequently a major factor in deciding between a prosthesis (tissue expander and/or implant), autologous tissue (e.g., transverse rectus abdominis myocutaneous [TRAM] or latissimus dorsi [LD] flap), or a combination (e.g., LD flap over an implant) for breast reconstruction and between immediate and delayed reconstruction *(13–15)*. However, this need often cannot be determined pre- or intraoperatively. Final pathologic assessment of the mastectomy specimens and axillary lymph node(s) commonly determines whether breast cancer patients will receive radiation therapy.

Reconstructive surgeons are often reluctant to perform immediate reconstruction in patients who are at increased risk for needing post-operative radiation therapy. The alternative choice is a delayed reconstruction; however, with a delayed reconstruction, the shape of the breast skin envelope is not preserved, and the final outcome may be less aesthetically successful than immediate reconstruction. In addition, delayed reconstruction subjects the patient to additional surgical procedure(s) and does not provide the psychologic benefit of having a reconstructed breast mound immediately following mastectomy *(10,11)*. Using a tissue expander to preserve the shape of the breast skin envelope as a temporary first step is one approach to this problem. This provides time for the patient and surgeon to decide what type of definitive reconstruction will be performed. This approach may be particularly helpful when there is concern whether the patient will receive post-operative radiation therapy. Another approach is to delay breast reconstruction for women who are at "higher risk" for receiving post-mastectomy radiation therapy.

Women contemplating post-mastectomy breast reconstruction should be advised to undergo a pre-mastectomy workup, which will provide the best possible assessment of their risk of nodal involvement. This should include a detailed physical examination, diagnostic mammography, and possibly ultrasonography of the breast and regional nodal basins with fine-needle aspiration biopsy of suspicious nodes. With information from this workup, the woman and surgeon, together, can make a more informed decision regarding the method and timing of reconstruction.

Breast reconstruction is a mix of reconstructive and aesthetic ideals. Breast reconstruction is much more than closing a chest wound or filling in a defect. How the reconstructed breast looks after completion of the reconstruction is important. In many patients, particularly those with large, pendulous breasts or small breasts without rounded contours, the symmetry of the reconstruction can be significantly improved by reducing or lifting the contralateral breast or by placing a subpectoral implant beneath it to give it a rounded shape.

There are three main forms of breast reconstruction: an expander/implant, an LD flap with or without a permanent implant, and a TRAM flap or related abdominal tissue flap. During the initial consultation, our patients are given the choice between these options, with a discussion of the pros and cons of each.

Expander/Implant Reconstruction

The use of a tissue expander followed by insertion of a saline- or silicone-filled prosthesis is the most common method of breast reconstruction in the United States. For patients who after discussion remain uncertain about the type of breast reconstruction to choose, this technique is the most advisable. This method has the lowest morbidity of the options available and does not prevent the use of other reconstructive techniques if the patient changes her mind in the future *(16)*. In addition, the tissue expander/implant technique is the least invasive option, maintains the shape of the breast skin envelope, and does not involve surgery outside the breast area.

Placement of a tissue expander at the time of mastectomy can be seen as the first step in a planned multi-step procedure that ultimately produces a fully reconstructed breast. Although this strategy "burns no bridges," choosing and performing the reconstructive option best suited for the patient as the primary procedure, whenever possible, reduces the potential need for additional operative procedures. Every attempt should be made to educate the patient about each available option, including a detailed comparison of the risks, complications, expected outcomes, and recovery times. Information sources that may be helpful to patients include written materials, diagrams, photographs, videos, and discussions with other patients who have had each procedure (including those who have had both positive and negative experiences). All this information may prove to be too much for some women, who are also having to deal with a newly diagnosed cancer; for them, delaying the final decision by placing an expander may provide enough emotional relief from having to make a decision to warrant the possible extra surgical step in their reconstruction. This issue has taken on more significance as the number of women who receive radiation after mastectomy grows. Temporarily placing the expander at the time of mastectomy allows a skin-sparing mastectomy to be performed, but prevents the risk of radiation damage to autologous tissue flaps.

The expander is a durable implant that has a built-in, self-sealing access port, much the same as an implanted venous access device for chemotherapy. The port allows a standard needle to be inserted through the partially denervated mastectomy flap to gradually add fluid to the expander. The expander is filled only partially when inserted to avoid placing undue tension on the mastectomy flaps, which will have been vascularly compromised by the removal of the underlying breast tissue that normally carries the primary blood supply to the breast skin. Inserting the expander only partially filled allows the skin to recover; typically, expansion begins in the office 1 to 3 weeks after surgery. The expander is replaced with a permanent implant later.

The expander/implant reconstruction has several advantages. Not only can this type of reconstruction be performed through the mastectomy incision, but it is the only type of reconstruction that does not require a donor site incision on another part of the body. The overall magnitude of surgery is less, and recovery is faster than autologous tissue flap reconstruction. Patients who have a tissue expander placed immediately after mastectomy usually spend the same amount of time in the hospital as mastectomy-only patients.

The use of an expander is limited by the quality and availability of the overlying soft tissues and skin of the breast. This type of reconstruction will not typically produce any ptosis (drooping) of the reconstructed breast. Therefore, procedures on the opposite breast are more commonly needed with expander/implant reconstruction than with LD or TRAM flap reconstruction. This reliance on the overlying tissue is the reason radiation has a relatively profound effect on this type of reconstruction. There is no question that the complication rate is higher with expander/implant reconstruction in patients that receive pre-operative or post-operative radiation therapy *(13)*. This leads to controversy regarding the advisability of performing an implant reconstruction in irradiated patients. Many believe it is acceptable as long as the patient is informed of the increased risk of a firm, sometimes painful breast mound that may necessitate implant removal and/or a second reconstruction with an LD flap plus implant or a TRAM flap. Many other reconstructive surgeons are reluctant to use tissue expander/implant reconstruction in patients who have had or will receive chest wall radiation therapy, particularly if an autologous tissue reconstructive option is available.

Another potential disadvantage of expander/implant reconstructions is the way the reconstructed breast looks and feels without clothing. Since the implant is composed of a silicone shell filled with saline or silicone gel, the reconstructed breast does not have the same feel and contour as a natural breast. The visual difference is minimized in bilateral reconstruction; the symmetric appearance of two implant-reconstructed breasts gives the illusion of a more natural result.

LD Flap with Implant

The LD flap represents the next level of reconstruction beyond an implant alone. The LD flap can be used with or without an implant underneath, depending on volume needs. LD reconstruction is most often chosen by patients who desire a more natural result and yet do not want to or cannot utilize abdominal tissue. The LD muscle is a powerful adductor of the arm, pulling the arm down, towards the body. Although there is rarely any noticeable weakness associated with harvest of the LD muscle, the strength of this muscle could be missed by athletes, so women should be asked if they are seriously involved in activities that require a strong downward pull of the arm (e.g., chin-ups, rock climbing, or competitive swimming).

When compared with the expander/implant option, the LD procedure often provides a superior aesthetic result *(17,18)*. Because the implant reconstruction (even with a LD flap) is associated with increased complications when radiation therapy is used, many surgeons are reluctant to perform this operation on a woman who is likely to receive postoperative radiation therapy. Although this flap may not be recommended prior to radiation, its use after radiation is well accepted. A major benefit of an LD flap plus implant reconstruction over a tissue expander/implant reconstruction is the ability to create a breast mound at the time of mastectomy (usually without the need for serial tissue expansion and/or expander-implant exchange).

When an LD flap is harvested for breast reconstruction, an elliptical paddle of skin is elevated along with the underlying muscle. The incision may be placed either horizontally, to hide under the bra line, or obliquely, to allow open-back clothing to be worn, or obliquely along the resting skin tension lines. The choice of the incision angle and location, as with the type of reconstruction, should be discussed with the patient so the surgery may be tailored as much as possible to her needs.

The muscle and skin unit are transposed from the back to the front, transferring the skin and soft tissue into the mastectomy defect to partially replace the breast tissue. The skin, nipple-areola, and biopsy sites that are removed by the mastectomy typically can be fully replaced with skin from the flap. The muscle and overlying skin paddle provides a thicker tissue layer over the implant, resulting in less implant palpability, a softer feel of the breast, a better overall aesthetic outcome, and a lower implant complication rate. However, the volume of the breast is rarely matched with soft tissue from the flap alone. Although an implant is still required to make up this volume difference, the tissue that is transferred decreases the size of implant required to match the opposite, leading to a more natural look and feel. The primary advantage of the LD flap over an expander/implant alone is thus that the skin is replaced, maintaining the natural skin envelope, a smaller implant is required, and more tissue covers the implant.

Abdominal Flaps

In many women, there is sufficient abdominal tissue, both skin and adipose tissue, to completely reconstruct the breast using an abdominal flap. This type of reconstruction results in the most natural look and feel of the three major types of reconstruction. The skin of the abdomen replaces the skin that is removed at the time of the mastectomy, recreating the natural skin envelope, an advantage shared by LD flap reconstruction. Abdominal flap procedures, as opposed to an LD flap, are ideal for patients who do not want to have an implant. Abdominal flaps are also more effective in recreating ptosis and reducing the likelihood that symmetry surgery will be needed on the opposite breast. In addition, a breast reconstructed with an abdominal flap will move and shift with position changes, in a manner that closely matches that of a natural breast. Furthermore, the flap will change volume with fluctuations in weight: the abdominal flap will increase in size with weight gain and decrease with weight loss. The magnitude of the change may closely match changes in the opposite breast.

There are significant trade-offs for the benefits obtained with an abdominal flap. This option represents the largest magnitude of surgical breast reconstruction procedures. There is a scar on the abdomen, extending across the lower abdominal crease. The abdominal wall may be weakened by the removal of or dissection through the rectus abdominis muscle; this possibility needs to be discussed with the patient. Patients who choose this option usually see the abdominal trade-off in a positive light: the abdominal flap is viewed much like an abdominoplasty, improving abdominal contour. Those who feel that the flattening of their abdomen and the sight of a scar on the abdomen will have an overall negative impact often choose another form of reconstruction.

The TRAM flap is the most traditional and best-known abdominal flap. This flap typically uses the entire rectus abdominis muscle on one side based on the superior epigastric vessels, which are an extension of the internal mammary vessels. The free TRAM flap uses only the lower portion of the rectus abdominis muscle supplied by the deep inferior epigastric blood vessels; these vessels are anastomosed to recipient vessels in the chest wall using microvascular techniques. The impact of various amounts of rectus abdominis muscle included with the flap transfer is, however, a controversial issue in plastic surgery today. The rectus abdominis muscle serves only as a carrier or conduit for blood flow to the skin and subcutaneous fatty tissues in the reconstructed breast. The muscle itself does not contribute significantly to the volume of the breast reconstruction. Therefore, various muscle-sparing flaps have been developed and are being investigated in an effort to minimize abdominal morbidity.

The deep inferior epigastric perforator (DIEP) flap is similar to the free TRAM flap except that additional dissection is done to leave the muscle on the abdomen (by intramuscular dissection of the blood supply to the abdominal skin) and only the skin, fat, and blood vessels of the lower abdomen are transferred. However, some surgeons feel that the dissection through the rectus abdominis muscle inherent in the DIEP flap denervates the muscle and leaves an abdomen in much the same condition as the free TRAM flap.

The superficial inferior epigastric artery (SIEA) flap involves transfer of the lower abdominal skin and fat, this time with the superficial blood vessels so that the rectus abdominis muscle and its overlying fascia is not incised or removed. From a donor site perspective, this is the best reconstruction *(19)*. However, not all women have an adequate superficial blood vessel system for the SIEA flap.

The advantage of the more advanced microvascular transfers is clear: less damage to the abdominal muscle and overlying fascia. They are, however, more complicated, and the vascular supply may not be as reliable. This means that more complicated reconstructions carry an increased risk for partial or total flap loss, as well as increasing the risk for return to the operating room for vessel repair. Finally, longer surgery and return trips to the operating room increase the potential for blood transfusion.

The most commonly used abdominal flap in the United States remains a single-pedicled TRAM flap based on a single (left or right) rectus abdominis muscle to supply blood flow via an uninterrupted connection to the superior epigastric artery. However, the blood supply provided by the superior epigastric artery is not always sufficient for the volume of tissue that may be required for a reconstruction. Increased blood flow may be obtained by performing a free TRAM flap. A free TRAM flap uses the larger-caliber inferior epigastric vessels along with only a portion of one side of the rectus abdominis muscle, the portion containing the main perforating vessels or connecting vessels to the skin and subcutaneous tissue. This tissue, along with the inferior epigastric vessels, is completely disconnected from its native circulation. This "free" flap is then placed on the chest, and the artery and vein are reconnected to blood vessels in the chest or axilla under microscopic magnification. A free TRAM flap has several advantages over a pedicled TRAM flap, including increased blood flow, less rectus abdominis muscle harvest, and less medial chest wall dissection *(20)*. The greater vascularity of the free, compared to the pedicled, TRAM flap also allows for a greater volume of flap tissue to be reliably used and may reduce the risk of partial-flap necrosis and fat necrosis. This is particularly beneficial for patients with compromised vascularity of the TRAM tissue, such as tobacco users. The free TRAM and its modifications are technically more challenging than a pedicled TRAM flap, and whether they can be performed depends on both the patient's vascular anatomy and the surgeon's familiarity with these procedures.

Reconstruction for Lumpectomy Defects

The combination of lumpectomy and radiation therapy is a well-established treatment for breast cancer. One of the main factors in deciding if a patient is a candidate for this breast-conserving therapy is the size of the tumor relative to the size of the breast. As the relative size of the excision increases, so does the resultant deformity. At some point, the deformity becomes so pronounced that a mastectomy becomes a more appropriate option. The point at which this occurs varies depending upon the patient's and surgeon's willingness to accept deformity in return for conservation of some remaining breast tissue and the nipple/areola, with its sensation. Reconstruction is an option when a large lumpectomy defect is anticipated *(21,22)*. The reconstruction may be either delayed-immediate or delayed. Delayed-immediate is surgery performed after final pathology but before radiation therapy. Usually this means 1–3 weeks after the extirpative procedure. Delayed reconstruction is performed after radiation, typically 6–12 months after, to allow for stabilization of the radiation effect on the tissues. As with post-mastectomy reconstruction, there are advantages to delayed-immediate reconstruction in most cases. The reconstruction is often combined with a lymph node dissection if that procedure is required. Thus, the sequence would be: (1) initial biopsy; (2) lumpectomy with or without sentinel node biopsy; and (3) reconstruction with or without lymph node dissection, after final pathology results are known.

Many methods are available for repair of partial breast defects. These can generally be divided into three groups: (1) rearrangement of remaining breast tissue; (2) transfer of additional autologous tissue; and (3) placement of a subpectoral implant.

Women with large breasts, especially those who would benefit from, or be accepting of, breast reduction can often be treated with a local rearrangement of tissue on the affected breast and a breast reduction for symmetry on the opposite side. Other local rearrangement options may also be available depending on individual anatomic considerations *(23)*.

Transferring new tissue into the defect offers the most potential to return the breast as closely as possible to its pre-lumpectomy state *(24)*. New tissue can be provided with an LD muscle flap *(25)*. This flap has multiple advantages; the most important is its reliability. It also is readily available at the time of axillary lymph node dissection and may even be harvested through an extension of the axillary incision with endoscopic assistance. When flap harvest is performed in this manner, there is no scar on the back. If the equipment and technical expertise to perform an endoscopic harvest are not available, a limited incision to harvest the LD muscle may be employed. Increased tissue volume may be obtained with a skin paddle. A TRAM flap also may be used to repair a partial breast defect, but its use is probably best reserved for mastectomy defects.

Finally, if the defect is centrally located, or deeply located, a subpectoral implant may suffice for post-lumpectomy reconstruction. The implant is usually placed in the submuscular position to minimize interference with post-operative mammograms. Although the implant may not be able to correct surface irregularities when placed submuscularly, it will be able to compensate for overall volume loss. An important part of this reconstruction option is a discussion of the increased risk of capsular contracture in patients who have received radiation. This increased risk must be understood by the patient.

Nipple/Areola Reconstruction

Reconstruction of the nipple and areola often represents the final step in the restoration of the breast. Several techniques have been described. We currently favor the use of a local flap of skin, fashioned into a nipple shape *(26)*. The newly created nipple and surrounding skin are tattooed 6–10 weeks after the nipple reconstruction to create the areola. This avoids creating a donor defect elsewhere in the body.

Head and Neck Cancers

This book also addresses repair of head and neck oncologic defects. The flap choice for head and neck reconstruction should be based on the characteristics of the resection defect, including the thickness or bulk of the tissue required, the need for a bone component, and the amount of skin required for oral lining. Smaller defects are usually closed primarily, or with local flaps *(27)*. As defects become larger, regional flaps (primarily pectoralis major flaps) are utilized. The pectoralis major flap is particularly useful in the neck because it reaches the site easily and its bulk is well tolerated. Excess stretching of the pectoralis major flap to reach higher into the oral cavity increases the risk of complications, especially fistula formation. For larger defects in the face and intraoral areas above the neck, free tissue transfer has replaced the pectoralis and other regional flaps *(28,29)*.

Free flap reconstruction has become much more commonly performed in the plastic surgery community. More experience with free flap reconstruction has resulted in a decrease in operative time, flap loss, and other complications. Most large centers now report free flap success rates greater than 95% in head and neck reconstruction *(30,31)*. With free flaps offering better functional results and improved aesthetic outcomes, most patients who undergo significant head or neck resections are candidates for immediate free flap reconstruction *(32,33)*.

The free radial forearm flap is an excellent choice for many head and neck defects, particularly when intraoral tissue is needed, because it provides thin, pliable, skin-containing tissue. Other good options when thin tissue is required are the anterolateral thigh flap and lateral arm flap. A free vertical rectus abdominis myocutaneous flap is a good choice when both bulk and intraoral lining are required, such as for total glossectomy defects. When intraoral defects, such as hemiglossectomy defects, do not significantly involve the floor of the mouth and/or base of the tongue, reconstruction can often be performed with primary closure, skin grafting, and/or secondary intention healing with a good functional outcome.

For mandibular reconstruction, the free fibula flap is the "workhorse" flap, owing to its long, bicortical vascularized bone; the ability to cut the bone into multiple individually vascularized segments, which are plated together to accurately restore the natural shape of the missing mandible; and the ability to include a thin skin paddle with the flap for intraoral lining. The use of a soft-tissue-only reconstruction (such as a free vertical rectus abdominis myocutaneous flap), however, is an acceptable alternative for posterior mandibular defects, particularly when the condyle is resected.

In facial reconstruction, excellent functional and aesthetic results can be achieved with a local flap by following two basic principles: replace missing tissue with "like" tissue (such as reconstructing lip defects with remaining lip tissue), and repair defects on the face using the "aesthetic subunit" principle when possible. Skin grafts can also be acceptable reconstructive options for facial defects. Full-thickness grafts taken from the head and neck region usually provide a better aesthetic outcome because they contract less and have a better color match than do split-thickness grafts and grafts harvested from other regions.

Intraoral Defects

Most large intraoral defects, including tongue resections of less than 70%, are best reconstructed with free radial forearm flaps. The radial forearm flap is preferably taken from the nondominant arm, as long as an Allen's test confirms adequate blood flow to the hand via the ulnar artery. This flap offers thin, pliable, and usually hairless tissue and is highly reliable in reconstructing intraoral defects. The donor site on the arm is closed with a skin graft, and post-operative complications are rare.

Providing sensation to intraoral flaps is an area of controversy and ongoing research. Kimata and coworkers reported increased sensitivity in free anterolateral thigh flaps and TRAM flaps used for intraoral reconstruction when the cutaneous nerves were anastomosed to a divided hypoglossal nerve or lingual nerve *(34)*. Their study demonstrated that the number and type of end sensory organs in the skin of the forearm are not the limiting factor in restoring intraoral sensibility.

Small intraoral defects that can be closed primarily without restricting jaw excursion or tongue mobility should be closed primarily*(27)*. Slightly larger defects may be left open to contract and re-epithelialize, but caution should be taken to ensure contracture does not limit jaw or tongue motion.

Mandibular Defects

Most anterior mandibular bony defects are now being reconstructed with microvascular fibula transfer *(30)*. The fibula offers strong, cortical bone of sufficient length to reconstruct any magnitude of mandibular resection. In addition, the bicortical nature of the fibula allows for the use of osseo-integrated implants for dental rehabilitation.

The fibula receives its vascular supply from the peroneal vessels. Just as the Allen's test is used to ensure that blood flow to the hand will be adequate after harvest of the radial artery, evaluation of pedal pulses is done to ensure that blood flow to the foot will remain adequate after removal of the peroneal artery with the fibula. If a patient has palpable dorsalis pedis and posterior tibial pulses, the risk of vascular compromise from harvest of the peroneal artery is low. If one or both of the pedal pulses are absent on the side of the planned fibula harvest, the peroneal vessel may be absent or severely diseased, or it may be the only vessel supplying the foot. In a patient without normal pedal pulses, an angiogram is indicated to evaluate the vascular supply of the legs and determine whether the fibula can be safely used.

When the fibula is not available, free tissue transfer from other bony sites may be possible. The iliac crest offers abundant bone, but the soft tissue component of flaps from this site is bulky, and the hip donor site defect is more problematic than the leg donor site defect after a fibula harvest. The scapula and radius, as part of the radial forearm flap, offer thin soft tissue and acceptable donor site morbidity, but the quality and amount of bone available for transfer are limited.

If the mandibular defect is lateral and/or posterior, it may be reconstructed with a plate and/or a soft tissue flap. However, anterior defects, even small ones, require bony reconstruction because plate-only reconstruction in this region has a very high failure rate and soft-tissue-only flaps do not maintain the anterior projection of the mandible. If radiation will not be given post-operatively and has not been given pre-operatively, then conventional, non-vascularized bone grafts may be considered.

Defects of Pharynx and Cervical Esophagus

Plastic surgeons become involved with cervical esophageal and pharyngeal reconstructions when flap reconstruction is needed instead of, or in addition to, more traditional procedures like gastric pull-up or colonic interposition. The classic flap used at these sites is a pectoralis major myocutaneous flap. This pedicled flap does not require microvascular anastomosis and thus adds little time to what is usually an already complicated resection and reconstruction procedure. This flap also may be used for patching defects, although not segmented ones. The flap's disadvantages are its less reliable blood supply and added bulk compared with free flap alternatives. The donor site defect may also be deforming for female patients.

Free tissue transfer brings added complexity but also offers significant advantages. For smaller defects, including smaller segmental esophageal defects, a radial forearm flap provides thin, well-vascularized tissue. This flap may be used as a patch or formed into a tube to replace a segment of the pharynx and/or esophagus.

Some surgeons feel that the free jejunal flap is the most versatile flap for reconstructing defects in this region *(35)*. This flap may be used as a patch or used for reconstruction of any size segment from the pharynx to esophagus at the thoracic inlet. A proximal segment of jejunum is harvested with a vascular pedicle from the superior mesenteric vessels.

Microvascular anastomosis to a branch of the external carotid artery and a suitably sized vein is facilitated by the exposure created for the tumor extirpation and neck dissection.

In recent years, free flaps that contain skin paddles, such as the radial forearm and anterolateral thigh flaps, have gained popularity for cervical esophageal reconstruction. These flaps are tubed to restore continuity between the pharynx and distal cervical esophagus. Some surgeons feel that tubed skin-containing free flaps have less donor site morbidity and better functional outcomes compared to a free jejunal flap reconstruction, including voice and swallowing rehabilitation.

Defects of Facial Skin and Soft Tissue

Defects of the skin and subcutaneous tissue of the head and neck can create both aesthetic and functional reconstructive challenges for plastic surgeons. The rich skin blood supply and laxity (especially in the elderly) in this region allow for many wounds to be closed primarily. However, patients with defects in certain locations of the face that may be closed primarily are sometimes better served by other methods because of the potential for distortion of key anatomic landmarks. Progressing from simple reconstructive options to a more complex solution is referred to as the "reconstructive ladder." Plastic surgeons are taught to first consider a simple option before deciding on a complex solution. Some defects are well suited to simple solutions, like primary closure or split- or full-thickness skin grafts. However, in certain locations skin grafts do not give an adequate aesthetic result in terms of contour and/or color. Local skin flaps, a step up the reconstructive ladder, frequently allow for closure of small wounds, often with good aesthetic results. Regional flaps based on known blood supplies allow for closure of larger defects. These larger flaps allow for the replacement of the "aesthetic subunits" of the nose or face as needed *(36)*. And at the complex top of the reconstructive ladder, free tissue transfer is used to cover large defects, especially when vital structures or tissues that cannot support a skin graft alone are exposed.

When the subunit principle is used in nasal reconstruction, horrifying deformities can be corrected with great success *(36)*. Small lesions can usually be closed by primary closure, skin grafting, or a local skin flap. An entire subunit or more can be covered with a forehead flap. The need to recreate the specialized layers of the nose (skin, cartilage, and nasal lining) makes nasal reconstruction a particularly challenging endeavor, usually requiring a multi-staged surgical approach. Three or four separate operations may be required to complete all elements of a nasal reconstruction.

Small defects of the lips may be closed primarily, but defects involving greater than approximately one-third of the upper or lower lip require tissue reconstruction. Because the lip is a specialized structure consisting of a muscular layer between skin and mucosal layers, it is best to try to recreate these layers. The Abbe flap is composed of a full-thickness segment from the unaffected lip based on the labial artery. The flap is transferred to the opposite lip with the labial artery pedicle still connected to the donor lip. This effectively sews segments of the upper and lower lip together. The vascular pedicle is then divided between 2 and 3 weeks after initial inset (once the flap tissue has developed new blood supply from the surrounding lip tissue). This restores the separation of the upper and lower lips, transferring a segment from one to the other (most commonly from the lower lip into a defect in the upper). Other, more complicated lip flaps have also been described, like the Karapandzic flap, which uses a rotation of lip and cheek tissue to replace missing lip tissue. With both of these techniques, no new lip tissue is added, just rearranged. This leads to a smaller oral opening, which can interfere with denture use. These methods are preferred because nothing is better than lip tissue, and to a point, a smaller oral opening is preferred to bringing in non-lip tissue. If the defect is so large and as to require replacement of lip tissue, a free flap is usually required.

Sarcoma

By incorporating plastic surgical flap reconstructions into the resection of sarcomas of the extremities, the amputation rate in sarcoma patients has been drastically reduced in the past several decades. Limb salvage procedures have been extended to tumors whose size or location had previously mandated amputation. The use of pedicled and free muscle and myocutaneous flaps enables closure of large wounds, allowing for earlier initiation of post-operative radiation therapy. Additionally, techniques such as tendon transfer and reconstruction of the blood vessels and nerves may be performed during limb salvage to improve functional rehabilitation.

Conclusion

Plastic surgical reconstruction has made a significant impact on the care of cancer patients. This introductory chapter highlights some of the reconstructive issues with the most common referrals to plastic surgery in a major cancer center: breast cancer, head and neck cancer, and sarcoma. Subsequent chapters will address these reconstructive issues in greater detail. Considerable reconstructive successes have also been achieved in numerous other areas of cancer treatment, including reconstruction of the vagina/perineum, lumbosacral area, chest/abdominal wall, scalp, ear, craniofacial region, and upper and lower extremities and repair of defects caused by radiation injury.

References

1. Albanell J, Baselga J. Systemic therapy emergencies. Semin Oncol 2000;27:347–361.
2. Disa JJ, Chang RR, Mucci SJ, Goldberg NH. Prevention of Adriamycin-induced full-thickness skin loss using hyaluronidase infiltration. Plast Reconstr Surg 1998;101:370–374.

3. Fenchel K, Karthaus M. Cytotoxic drug extravasation. Antibiot Chemother 2000;50:144–148.
4. Kassner E. Evaluation and treatment of chemotherapy extravasation injuries. J Pediatr Oncol Nurs 2000;17:135–148.
5. Vandeweyer E, Heymans O, Deraemaecker R. Extravasation injuries and emergency suction as treatment. Plast Reconstr Surg 2000;105:109–110.
6. Larson D. Treatment of tissue extravasation by antitumor agents. Cancer 1982;49:1796–1799.
7. Alderman AK, Wilkins EG, Lowery JC, Kim M, Davis JA. Determinants of patient satisfaction in postmastectomy breast reconstruction. Plast Reconstr Surg 2000;106:769–776.
8. Goin M, Goin J. Midlife reactions to mastectomy and subsequent breast reduction. Arch Gen Psychiatry 1981;38:225–227.
9. Mock V. Body image in women treated for breast cancer. Nurs Res 1993;42:153–157.
10. Contant C, van Wersch A, Wiggers T, Wai R, van Geel A. Motivations, satisfaction, and information of immediate breast reconstruction following mastectomy. Patient Educ Couns 2000;40:201–208.
11. Stevens L, McGrath M, Druss R, Kister S, Gump F, Forde K. The psychological impact of immediate breast reconstruction for women with early breast cancer. Plast Reconstr Surg 1984;73:619–628.
12. Brandberg Y, Malm M, Blomqvist L. A prospective and randomized study, "SVEA," comparing effects of three methods for delayed breast reconstruction on quality of life, patient-defined problem areas of life, and cosmetic result. Plast Reconstr Surg 2000;105:66–74; discussion 75–76.
13. Spear SL, Onyewu C. Staged breast reconstruction with saline-filled implants in the irradiated breast: recent trends and therapeutic implications. Plast Reconstr Surg 2000;105:930–942.
14. Tran NV, Evans GR, Kroll SS, et al. Postoperative adjuvant irradiation: effects on transverse rectus abdominis muscle flap breast reconstruction. Plast Reconstr Surg 2000;106:313–317; discussion 18–20.
15. Zimmerman RP, Mark RJ, Kim AI, et al. Radiation tolerance of transverse rectus abdominis myocutaneous-free flaps used in immediate breast reconstruction. Am J Clin Oncol 1998;21:381–385.
16. Collis N, Sharpe DT. Breast reconstruction by tissue expansion. A retrospective technical review of 197 two-stage delayed reconstructions following mastectomy for malignant breast disease in 189 patients. Br J Plast Surg 2000;53:37–41.
17. Gerber B, Krause A, Reimer T, Muller H, Friese K. Breast reconstruction with latissimus dorsi flap: improved aesthetic results after transection of its humeral insertion. Plast Reconstr Surg 1999;103:1876–1881.
18. Slavin SA, Schnitt SJ, Duda RB, et al. Skin-sparing mastectomy and immediate reconstruction: oncologic risks and aesthetic results in patients with early-stage breast cancer. Plast Reconstr Surg 1998;102:49–62.
19. Arnez ZM, Khan U, Pogorelec D, Planinsek F. Breast reconstruction using the free superficial inferior epigastric artery (SIEA) flap. Br J Plast Surg 1999;52:276–279.
20. Ross AC, Rusnak CH, Hill MK, et al. An analysis of breast cancer surgery after free transverse rectus abdominis myocutaneous (TRAM) flap reconstruction. Am J Surg 2000;179:412–416.
21. Clough KB, Cuminet J, Fitoussi A, Nos C, Mosseri V. Cosmetic sequelae after conservative treatment for breast cancer: classification and results of surgical correction. Ann Plast Surg 1998;41:471–481.

22. Clough KB, Kroll SS, Audretsch W. An approach to the repair of partial mastectomy defects. Plast Reconstr Surg 1999;104:409–420.
23. Gabka CJ, Baumeister RG, Maiwald G. Advancements of breast conserving therapy by onco-plastic surgery in the management of breast cancer. Anticancer Res 1998;18:2219–2224.
24. Papp C, Wechselberger G, Schoeller T. Autologous breast reconstruction after breast-conserving cancer surgery. Plast Reconstr Surg 1998;102:1932–1936; discussion 37–38.
25. Kat CC, Darcy CM, O'Donoghue JM, Taylor AR, Regan PJ. The use of the latissimus dorsi musculocutaneous flap for immediate correction of the deformity resulting from breast conservation surgery. Br J Plast Surg 1999;52:99–103.
26. Few JW, Marcus JR, Casas LA, Aitken ME, Redding J. Long-term predictable nipple projection following reconstruction. Plast Reconstr Surg 1999;104:1321–1324.
27. McConnel FM, Pauloski BR, Logemann JA, et al. Functional results of primary closure vs flaps in oropharyngeal reconstruction: a prospective study of speech and swallowing. Arch Otolaryngol Head Neck Surg 1998;124:625–630.
28. Kroll SS, Evans GR, Goldberg D, et al. A comparison of resource costs for head and neck reconstruction with free and pectoralis major flaps. Plast Reconstr Surg 1997;99:1282–1286.
29. Choi JO, Choi G, Chae SW, Jung KY. Combined use of pectoralis major myocutaneous and free radial forearm flaps for reconstruction of through-and-through defects from excision of head and neck cancers. J Otolaryngol 1999;28:332–336.
30. Schusterman MA, Miller MJ, Reece GP, Kroll SS, Marchi M, Goepfert H. A single center's experience with 308 free flaps for repair of head and neck cancer defects. Plast Reconstr Surg 1994;93:472–478; discussion 79–80.
31. Truelson JM, Leach JL, Close LG. Reliability of microvascular free flaps in head and neck reconstruction. Otolaryngol Head Neck Surg 1994;111:557–560.

2

The Principles of Cancer Reconstruction

Margo Herron and Michael W. Neumeister

The surgical management of various types of cancer offers some of the most challenging opportunities in reconstruction that plastic surgeons can face. Although obtaining adequate surgical margins should never compromise the gold standards of treatment, care should be taken to preserve functional and specialized tissue whenever possible, keeping the reconstruction plan in mind from the onset of the operation. The principles of cancer reconstruction are rather broad, but can be better understood by dividing them into five key points: evaluation of the defect, the surgical goals, surgical options, the operative procedure, and finally outcome analysis. It is not only the size, location, and properties of the resected tissue that are important, but also the overall health of the patient, the pre-morbid body habitus, and the potential detrimental effects on the donor site that lend information to plastic surgeons, allowing them to formulate a reconstructive option for the patient that offers the best possible outcome *(1)*.

A thorough evaluation of the defect is essential to (1) restore contour, (2) provide stable coverage at the defect, and (3) restore function *(2)*. A series of critical questions need to be answered to help identify which type of closure is best suited for any given resection (Table 2.1). There are various techniques of reconstruction that have application in the management of cancer resection. The smaller the resection defect, the more likely primary closure or local tissue rearrangement can be applied. This is seen routinely following excision of small skin cancers found on the trunk, extremities, or on the head and neck. Wounds closed under tension are prone to dehiscence or widening of the scar *(3)*. Dead space should be obliterated and all necrotic material debrided to avoid complications such as infection, hematoma, seroma, or skin and flap compromise *(4)*. If closure is to be accomplished with vascularized tissue, the various flaps need to be evaluated based on their composition, vascular supply, proximity to the wound, and movement (Table 2.2) *(1)*.

Defining the surgical goals for any given defect seems like a rather intuitive statement. Its importance, however, cannot be overemphasized. Put simply, the goals will define the type of reconstruction necessary to obtain the most appropriate closure. The "reconstructive ladder" includes

Table 2.1. Principles of Cancer Reconstruction

1. What is missing?
2. What function is lost?
3. Does the flap need to restore everything that is lost?
4. Which flap will provide the best contour?
5. Is vascularized bone, tendon, or nerve needed?
6. Is sensation in the flap required?
7. What amount of tissue is required for the reconstruction?
8. What will provide the best result: local, regional, distant, or free flap?
9. What type of reconstruction will provide the least donor site morbidity?
10. Which flap is more reliable?
11. What is the best color match?
12. Is a hair-bearing flap required?
13. Where are the recipient vessels?
14. Are vein grafts or vascular loops required?
15. Is radiation a factor either before or after surgery?
16. Is a staged procedure required?

progressively more complex procedures ranging from primary closure to skin grafts, local flaps, regional flaps, distant flaps, and ultimately to free tissue transfer. The optimal closure to restore form and function often dictates using the "reconstructive elevator," moving directly to free tissue transfer (the most complex option) at times *(1,2)*. For example, a through

Table 2.2. Classification of Flaps

Composition	Proximity to Wound
Fasciocutaneous	Local
Musculocutaneous	Regional
Osseocutaneous	Distant
Fascial	
Muscle	**Movement**
Osseous	Advancement
Bowel	Transposition
Omentum	Rotation
	Interpolation
Vascularity	Neurovascular pedicle
Random pattern	Free flap
Axial	
Antegrade/retrograde	
Island flap	
Free flap	
Perforator	

and through defect of the cheek and oral commissure may be readily closed with a folded, pedicled pectoralis major flap, but would leave a bulky, poorly contoured reconstruction. Alternatively, a free radial forearm harvested with the palmaris longus tendon would permit a better contour with commissure reconstruction. The palmaris longus tendon acts as a sling to support the commissure, preventing oral incontinence (Figure 2.1) *(5)*. Goals, therefore, should include closure, restoration of function, contour and symmetry balance, color match, and reliability. Another aspect of closure involves the concept of restoration of all tissues that have been resected *(1,2)*. It may not be necessary or advisable, in many cases, to reconstruct all of the missing tissues, including muscle, nerves, tendons, bone, or other specialized organs. The reconstruction of these tissues may in fact be detrimental to the patient, as it may only lead to donor site morbidity with scarring and loss

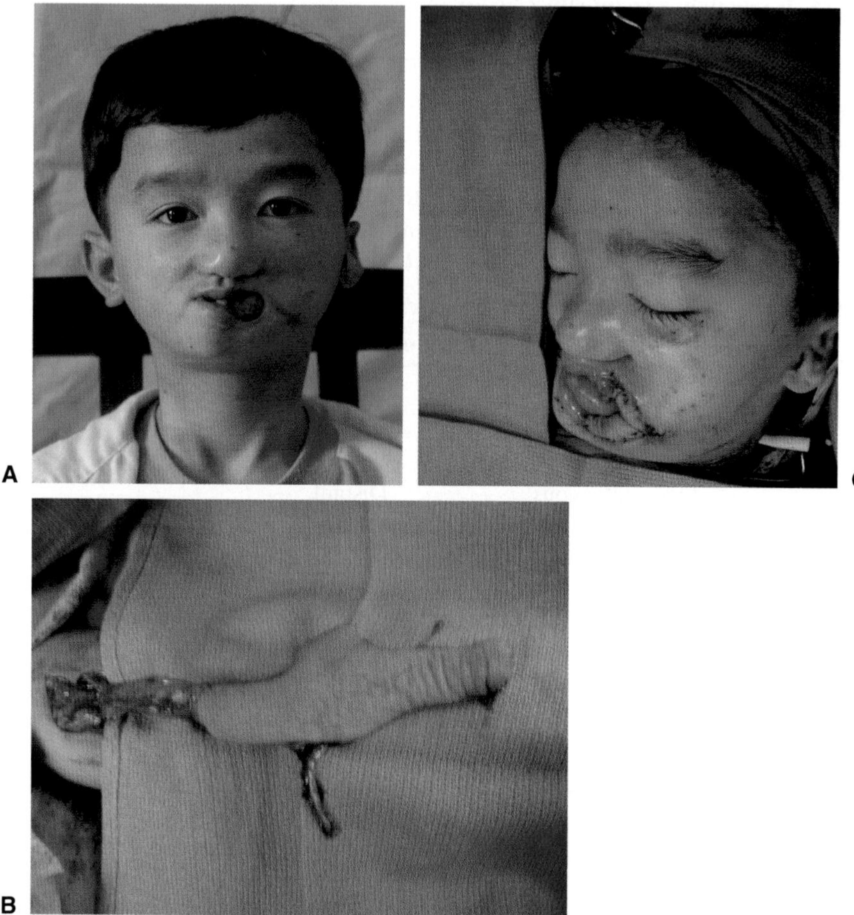

Figure 2.1. (**A**) A defect on the lateral aspect of the commissure requires soft tissue and support. (**B, C**) An appropriate flap that is thin and pliable that can be supported with the palmaris longus tendon is the radial forearm flap.

of function of other body parts. Some cancer resections may only be palliative, and the morbidity of composite reconstruction may not be warranted because by the time function is restored to the operative site, the patient may have succumbed to the disease. For instance, a palliative resection of a mandible and floor of the mouth may warrant a regional flap and reconstruction plate rather than an osteocutaneous flap. The surgical oncologist and the plastic surgeon need to work as a coordinated team with similar goals and sound communication to best treat such patients. If, on the other hand in the previous case, the patient resection deficit warrants a more definitive reconstruction, then further goals need to be defined. Now, the patient requires a vascularized bone flap and intra-oral lining. If dental rehabilitation with osseointegrated implants is planned, a free osteocutaneous flap such as a fibula or iliac crest should be used to allow intra-oral lining and enough bone stock for the implants (Figure 2.2). A radial forearm osteocutaneous flap would not provide enough bone for the osseointegrated implants and would therefore be a less than optimal choice for the reconstruction *(6,7)*. Similarly, a wide resection of a sarcoma in the forearm of an elderly patient would not warrant nerve and tendon graft reconstruction along with soft tissue coverage, as the likelihood of restoration of function is essentially negligible. Expendable tendon transfers and soft tissue coverage would be more appropriate for the aforementioned patient, with less likelihood of the need for secondary procedures. The goals of the treatment are therefore defined at least in part by a number of factors intrinsic to the nature of the cancer, to the resultant defect, and to the entirety of the patient.

The evaluation of the resection defect therefore requires a logical, comprehensive approach to provide optimal results and patient satisfaction. Many times, the reconstructive efforts necessitate three-dimensional planning. The donor tissue is shaped and contoured to the defect in all planes. In head and neck cancer reconstruction, for instance, it is not uncommon for the resection to include a portion of the maxilla, the palate, the maxillary sinus, and part of the nose. The reconstructive option, then, may include a flap that requires three distinct skin paddles to provide lining for the nose, the palate, and the overlying skin (Figure 2.3) *(8)*. Other defects, on the other hand, may not need multiple skin paddles. A myocutaneous flap, used in a similar fashion, may suffice where the skin paddle is used for external skin closure and the intra-oral exposed muscle is allowed to (mucosalize re-epithelize with oral mucosa) over time. The choice of flap depends on certain characteristics and requirements of the defect and the patient, as well as the surgeon's preference. Patient factors such as available donor sites, body habitus, history of tobacco use, previous surgeries, co-morbid medical conditions, and the nature of the recipient site influence the type of flap to be used in any given situation. The surgeon's experience with certain flaps, as well as their preference, will also play a role in the type of reconstruction performed. Many times, patients may have had previous surgeries that may interfere with certain donor sites. A previous thoracotomy may prevent

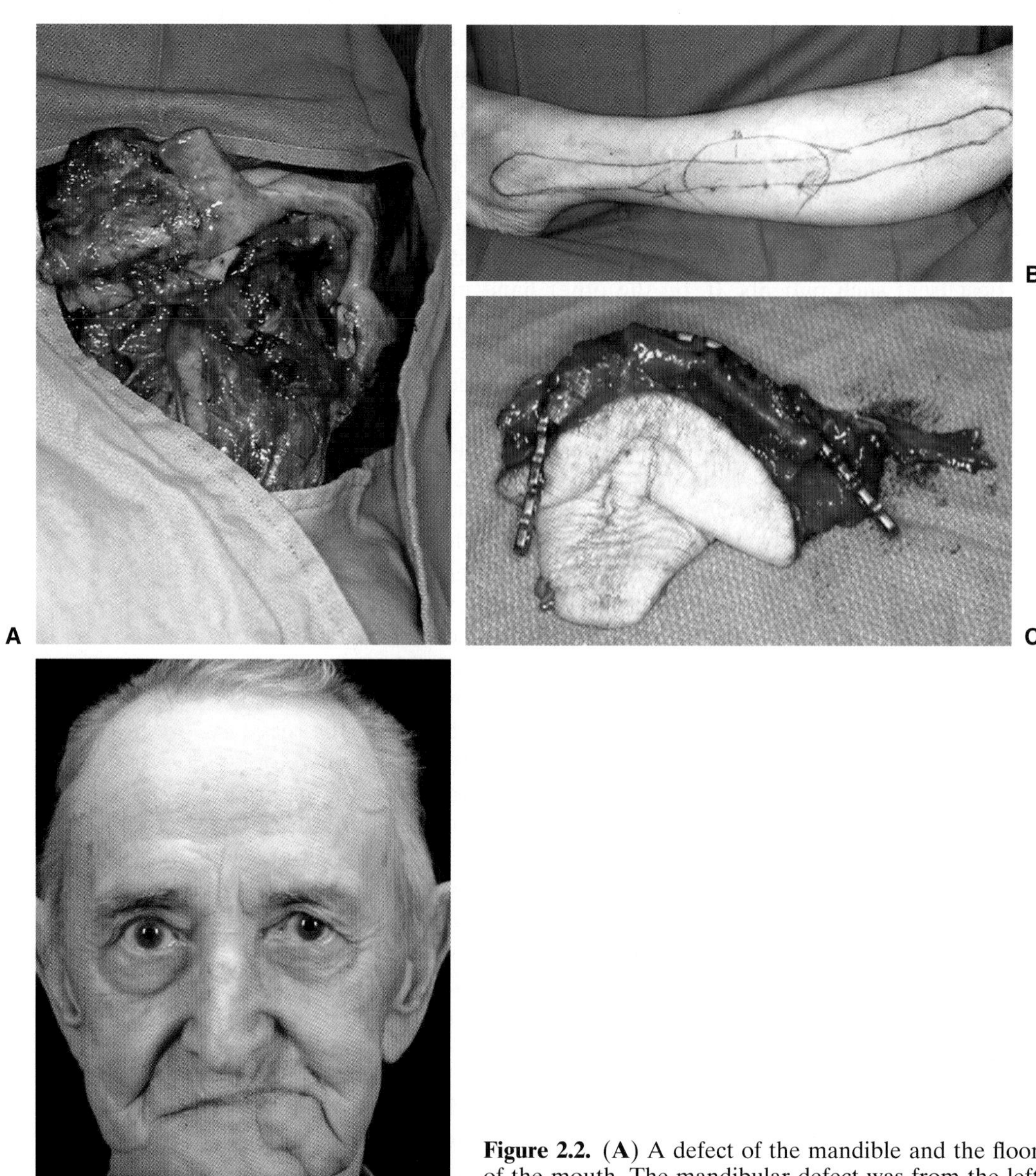

Figure 2.2. (**A**) A defect of the mandible and the floor of the mouth. The mandibular defect was from the left parasymphseal to the right body of the mandible. (**B, C**) A fibular osteocutaneous flap is designed in contoured through osteotomies to fit the mandible defect. The skin paddle provides coverage of the floor of the mouth. (**D**) Final result providing good contour of the mandible.

the use of the latissimus dorsi (LD) flap because the incision has disrupted the thoracodorsal vessels, as well as the muscle itself *(9)*. Other scars on the recipient sites may render these flaps unreliable, and therefore an alternative flap must be chosen. The patient's body habitus also plays an important role. In extremely obese patients, certain myocutaneous and fasciocutaneous flaps may be too bulky and non-maleable. Such flaps, not only result in significant donor site contour defecits, but also the compromise the contour of the recipient site. Conversely, extremely thin patients may not have enough tissue for fasciocutaneous flaps to appropriately fill certain contour defects.

After some cancer resections, the resultant bed is well vascularized and would accept a split-thickness skin graft or a full-thickness skin graft. The decision to use such grafts is dependent on the judgment of the surgeon relative to the goals of reconstruction. For instance,

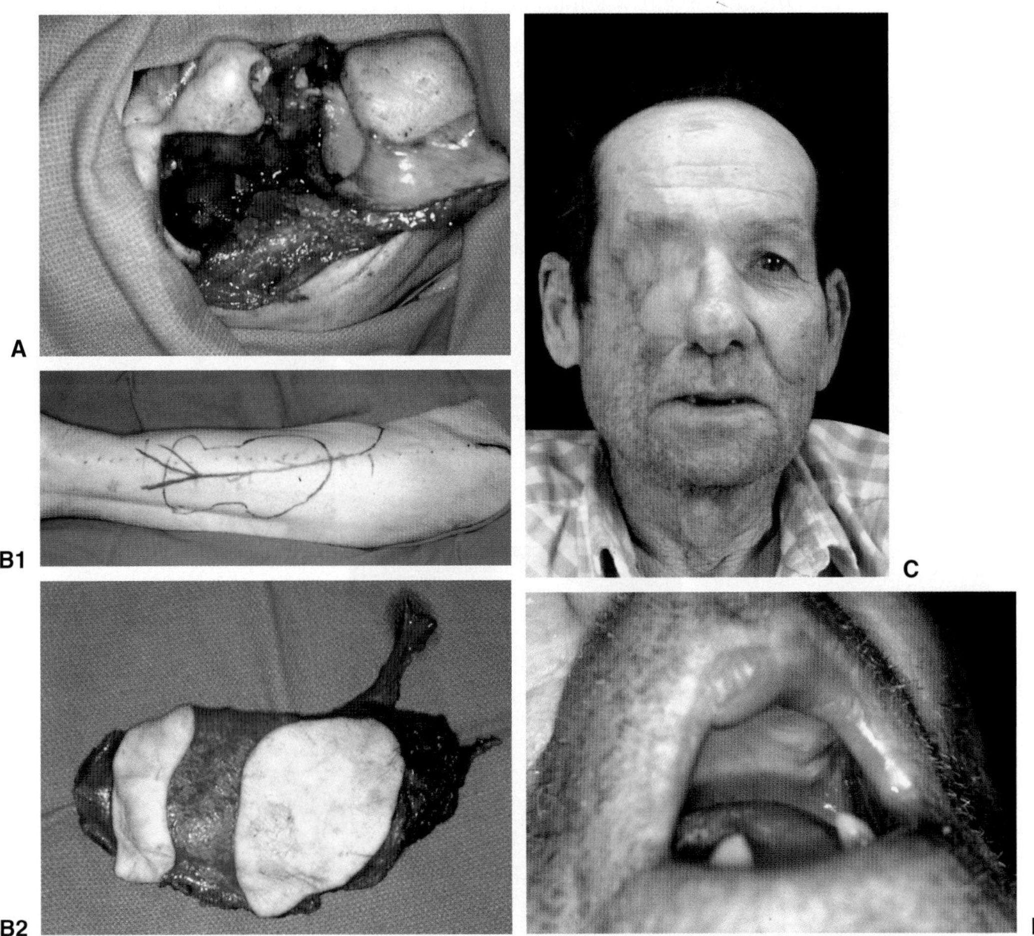

Figure 2.3. (**A**) A complex defect of the face involving the orbit, nose, palate and external skin. (**B1, B2**) Intralateral thigh flap is utilized to provide adequate coverage. The skin paddles are designed to support the palate, nose and external lining. (**C, D**) Final result with obliteration of the defect and adequate coverage of the skin and palate.

split-thickness skin grafts over exposed muscle in the forearm following cancer resection are acceptable because function is not compromised, and the residual contour is minimal. A split-thickness skin graft on the lower eyelid, however, may result in a cicatricial ectropion and contour deformities *(10–12)*. Improved functional and aesthetic results for these defects are often achieved with local flaps from adjacent tissues. Such flaps would include V-Y, transposition, rhomboid, rotation, or advancement flaps *(13)*. Regional flaps, such as the forehead flap, are extremely valuable staged reconstructions of nasal defects because of the relative abundance of forehead tissue and because of the similar color and texture of these two anatomical structures (Figure 2.4) *(14)*. Almost all skin above the clavicle has similar color and is generally darker than skin from other areas in the body. Reconstruction of defects above the clavicle offers a better final appearance if the donor site can be harvested within this region as well. Even full-thickness skin grafts taken from the supraclavicular, pre-auricular, or post-auricular areas will blend in to greater extent when applied to facial defects compared to full-thickness

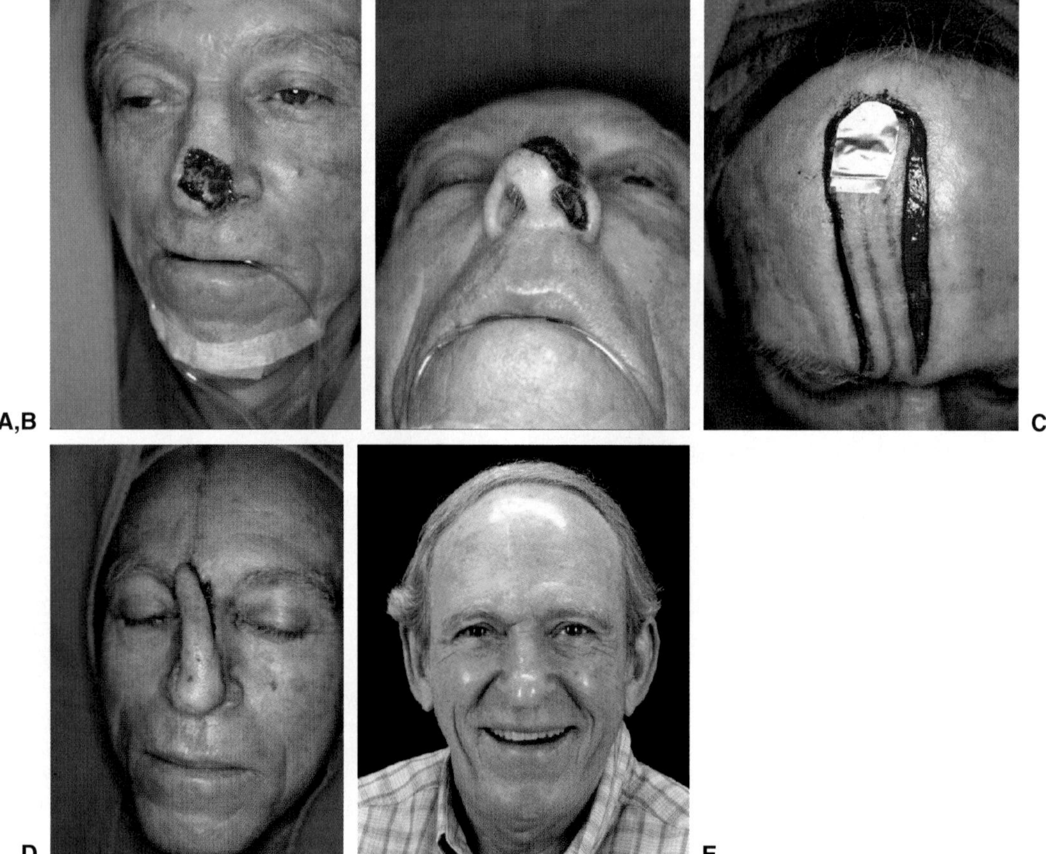

Figure 2.4. (**A, B**) Nasal defect with exposed cartilage. (**C**) A forehead flap is designed on the right supratrochlear vessels. (**D**) The flap is transposed to cover the defect while the donor site is closed primarily. (**E**) Final result after division and inset and maturation of the flap on the nose.

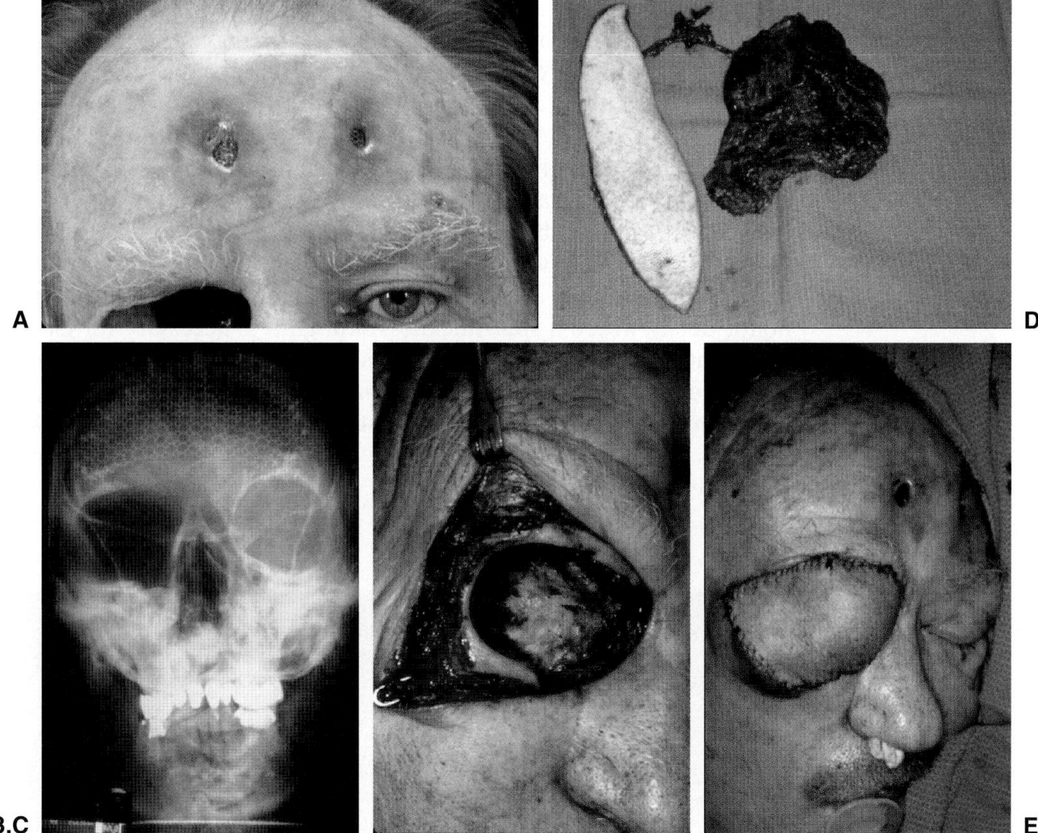

Figure 2.5. (**A, B, C**) A long standing defect of the forehead with exposed mesh draining sinus from a previous orbital exoneration is noted. (**D**) A chimeric flap involving the latissimus and scapular flap has been elevated on one pedicle. (**E**) The mesh is removed, the muscle portion of the flap is used to provide vascularized coverage underneath the forehead skin while the scapular flap provides adequate obliteration of the orbit.

graft harvested from other donor sites. Split-thickness skin grafts have the advantage of more reliable engraftment and ample donor sites. Full-thickness skin grafts, on the other hand, offer of the advantage of limited secondary contraction and the potential for partial sensory re-innervation. Unfortunately, both full- and split-thickness grafts may result in pigmentation changes, unpredictable contraction, or loss of the graft secondary to infection, hematoma, seroma, or shearing *(10–12)*. To prevent secondary joint contracture in the extremities, reconstruction of resection defects over flexion creases are better served with a flap from local, regional, or distant areas.

Despite a variety of donor sites now available in the armamentarium for reconstruction, plastic surgeons should capitalize on the inherent characteristics of each site. For instance, the scapular flap provides an abundant skin paddle that is easily pliable and able to conform to the three-dimensional defects. This flap can also be harvested as an osteocutaneous flap or as a chimeric flap incorporating the serratus anterior muscle and/or the LD muscle on a single pedicle (Figure 2.5) *(15–16)*.

The vascular pedicle itself is rather long and the vessel diameters are relatively large. Although these characteristics make the scapular flap rather appealing, the donor site often lends itself to inconvenient positioning of the patient, a prominent scar on the back, a high incidence of seroma formation, and a limit on the width and length of the flap *(17)*. The anterolateral thigh flap, on the other hand, can provide an enormous skin paddle incorporating muscle and/or fascia, and has a very long pedicle with large caliber vessels (Figure 2.6). The flap does not typically have an osseous component, however. The lateral leg can be closed primarily if a small flap is harvested. Larger flaps can leave a significant donor defect where a split-thickness skin graft is necessary for closure. The contour of the defect is matched to donor site characteristics to minimize secondary procedures yet maximize the goals of the reconstruction (Figure 2.7) *(18)*. The reconstructive surgeon, then, must weigh the pros and cons of each donor site and match them to the recipient site's specific requirements.

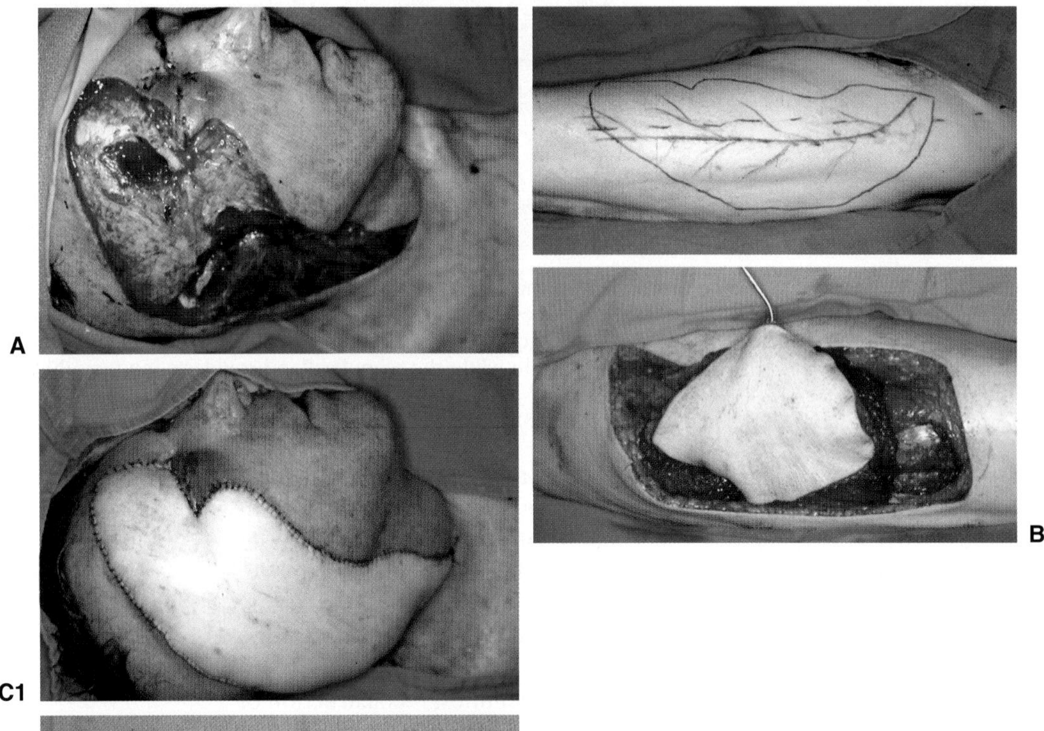

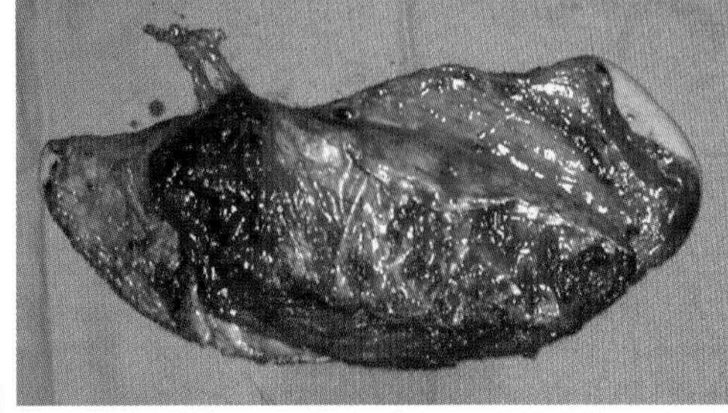

Figure 2.6. (**A**) A large defect of a scull base and lateral scull was a results from an excision of a squamous cell carcinoma. (**B**) An anterolateral thigh flap is designed to provide a large amount of coverage. The vastus lateralis is harvested with the flap to fill in the dead space. (**C**) The anterolateral thigh flap can be harvested as a myocutaneous flap is the muscle is required to obliterate space it can be contoured to fit extremely large defects.

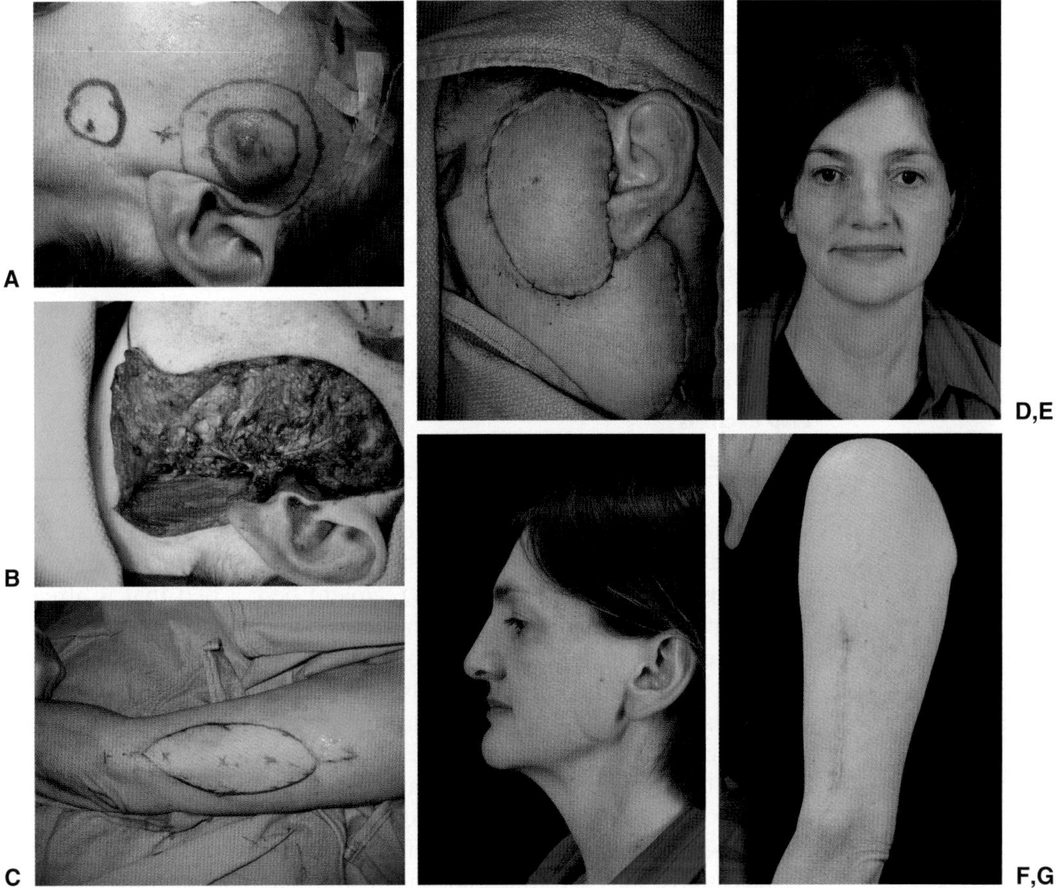

Figure 2.7. (**A**) A malignant melanoma over the superficial parotid requires wide excision and superficial parotidectomy. (**B**) A large defect with exposed facial nerve and contour irregularity is a result of the cancer resection. (**C**) A lateral arm flap which would provide appropriate bulk is fashioned based on the posterior radial collateral artery. (**D, E**) The flap is inset on the face following anastomosis in the neck. Good contour is noted. (**F**) Lateral view illustrating the contour of a well designed flap in sensitive areas. (**G**) The donor site is acceptable.

Two specific detrimental extrinsic factors, patient's tobacco use and pre- or post-operative radiation therapy, have significant ramifications on the choice of reconstruction, as well as the ultimate outcome following reconstruction. There are many detrimental effects of smoking on the vascularity and viability of tissue (Table 2.3). Patients who use tobacco are not only at risk for the development of the cancer requiring reconstruction, but also for partial flap loss owing to necrosis. Wound healing complications at the donor site as well as the recipient site are much more prevalent in smokers than non-smokers *(3–4,19–20)*. Similarly, radiation has an extremely profound influence on the ability of tissues to heal following surgery. Radiation ultimately results in endarterits obliterans, relative ischemia, and tissue fibrosis (Table 2.4) *(3–4,21)*. As a general principle, the chronic skin changes that result from the radiation should alert the surgeon to excise this tissue and replace it with new

Table 2.3. Effects of Smoking on Flaps *(19–20)*

Vasoconstriction
Increased platelet adhesions
Decreased proliferation of red blood cells, fibroblasts, and macrophages
Decreased oxygen transport and metabolism
Increased nicotine, hydrogen cyanides, and carbon monoxide levels
Fat necrosis
Delayed wound healing
Wound infections
Poor scaring
Wound dehiscence
Flap necrosis
Skin sloughing

vascularized tissue either as a pedicled flap or a free flap (Figure 2.8). Skin grafts in these areas are not as reliable because they necessitate procuring a blood supply from the recipient bed; a bed that is already compromised. The skin graft is prone to poor engraftment and subsequent break down, leading to prolonged wound healing complications. *(3–4,22)*. Post-operative radiation also has detrimental effects on the flap reconstruction. Radiation results in fibrosis and shrinkage of the flap, leading to a negative impact on the contour, position, and function of the flap. With the effects of post-operative radiation in mind, the surgeon has a few choices. If possible in this circumstance, the flap reconstruction should be delayed. This is exemplified in breast reconstruction, where reconstructive surgery following mastectomy should be delayed until after the radiation treatments have finished. This decreases radiation's potential compromising effects on the final aesthetic outcome *(23–25)*.

Table 2.4. Early/Late Effects of Radiation *(21–25)*

Early	Late
nuclear chronatin dumping	endarteritis obliterans
nuclear swelling	tissue fibrosis
mitochondrial and endoplasmic reticular degeneration	tissue ischemia
cellular necrosis	hyperpigmentation
mitotic inhibition	flap contracture
generation of free radicals	fat necrosis
erythema	
skin desquamation	
ulceration	
hemorrhage	
necrosis	
infection	
dehiscence	

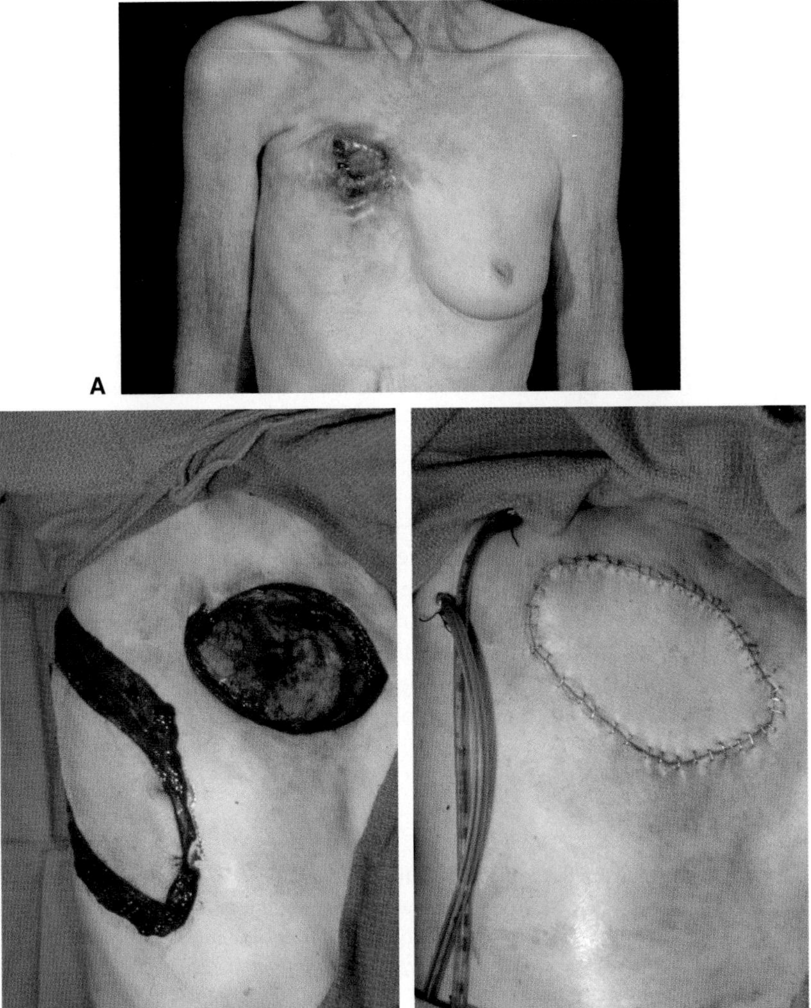

Figure 2.8. (**A**) Radiation osteonecrosis on a non-healing ulcer following a mastectomy and radiation therapy for breast cancer. (**B**) A latissimus dorsi myocutaneous flap is elevated following resection of the damaged irradiated tissue on the chest wall. (**C**) The latissimus flap is inset providing good stable vascularized coverage to the defect. The flap was harvested as a pedicle.

There are times when cancer reconstruction does not require the transfer of other tissue. Tissue expansion of local or adjacent tissues may meet the needs of adequate soft tissue coverage in certain circumstances. Nowhere is this more evident than in breast reconstruction, where tissue expansion beneath the pectoralis major muscle can provide an adequate pocket suitable for implants to restore breast form and contour (Figure 2.9) *(26)*. Secondary tissue expansion can be used to correct contour deformities, areas of scarring, alopecia, contractures, and unstable skin graft sites following the primary reconstruction *(27–28)*. The principles of tissue expansion have been well described, but it is usually performed as a secondary procedure rather than as the primary tumor resection and reconstruction procedure.

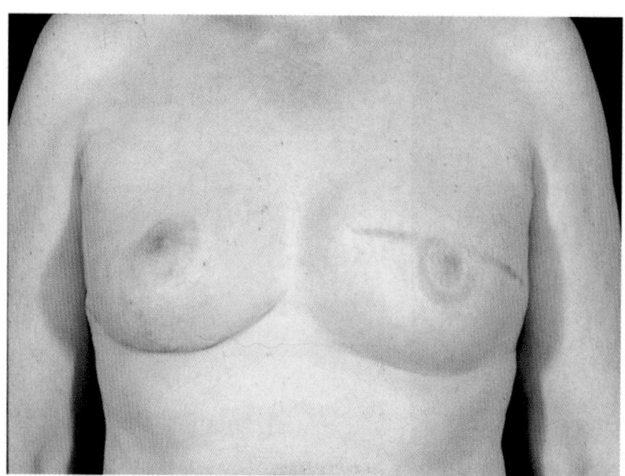

Figure 2.9. Implant reconstruction following a mastectomy. The implant is placed underneath the pectoralis major muscle to provide stable coverage for the implant.

The surgical resection of cancer can have a number of physical and psychological ramifications for patients. The reconstructive surgeon has the responsibility to coordinate the care of the patient to optimize the definitive contour and functional restoration. An accurate evaluation of the patient's medical history, the patient's expectations and goals, the resection defect, and the functional reconstruction goals are all very important components involved in the principles of cancer reconstruction.

References

1. Mathes S, Hansen S. Flap classification and application. In: Mathes S, Hentz V, eds. *Mathes plastic surgery*. Philadelphia: Saunders; 2006:365–378.
2. Mathes S, Nahai F. Flap selection: analysis of function, modifications, applications. *Reconstructive surgery: principles, anatomy and technique.* New York: Churchill Livingstone; 1997:37–160.
3. Broughton G, Janis J, Attinger C. Wound healing: an overview. Plas Reconstr Surg 2006;117:1e-S–32e-S.
4. Attinger C, Janis J, Steinberg J, et al. Clinical approach to wounds: debridgement and wound bed preparation including the use of dressings and wound-healing adjuvants. Plas Reconstr Surg 2006;117:72S–109S.
5. Furuta S, Sakaguchi Y, Iwasawa M, et al. Reconstruction of the lips. Oral commisure, and full-thickness cheek with a composite radial forearm palmaris longus free flap. Ann Plas Surg 1994;33:544–547.
6. Urken ML, Buckbinder D, Costantino PD. Oromandibular reconstruction using microvascular composite flaps: report of 210 cases. Arch Otolaryngol Head Neck Surg 1998;124:46–55.
7. Cordeiro P, Disa J, Hidalgo D, et al. Reconstruction of the mandible with osseous free flaps: a 10-year experience with 150 consecutive patients. Plas Reconstr Surg 1999;104:1314–1320.
8. Sakuraba M, Kimata Y, Ota Y, et al. Simple maxillary reconstruction using free tissue transfer and prostheses. Plas Reconstr Surg 2003;111:594–598.
9. Quillen CG. Latissimus dorsi myocutaneous flaps in head and neck reconstruction. Plast Reconstr Surg 1979;63:664–670.
10. Ratner D. Skin grafting from here to there. Dermatol Clin 1998;16(1):75–90.

11. Fifer R, Pieper D, Hawtorf D. Contraction rates of meshed, nonexpanded split-thickness skin grafts versus split-thickness sheet grafts. Ann Plast Surg 1993;31:162.
12. Paletta C, Pokorny J, Rumbolo P. Skin grafts. In: Mathes S, Hentz V, eds. *Mathes plastic surgery*. Philadelphia: Saunders; 2006:293–316.
13. Place M, Herber S, Hardesty R. Basic techniques and principles in plastic surgery. In: Aston S, Beasley R, Thorne C, eds. *Grabb and Smith's plastic surgery, fifth edition*. Philadelphia: Lippincott-Raven; 1997:20–25.
14. Mazzola RF, Marcus S. History of total nasal reconstruction with particular emphasis on the folded forehead flap technique. Plast Reconstr Surg 1983;72:408–414.
15. Yamamoto Y, Nohira K, Minakawa H, et al. The combined flap based on a single vascular source: a clinical experience with 32 cases. Plast Reconstr Surg 1996;97:1385–1390.
16. Aviv J, Urken M, Vickery C, et al. The combined latissimus dorsi-scapular free flap in head and neck reconstruction. Arch Otolaryngol Head Neck Surg 1991;117:1242–1250.
17. Bidros R, Metzinger S, Guerra A. The thoracodorsal artery perforator-scapular osteocutaneous (TDAP-SOC) flap for reconstruction of palatal and maxillary defects. Ann Plast Surg 2005;54:59–65.
18. Kimata Y, Uchiyama K, Satoshi E, et al. Anteriorlateral thigh flap donor-site complications and morbidity. Plast Reconstr Surg 2000;106:584–589.
19. Krueger JK, Rohrich RJ. Clearing the smoke: the scientific rationale for tobacco abstention with plastic surgery. Plast Reconstr Surg 2001;108:1063–1073.
20. Selber J, Kurichi J, Vega S, et al. Risk factors and complications in free tram flap breast reconstruction. Ann Plast Surg 2006;56:492–497.
21. Lopez E, Guerrero R, Nunez M, et al. Early and late skin reactions to radiotherapy for breast cancer and their correlation with radiation-induced DNA damage in lymphocytes. Breast Cancer Res 2005;7:R690–R698.
22. Tadjalli H, Evans G, Gurlek A, et al. Skin graft survival after external beam irradiation. Plast Reconstr Surg 1999;103:1902–1908.
23. Bristol S, Lennox P, Clugston P. A comparison of ipsilateral pedicled TRAM flap with and without previous irradiation. Ann Plast Surg 2006;56:589–592.
24. Rogers NE, Allen RJ. Radiation effects on breast reconstruction with the deep inferior epigastric perforator flap. Plast Reconstr Surg 2002;109:1919–1924.
25. Kroll SS, Robb GL, Reece GP, et al. Does prior irradiation increase the risk of total or partial free-flap loss? J Reconstr Microsurg 1998;14:263–268.
26. Cordeiro P, McCarthy C. A single surgeon's 12-year experience with tissue expander/implant breast reconstruction: Part I. A prospective analysis of early complications. Plast Reconstr Surg 2006;118:825–831.
27. Spence R. Experience with novel uses of tissue expanders in burn reconstruction of the face and neck. Ann Plast Surg 1992;28:453–464.
28. LoGiudice J, Gosain A. Pediatric tissue expansion: indications and complications. Plast Surg Nurs 2004;24:20–26.
29. Lamberty B, Cormack G. Fasciacutaneous system. *The arterial anatomy of skin flaps*. New York: Churchill Livingstone; 1994:119–129.

3

Breast Reconstruction

Timing and Coordination with Adjuvant Therapy

Steven J. Kronowitz and Geoffrey L. Robb

Recent developments in the management of breast cancer, including axillary sentinel lymph node biopsy and the increasing use of both postmastectomy radiation therapy (PMRT) and adjuvant and neoadjuvant chemotherapy, have had a significant impact on breast reconstruction. The interplay and sequencing of these diagnostic and treatment modalities in patients with breast cancer has become an important issue.

This chapter will address the clinical dilemma of predicting which patients will require PMRT, current indications for PMRT, technical problems associated with the delivery of PMRT after immediate breast reconstruction, aesthetic outcomes in patients treated with PMRT after immediate breast reconstruction, the effects of adjuvant and neoadjuvant chemotherapy on breast reconstruction, and important considerations for the multi-disciplinary breast cancer team.

The Impact of Axillary Sentinel Node Biopsy on the Timing of Breast Reconstruction

The current recommendation when a sentinel node is found to be positive is to perform a completion level I and II axillary node dissection, because additional nodes will be involved in up to 40% of such patients *(1,2)*. Current practice dictates that if the intraoperative assessment of the sentinel lymph node is positive, a completion level I and II axillary nodal dissection is performed at the time of the initial operation. Unfortunately, the intraoperative examination of sentinel lymph nodes with frozen section analysis, imprint cytology techniques, or both does not reveal all micrometastases *(3,4)*. Conducting an axillary lymph node dissection after sentinel node biopsy and immediate autologous breast reconstruction have taken place can compromise the blood supply to the reconstructed breast, particularly the thoracodorsal vascular system, parts of which are often used as recipient vessels for a free transverse rectus abdominis myocutaneous

(TRAM) flap or as a vascular pedicle for a latissimus dorsi myocutaneous flap *(5)*.

Several recent studies *(5,6)* have evaluated clinicopathologic factors that may help identify preoperatively which clinically node negative patients are at risk for undetectable micrometastatic axillary disease. A recent report from our institution *(5)* demonstrated that patients who were 50 years of age or younger, patients who had tumors larger than 2 cm, and patients who had lymphovascular invasion detected in the initial biopsy specimen were at higher risk for harboring axillary metastases. However, although these factors can help identify high-risk patients, the ability to consistently predict and quantify axillary involvement before surgery is limited.

As use of the axillary sentinel node biopsy technique in conjunction with breast reconstruction continues to increase (Figure 3.1), our current approach to immediate breast reconstruction should be reevaluated for patients at high risk of axillary involvement to avoid possibly compromising the vascularity to the reconstructed breast. In a study published in 2002 *(5)*, we proposed an algorithm for decision-making for breast reconstruction in clinically node-negative breast cancer patients (Figure 3.2) *(5)*. Although risk of an immediate breast reconstruction could be avoided simply by performing an initial complete level I and II axillary dissection because all nodes will be removed without the worry about coming back for more axillary surgery, this practice could impose significant surgical morbidity (lymphedema and shoulder dystocia) on patients whose axillary nodes may turn out to be negative for disease on permanent pathologic analysis *(7)*. Delayed breast reconstruction may also be an option; however, immediate breast reconstruction has well-recognized benefits in terms of aesthetics and lessening the psychological effects of mastectomy *(8)*. Although postoperative axillary radiation may be a consideration for locoregional control when the sentinel

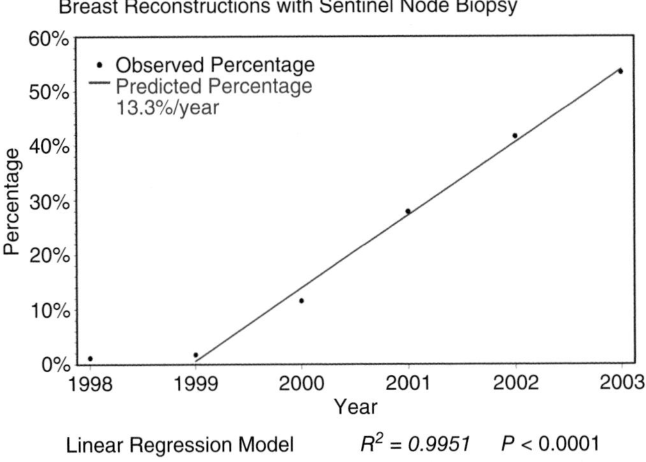

Figure 3.1. The increasing use of sentinel node biopsy in combination with breast reconstruction at M. D. Anderson Cancer Center.

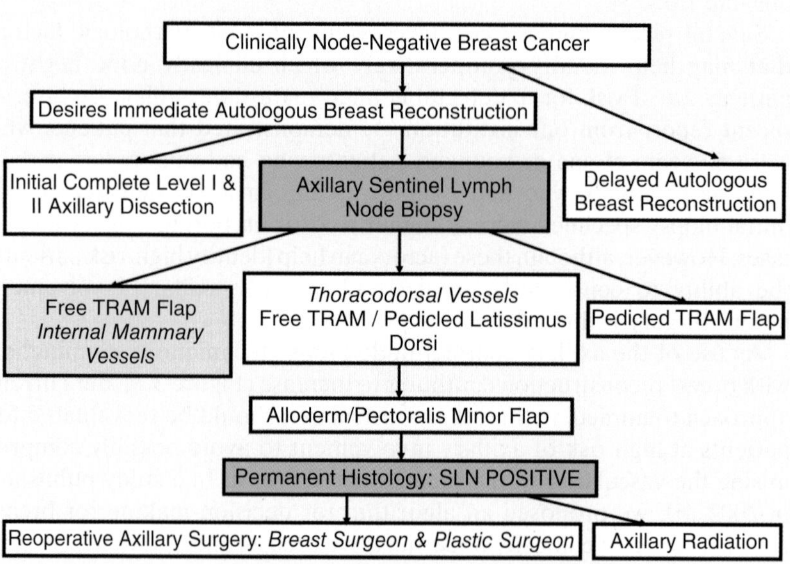

Figure 3.2. An algorithm for decision-making in clinically node-negative breast cancer patients who desire autologous breast reconstruction and sentinel node biopsy. TRAM, transverse rectus abdominis myocutaneous flap; LD, latissimus dorsi myocutaneous. Reproduced with permission from *(5)*.

node is found to be positive on permanent histopathologic analysis, it does not provide the important prognostic information obtained from the additional nodal tissue *(9)*. When immediate breast reconstruction is performed with either a microvascular TRAM flap (with the most commonly used recipient vessels being the thoracodorsal artery and vein) or a pedicled latissimus dorsi myocutaneous flap, the vascular pedicle may be at risk if subsequent axillary surgery is required. An alternative to use of these vessels for immediate autologous breast reconstruction in patients undergoing mastectomy and axillary sentinel node biopsy, which may minimize the risk of vascular damage on reoperation, includes use of the internal mammary artery and vein as recipient vessels for a microvascular or a pedicled TRAM flap *(5)*. With the use of axillary sentinel node biopsy now routine at our institution, the internal mammary vessels are often our first choice in immediate microvascular TRAM flap breast reconstruction to avoid the potential for vascular injury to the TRAM flap if subsequent axillary surgery is required.

Another confounding factor is the possible need for postoperative axillary radiation when the sentinel node is found to be positive *(9)*. At the time of surgery, it is not known whether postoperative radiation will be required, because findings from the pathologic examination of the additional tissue are not available until several days after the surgery. Therefore, if the intraoperative examination reveals a positive sentinel node, the decision of whether to proceed with an immediate breast reconstruction or to delay reconstruction until after the results of the permanent pathology are known will need to have been made beforehand by the multi-disciplinary breast cancer team and the patient. At our institution, the decision of whether to proceed with breast reconstruction if the sentinel node is positive or to delay the reconstruction is greatly influenced by existing treatment guidelines *(5)*.

The Influence of the Need for PRMT on the Timing of Breast Reconstruction

The increasing use of PMRT in patients with early-stage breast cancer, along with the inability to determine preoperatively which patients will require PMRT, has increased the complexity of planning for immediate breast reconstruction. There are two potential problems with performing an immediate breast reconstruction in a patient who will require PMRT. First, an immediate breast reconstruction may interfere with the delivery of PMRT. Second, PMRT can adversely affect the aesthetic outcome of an immediate breast reconstruction. Because the potential need for PMRT is one of the most important considerations affecting the timing and technique of breast reconstruction, the multi-disciplinary breast team must work together in planning surgery for patients with breast cancer who desire reconstruction after mastectomy. The preoperative consultation with the patient should include emphasis on the potentially adverse effects that radiation treatment can have on aesthetic outcome of an immediate breast reconstruction *(10)* and on the technical problems with delivery of radiation to a reconstructed breast *(11)*.

Recently, both the American Society for Therapeutic Radiology and Oncology *(9)* and the American Society of Clinical Oncology *(12)* published consensus statements regarding PMRT. Both groups currently recommend PMRT in patients with four or more positive lymph nodes or advanced tumors. However, on the basis of recent prospective, randomized controlled trials (the so-called Danish and Canadian trials *[13,14]*) that demonstrated superior locoregional control, disease-free survival, and overall survival in breast cancer patients with T1 or T2 disease and one to three positive lymph nodes with the addition of PMRT to mastectomy and chemotherapy, both societies have emphasized the need for additional prospective data concerning the use of PMRT in these patients. In the future, depending on the outcome of ongoing trials, PMRT may be widely recommended in patients with early-stage breast cancer. Some institutions have already instituted routine PMRT in patients with early-stage disease.

The Difficulties with Radiation Delivery after Immediate Breast Reconstruction

An important issue in immediate breast reconstruction is whether the reconstructed breast will impair the delivery of PMRT. Immediate breast reconstruction can cause technical problems with the design of the radiation fields for PMRT *(15,16)*. The previously mentioned randomized trials that reported a survival advantage with PMRT *(13,14)* included the internal mammary nodes within the radiation fields. To treat these areas and minimize the dose to the heart and lungs, a separate electron beam on the medial chest wall may be required to match the laterally placed opposed tangent fields *(15)*. Some anatomic configurations make it difficult to successfully deliver PMRT using such a separate medial electron-beam field *(16)*. The sloping contour of a reconstructed breast may lead to an imprecise geometric matching of the medial and lateral radiation fields. Alternative radiation fields may result in either exclusion of the internal mammary nodes or increased irradiation of normal tissues. It is important to discuss these issues with the treating radiation oncologist so that a unified treatment plan can be instituted.

The Adverse Affects of PMRT on the Aesthetic Outcome of an Immediate Breast Reconstruction

Our experience at The University of Texas M. D. Anderson Cancer Center *(10,17,18)* and many of the other experiences reported in the literature *(17,19–22)* indicate that autologous tissue is preferable for breast reconstruction in patients who have received PMRT, and that consideration to delay breast reconstruction should be discussed with patients who are known preoperatively to require PMRT. There are other centers, most notably Memorial Sloan Kettering in New York, who believe that satisfactory breast reconstruction can be obtained in radiated patients with the use of tissue expanders and permanent silicone or saline implants. Unfortunately, evaluation of complication rates and aesthetic outcomes is extremely difficult because of significant variation in the sequencing of PMRT and reconstruction, the administration of systemic therapy, the duration of follow-up, and the techniques of radiation delivery and breast reconstruction.

In 1997, Williams and colleagues *(22)* from Emory University compared outcomes of pedicled TRAM flap breast reconstruction in 19 patients who received PMRT after reconstruction and 108 patients who received PMRT before reconstruction with outcomes in 572 patients who underwent TRAM flap breast reconstruction without PMRT. At a mean follow-up time after reconstruction of 47.6 months, 52.6% of the patients who received PMRT after TRAM flap reconstruction demonstrated postirradiation changes, and 31.6% required surgical intervention.

Spear and Onyewu *(19)* published a review in 2000 evaluating the effects of irradiation on outcomes after two-stage breast reconstruction with saline-filled implants. These authors retrospectively compared 40 patients who underwent two-stage saline-filled-implant breast reconstruction followed by irradiation with 40 other patients who underwent the same reconstruction procedure without irradiation. The incidence of complications was significantly higher in the irradiated group than in the control group (52.5 versus 10%; $p = 0.001$). Of the irradiated patients, 32% had symptomatic capsular contractures, whereas no contractures occurred in the control group. A total of 47% of the 40 irradiated breasts needed flap procedures, whereas only 10% of the nonirradiated breasts needed flaps. Evaluating and using this data requires careful patient education. Women in this situation may still feel that they prefer a chance at the less invasive surgery involved in implant reconstruction.

In 2001, investigators at our institution published a retrospective study *(10)* comparing immediate and delayed free TRAM flap breast reconstruction in patients receiving PMRT. In this study, 32 patients had immediate TRAM flap reconstruction before X-ray therapy (XRT), and 70 patients had PMRT before TRAM flap reconstruction. The mean follow-up times after the end of treatment for the immediate and delayed reconstruction groups were 3 and 5 years, respectively. The incidence of early flap complications (vessel thrombosis and partial or total flap loss) did not differ significantly between the two groups. However, the incidence of late complications (fat necrosis, flap volume loss, and flap contracture) was significantly higher in the immediate reconstruction group than in the delayed reconstruction group (87.5 versus 8.6%; $p = 0.001$). Furthermore, 28% of the patients with immediate reconstruction required an additional flap to correct the distorted contour that resulted from flap shrinkage and severe flap contracture after PMRT.

In 2002, Rogers and Allen *(23)* published the results of a study on the effects of PMRT on breasts reconstructed with a deep inferior epigastric perforator (DIEP) flap. In this study, a matched-pairs analysis was performed of 30 patients who had breast reconstruction with a DIEP flap and PMRT and 30 patients who underwent DIEP flap reconstruction without PMRT. Patients who received PMRT had higher incidences of fat necrosis in the DIEP flap (23.3 versus 0%; $p = 0.006$), fibrosis and shrinkage (56.7 versus 0%; $p = 0.001$), and flap contracture (16.7 versus 0%; $p = 0.023$).

In 2005, Spear and colleagues *(24)* found that patients who had TRAM flap reconstruction before irradiation had worse aesthetic outcomes, symmetry, and contractures than did patients who underwent irradiation before TRAM flap breast reconstruction. These authors recommended that TRAM flap reconstruction be postponed in patients known or expected to require PMRT.

The Effect of the Clinical Stage of Breast Cancer on the Timing of Breast Reconstruction

PMRT is given to some patients after mastectomy to reduce the risk of local-regional recurrence in high-risk patients. Currently, indications for PMRT include large tumor size or direct skin involvement (T3 or T4 tumors) or documented lymph node involvement in four or more lymph nodes. Therefore, the stage of the breast cancer is critical in reconstructive planning. Patients with clinical stage I breast cancer are considered to be at low risk for requiring PMRT and are therefore considered candidates for immediate breast reconstruction using any of the available approaches.

Some patients with clinical stage II breast cancer have a borderline elevated risk of requiring PMRT, and thus these are the patients for whom it is most difficult to formulate recommendations regarding breast reconstruction timing *(25,26)*. It is essential that these patients have a careful preoperative evaluation for risk factors for occult axillary nodal involvement (age younger than 50 years, lymphovascular invasion in the initial biopsy specimen, and T2 tumor) *(5)*. In patients with any of these risk factors, it may be preferable to avoid the use of breast implants, to perform delayed reconstruction, or to use a delayed-immediate approach (described in next section).

In patients with clinical stage III breast cancer (locally advanced), it may be preferable to delay reconstruction until after mastectomy and PMRT to avoid potential problems with radiation delivery and to avoid the possibility of adverse affects of PMRT on an immediately reconstructed breast *(10,17,18,20–22,24,25)*. Breast reconstruction has not been found to delay diagnosis or decrease survival in patients who present with stage III disease and later develop a local recurrence *(27)*.

The Evolving Options for the Sequencing of Breast Reconstruction and Adjuvant Therapy

Immediate Breast Reconstruction

Immediate breast reconstruction is usually reserved for patients with clinical stage I breast cancer and some patients with clinical stage II breast cancer who do not have an increased risk of requiring PMRT. Unfortunately, although the risk of requiring PMRT can be predicted before surgery, the need for PMRT cannot be definitively determined until the final pathologic evaluation is complete.

Immediate breast reconstruction offers many advantages over delayed reconstruction, including a better aesthetic outcome owing to preservation of the breast skin envelope (Figure 3.3) *(28)* and the psychological benefit of awakening from mastectomy with a reconstructed breast *(29)*. Immediate breast reconstruction also enables athletic patients with active lifestyles to more easily resume their daily activities.

Delayed Breast Reconstruction

Many of the aesthetic outcomes of delayed reconstruction, even when it is performed by experienced surgeons, are satisfactory at best *(28,29)*. However, patients who undergo delayed reconstruction after PMRT may be the most appreciative because they have had to experience the difficulties of not having a breast. The retained, irradiated, and scarred breast skin located between the mastectomy scar and the inframammary fold is usually resected at the time of delayed reconstruction because it is inflexible and does not allow for the reconstruction of a curved and

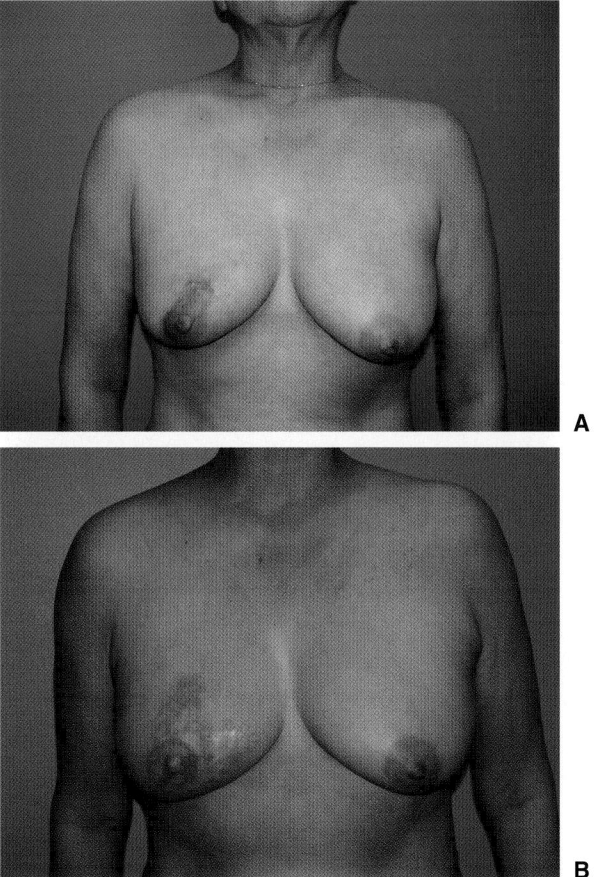

Figure 3.3. Immediate breast reconstruction using a microvascular TRAM flap in a 56-year-old woman with a right-sided breast cancer. **(A)** Preoperative view. **(B)** 1 year after a right total mastectomy, right axillary sentinel lymph node biopsy, and immediate breast reconstruction with a left microvascular TRAM flap (the internal mammary artery and vein served as recipient vessels). The patient required no revision procedures. She underwent nipple reconstruction and areola tattooing.

ptotic-appearing breast (Figure 3.4A). This not only requires a much larger volume of flap tissue owing to the need for skin replacement, but also requires the entire three-dimensional contour of the breast to be recreated (Figure 3.4B). The need to replace the inferior breast skin means that more flap skin is visible; this appearance is often referred to by patients as the "patch look" (Figure 3.4C). Because of the increased skin requirements, often three-quarters of the TRAM flap must be used to reconstruct the breast, leaving inadequate tissue for bilateral reconstruction. With delayed breast reconstruction, we also rely more significantly on the ability to perform a contralateral mastopexy (breast lift) to obtain symmetry, because it is more difficult to match the ptotic shape of a contralateral native breast (Figure 3.4C).

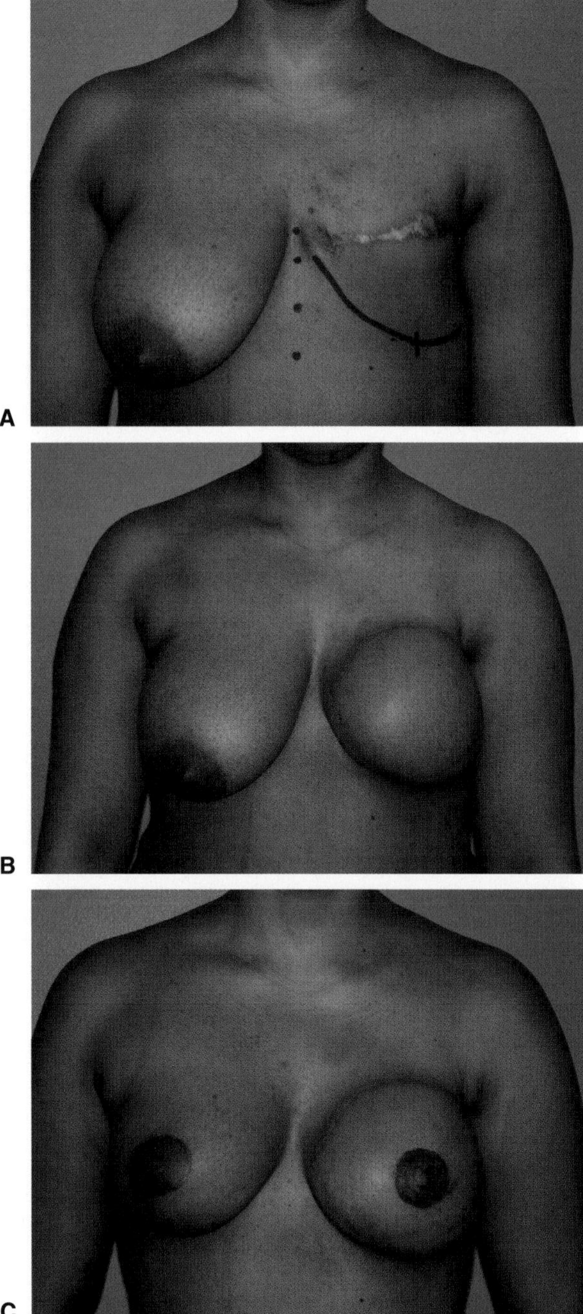

Figure 3.4. Delayed reconstruction after PMRT. **(A)** A 35-year-old woman who had undergone a left modified radical mastectomy presented for delayed reconstruction several years after PMRT; **(B)** 6 months after delayed reconstruction of the left breast with a right microvascular TRAM flap; **(C)** 3 months later, after a right vertical mastopexy for symmetry and a left nipple and areola reconstruction.

Delayed-Immediate Breast Reconstruction

At our institution, patients with clinical stage II breast cancer are evaluated by a multi-disciplinary breast cancer team (Figure 3.5), which includes a radiation oncologist. Patients who are deemed to be at increased risk for conditions necessitating PMRT and who desire breast reconstruction are considered eligible for a recently implemented two-stage approach, "delayed-immediate breast reconstruction" (Figure 3.6). Stage 1 consists of skin-sparing mastectomy with insertion of a completely filled textured saline tissue expander to preserve the shape and dimensions of the breast skin envelope until the results of the permanent pathology are known. After review of permanent sections, patients who do not require PMRT undergo delayed-immediate reconstruction (stage 2), and patients who require PMRT complete this therapy and then undergo a skin preserving approach to delayed reconstruction. We prefer to perform stage 2 of delayed-immediate reconstruction (definitive reconstruction) within approximately 2 weeks after mastectomy to avoid delays in the initiation of chemotherapy and to preserve the elasticity of the breast skin. In patients who require PMRT, we usually perform

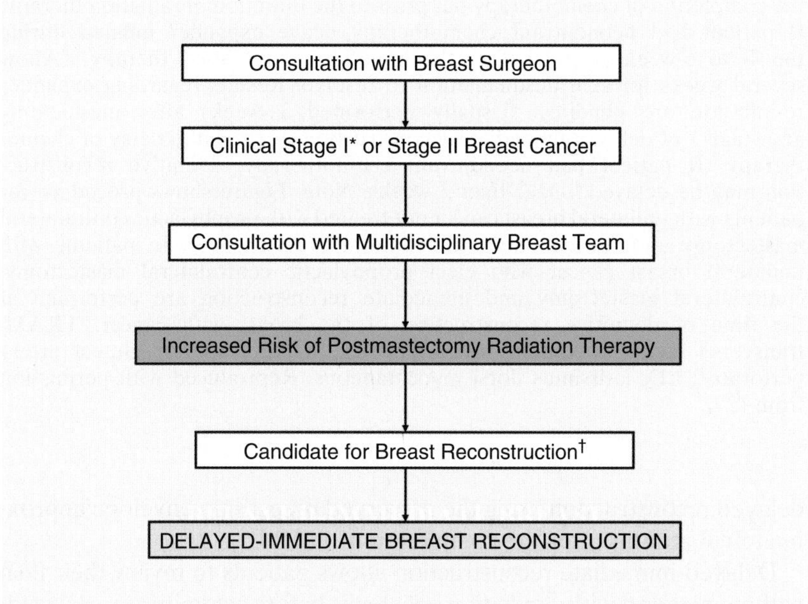

Figure 3.5. Clinical decision-making in patients with clinical stage II breast cancer who desire reconstruction after mastectomy. *Patients with multi-centric breast cancer by ultrasonography or extensive microcalcifications by mammography in whom it is unclear the extent of invasive breast cancer and are clinical stage I have been considered eligible for delayed-immediate breast reconstruction. †Increased risk defined as T2 tumor, T2 tumor with one positive lymph node, T2 tumor with positive biopsy margins, T2 tumor but possibly T3 tumor because of extensive calcifications consistent with ductal carcinoma in situ, T2 tumor either before or after neoadjuvant therapy, or T2 tumor with lymphovascular invasion on initial biopsy. Reproduced with permission from *(30)*.

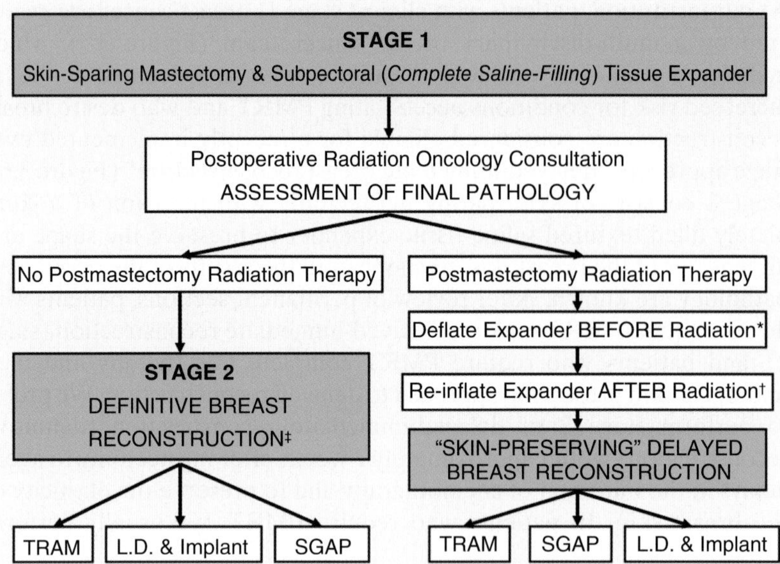

Figure 3.6. Schema for delayed-immediate breast reconstruction. *After the completion of chemotherapy but prior to the initiation of radiation therapy. If patient had neoadjuvant chemotherapy, leave expander inflated during the 4- to 6-week period before the initiation of radiation therapy. †Allow several weeks for skin desquamation to resolve. Results regarding expander re-inflation are pending. ‡Usually performed 2 weeks after mastectomy and stage 1 of delayed-immediate reconstruction to prevent a delay of chemotherapy. If patient had neoadjuvant chemotherapy, definitive reconstruction may be delayed longer than 2 weeks. Note: Figure shows procedure for patients with unilateral breast cancer not treated with prophylactic contralateral mastectomy and for patients with bilateral breast cancer. In patients with unilateral breast cancer who elect prophylactic contralateral mastectomy, contralateral mastectomy and immediate reconstruction are performed at the time of definitive reconstruction of the breast with cancer. TRAM, transverse rectus abdominis myocutaneous; SGAP, superior gluteal artery perforator; LD, latissimus dorsi myocutaneous. Reproduced with permission from *(30)*.

delayed reconstruction using the preserved breast skin envelope approximately 6 months after the completion of PMRT.

Delayed-immediate reconstruction allows patients to review their final pathology report with a radiation oncologist before committing to delayed-immediate or delayed reconstruction, placement of the fully inflated expander in stage 1 prevents retraction of the mastectomy skin and loss of breast shape, it also affords the opportunity to revise the inframammary fold and debride any nonviable mastectomy skin prior to insetting of an autologous tissue flap, and it can be adapted to any clinical practice and modified to comply with various institutional guidelines for PMRT.

With the delayed-immediate approach, patients who do not require PMRT can achieve aesthetic outcomes similar to those of immediate reconstruction (Figure 3.7), and patients who require PMRT can avoid

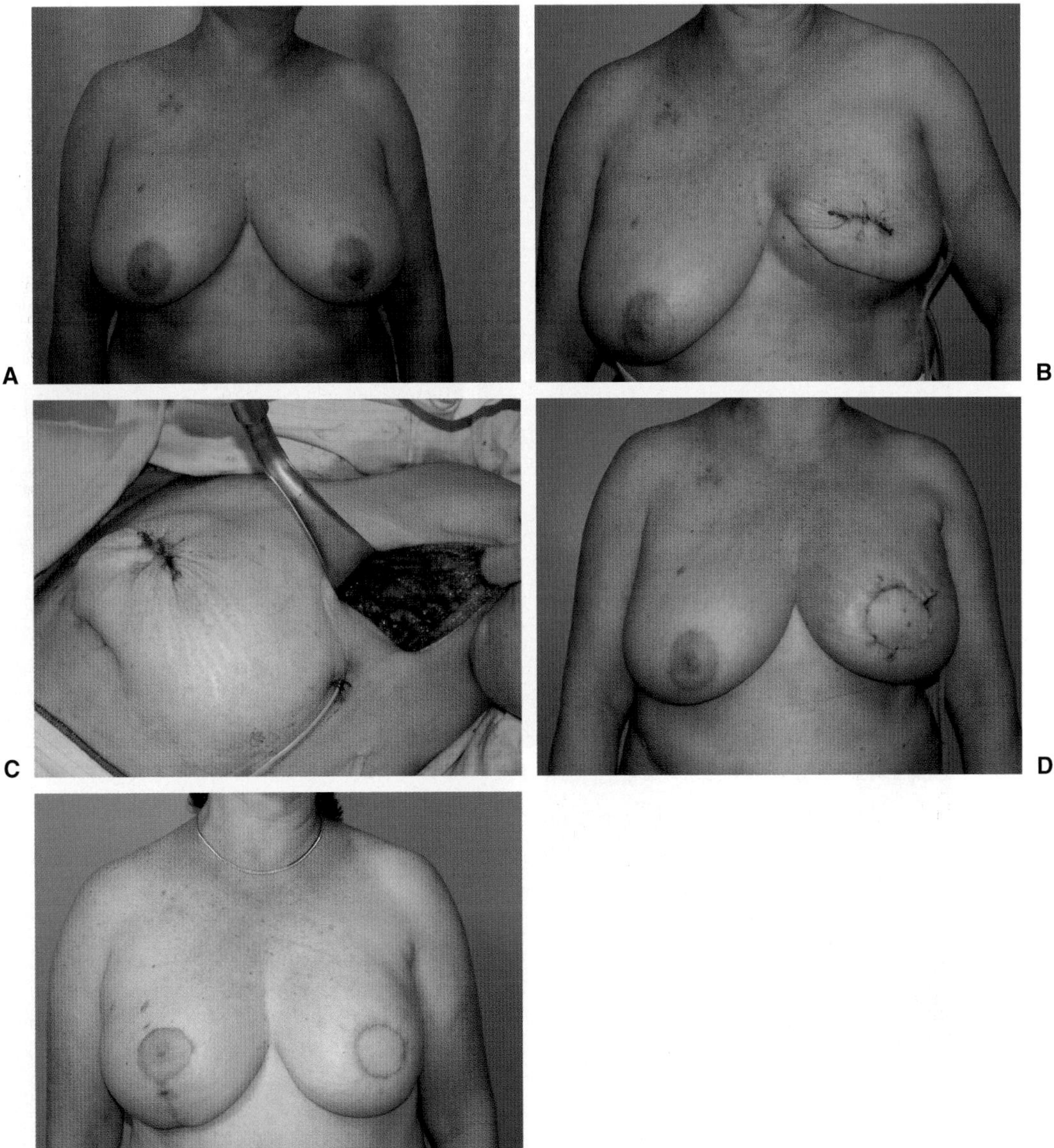

Figure 3.7. Delayed-immediate breast reconstruction in a 55-year-old woman with multi-centric left breast cancer. **(A)** Preoperative view after neoadjuvant chemotherapy; **(B)** 4 weeks after a left skin-sparing total mastectomy with axillary sentinel lymph node biopsy and subpectoral placement of a textured saline tissue expander expanded to the manufacturer's suggested intraoperative saline-fill volume of 700 cc; **(C)** Intraoperative view during complete axillary lymph node dissection performed 10 days after mastectomy; **(D)** 10 days after TRAM flap reconstruction; **(E)** 13 months after TRAM flap reconstruction and 6 months after a left vertical breast reduction for symmetry.

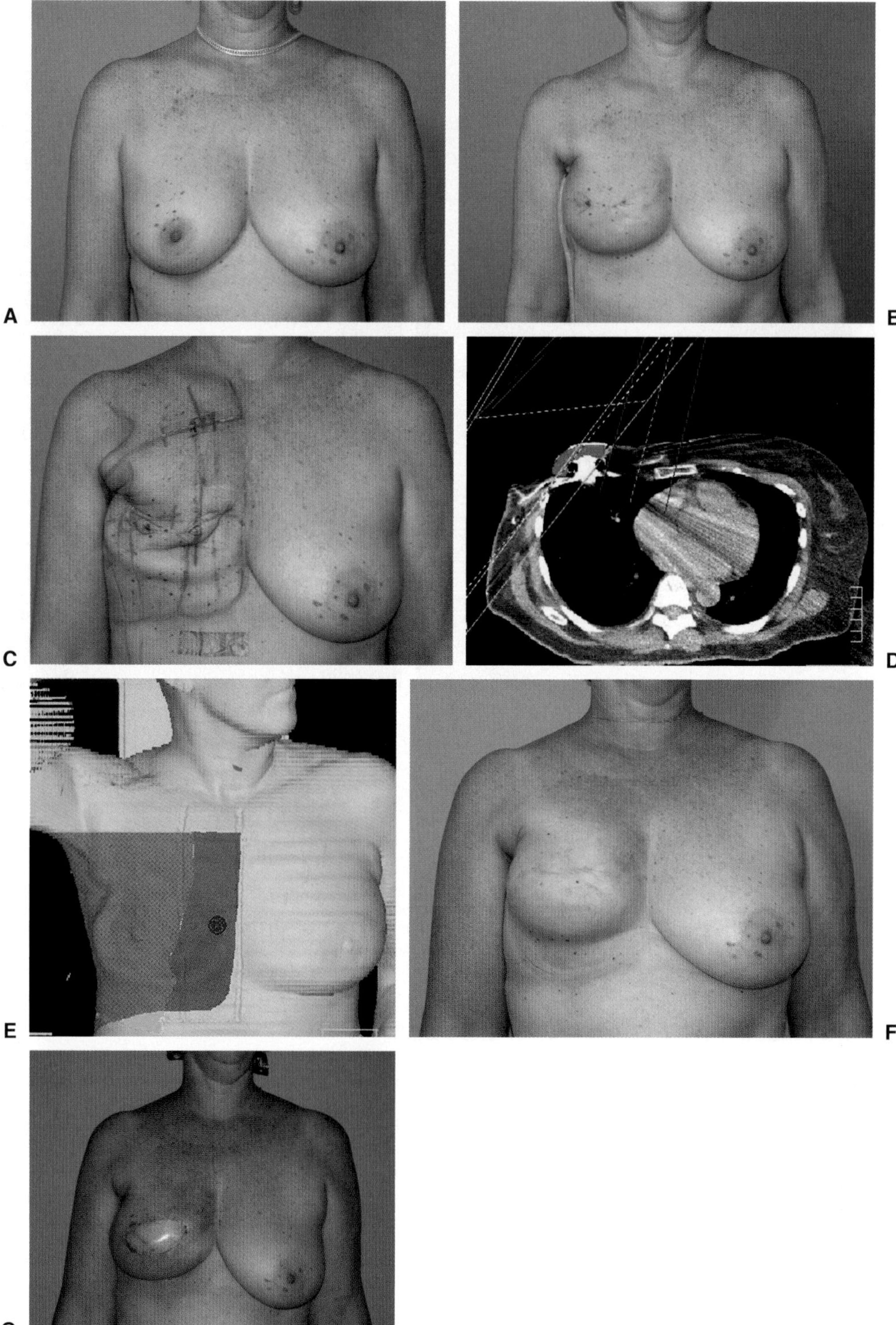
A
B
C
D
E
F
G

Figure 3.8. "Skin-preserving" delayed free microvascular TRAM flap reconstruction after stage 1 of delayed-immediate reconstruction and postmastectomy XRT in a 52-year-old woman with a clinical stage II (T2N1M0) right breast cancer. **(A)** Preoperative view after neoadjuvant chemotherapy. **(B)** Postoperative view 3 weeks after right skin-sparing modified radical mastectomy and stage 1 of delayed-immediate reconstruction with placement of a subpectoral textured saline tissue expander with an intraoperative saline-fill volume of 600cc. The permanent pathology after mastectomy upstaged the patient to stage III (T2N2M0). **(C, D, E)** Prior to the start of postmastectomy radiation therapy, the patient had complete deflation of the expander with removal of 600cc in our clinic. Complete deflation of the expander during postmastectomy radiation therapy allows for treatment of the internal mammary lymph nodes without excessive injury to the heart and lungs and avoids non-uniform radiation dose distribution. Shown is the three-dimensional planning used for the design of the radiation treatment fields using CT (axial and three-dimensional images) **(F)** Several weeks after the completion of postmastectomy radiation therapy, the tissue expander was progressively re-inflated to the pre-deflation volume of 600cc. **(G)** At 7 months after completion of the postmastectomy radiation therapy, the patient underwent a "skin-preserving" delayed breast reconstruction with a microvascular TRAM flap. Postoperative view 14 days after breast reconstruction. No breast revision or contralateral symmetry procedure has been performed.

problems associated with PMRT after an immediate breast reconstruction. Delayed-immediate reconstruction offers the opportunity for a better aesthetic outcome than is achieved with standard delayed reconstruction. Specifically, re-expansion of the mastectomy skin after PMRT (Figure 3.8) provides additional usable breast skin to perform delayed breast reconstruction. Delayed-immediate reconstruction provides an additional option that broadens patients' treatment choices and allows patients to participate fully in treatment and reconstruction decisions.

Although the delayed immediate reconstruction has been successfully used, others have followed a similar but different approach. If it is acceptable to the woman and the radiation oncologist, the expander that is placed at the time of mastectomy can be left in place with a moderate fill volume during the entire course of postoperative chemotherapy and radiation therapy. This allows the woman to have the benefits of immediate reconstruction and allows her to delay the next step of her reconstruction until all of her other therapies have been completed.

Coordinating Adjuvant or Neoadjuvant Chemotherapy Along with Breast Reconstruction

An increasing number of breast cancer patients with stage I disease are being treated with adjuvant (postoperative) chemotherapy. Concerns have been raised that the cytotoxic and myelosuppressive effects of chemotherapy may result in poor wound healing or an increased incidence of postoperative wound infections *(31–32)* after breast reconstruction. Concerns have also been raised that complications of immediate breast reconstruction may interfere with the subsequent administration of adjuvant chemotherapy *(33–36)*. Most studies of chemotherapy in patients treated with breast reconstruction have found no significant prolonged problems with wound healing *(33–36)*, no delays in the initiation or resumption of chemotherapy as a result of wound-healing problems or infections *(33–36)*, and no need for premature cessation of chemotherapy as a result of wound-healing problems *(33–35)*.

A study by Yule et al. *(33)* evaluated 46 patients who underwent immediate breast reconstruction with tissue expanders and subsequent permanent implants. A group of 23 patients received adjuvant chemotherapy, and 23 did not. The authors reported no statistically significant differences in wound healing, wound infection, or capsular contracture between the patients treated with chemotherapy and those who did not receive chemotherapy. Several studies *(34,35)* have shown that patients who undergo immediate breast reconstruction are not predisposed to delays in the initiation of adjuvant chemotherapy compared with patients who have mastectomy without reconstruction. Schusterman et al. *(37)* compared the free TRAM flap with the pedicled TRAM flap in patients requiring postoperative chemotherapy and found that 29% of patients who underwent reconstruction with a pedicled TRAM flap had a delay in the start of chemotherapy, compared with only 14% of the patients who underwent reconstruction with a free TRAM flap. In another study, by Caffo et al. *(36)*, patients who underwent immediate breast reconstruction did not require more frequent adjustments in the dose intensity of their chemotherapy as compared with patients who underwent mastectomy without reconstruction. Caffo et al. also observed that the interval between surgery and the start of expander inflation was not influenced by chemotherapy.

Neoadjuvant (preoperative) chemotherapy is being used with increasing frequency in breast cancer patients with stage II and III disease. The effect of neoadjuvant chemotherapy on surgical outcome is of particular concern in these patients, as is the potential for wound-healing problems that may delay any subsequent adjuvant therapy. As the interval between chemotherapy and surgery increases, the impact on wound healing diminishes *(38)*—the white blood cell count nadir occurs at 10 to 14 days after the last chemotherapy treatment—and recovery occurs by 21 days *(39)*. It is clinically recognized that an absolute neutrophil count less than 500 cells/mm^3 is detrimental to wound healing and wound strength *(40)*. Wound healing can usually occur normally when the white blood cell count is greater than 3000 cells/mm^3 *(40)*. Therefore, the timing of mastectomy with immediate breast reconstruction after neoadjuvant chemotherapy is important to avoid wound-healing problems.

Deutsch et al. *(41)* evaluated 31 patients who underwent immediate reconstruction with a TRAM flap after neoadjuvant chemotherapy. Of these, 17 patients had postoperative complications, but only two had a delay in the start of adjuvant chemotherapy. Seven patients were smokers, five of whom had complications. Both delays in chemotherapy occurred in smokers. Neither delay was longer than 6 weeks after the normal 4-week interval. The authors found no correlation between the number of preoperative chemotherapy cycles, interval from chemotherapy to surgery, or stage of disease and surgical outcome. There was no statistically significant difference in the incidence of complications between pedicled and free TRAM flap reconstructions. The authors concluded that immediate breast reconstruction with the TRAM flap can be performed safely in patients who receive neoadjuvant chemotherapy but that the combination of neoadjuvant chemotherapy and smoking may significantly increase the risk of complications.

Important Considerations for the Multi-Disciplinary Breast Cancer Team

The multi-disciplinary breast team should educate patients about breast reconstruction and increase their awareness of the interplay among the currently evolving diagnostic and treatment modalities. All patients who are candidates for immediate breast reconstruction should be made aware that if it is determined after reconstruction that PMRT is required, the presence of the reconstructed breast could decrease the quality of the aesthetic outcome *(10,17–23,28,42–44)* and cause technical difficulties with radiation delivery *(15,16)*. However, patients should also be made aware that the aesthetic results of delayed breast reconstruction are often less optimal than those of immediate reconstruction *(8,28)*. Throughout the patient education process, it is prudent to obtain appropriate patient consent and document it in the medical record.

Careful planning prior to surgery is required to minimize adverse effects of PMRT on breast reconstruction, which can result in significant patient dissatisfaction. During planning for immediate breast reconstruction, it is imperative to carefully review the stage of disease and the likelihood that the patient will require PMRT. If PMRT is planned, the risks associated with the use of an implant for breast reconstruction should be fully discussed, including the increased risk of capsular contracture and the increased need for change to or addition of a tissue flap to complete the reconstruction *(18,20,21,42,45)*. Capsular contracture can distort the appearance of the reconstructed breast and cause chronic chest wall pain and tightness *(43)*. Furthermore, the addition of a latissimus dorsi flap prior to radiation does not protect against the negative effects of radiation on breast implants *(18)*. Even though autologous tissue alone is preferred in an irradiated patient, autologous reconstructions can also be adversely affected by PMRT *(10,17,19,22,23,28)*. Contracture of the breast skin and atrophy of the flap *(43)* can result in anatomic distortion of the reconstructed breast that can progress over time, resulting in displacement of the flap superiorly *(43)*. Improving asymmetry can be extremely difficult *(43)*, and although a local flap may occasionally correct a small contour deformity, often an additional flap is required to restore breast shape and allow adequate healing.

In all cases of decision-making about possible postoperative XRT and whether or not to perform immediate breast reconstruction, the situation should be discussed at a multi-disciplinary conference or addressed between the various medical, surgical, and radiation teams, with active participation by the patient. Our institution's multi-disciplinary philosophy is to avoid immediate breast reconstruction in patients who will definitely require or have a high likelihood of requiring PMRT. At M. D. Anderson Cancer Center, we often utilize, "delayed-immediate breast reconstruction," for patients who are at high-risk for requiring PMRT. In this approach, we delay immediate reconstruction until after review of the final pathology report on the mastectomy specimen and the axillary lymph nodes. With the now routine use of axillary sentinel node biopsy in breast cancer patients, we now commonly use the internal mammary vessels as our first choice in immediate free TRAM breast reconstruction *(5)*, which in addition to other benefits has eliminated the potential for vascular injury to the reconstructed breast when the sentinel lymph node is found to be positive on review of permanent sections and additional axillary nodal surgery is required *(5)*. As the indications for PMRT and other treatment modalities continue to change, plastic surgeons will have to adapt their approach to breast reconstruction to maintain an appropriate balance between minimizing the risk of recurrence and providing the best possible aesthetic outcome.

References

1. Giuliano AE, Jones RC, Brennan M, et al. Sentinel lymphadenctomy in breast cancer. J Clin Oncol 1997;15:2345–2350.
2. Van Diest PJ, Torrenga H, Borgstein PJ, et al. Reliability of intraoperative frozen section and cytological investigation of sentinel lymph nodes in breast cancer. Histopathology 1999;35:14–18.
3. Wiser MR, Montgomery LL, Susnik B, et al. Is routine intraoperative frozen-section examination of sentinel lymph nodes in breast cancer worthwhile? Ann Surg Oncol 2000;7:651–655.
4. Turner RR, Hansen NM, Stern SL, Giuliano AE. Intraoperative examination of the sentinel lymph node for breast carcinoma staging. Am J Clin Pathol 1999;112:627.
5. Kronowitz SJ, Chang DW, Robb GL, et al. Implications of axillary sentinel lymph node biopsy in immediate autologous breast reconstruction. Plast Reconstr Surg 2002;109:1888.
6. Katz A, Strom EA, Buchholz TA, et al. Locoregional recurrence patterns after mastectomy and doxorubicin-based chemotherapy: implications for postoperative irradiation. J Clin Oncol 2000;18:2817.
7. Ivens D, Hoe AL, Podd TJ, et al. Assessment of morbidity from complete axillary dissection. Br J Cancer 1992;66:136–138.
8. Miller MJ. Immediate breast reconstruction. Clin Plast Surg 1998;25: 145–156.
9. Harris J, Halpin-Murphy P, McNeese M, et al. Consensus statement on post-mastectomy radiation therapy. Int J Radiat Oncol Biol Phys 1999;44:989.
10. Tran NV, Chang DW, Gupta A, Kroll SS, Robb GL. Comparison of immediate and delayed TRAM flap breast reconstruction in patients receiving postmastectomy radiation therapy. Plast Reconstr Surg 2001;108:78.
11. Buchholz TA, Strom EA, Perkins GH, et al. Controversies regarding the use of radiation after mastectomy in breast cancer. Oncologist 2002;7:539–546.
12. Recht A, Edge SB, Solin LJ, et al. Postmastectomy radiotherapy: clinical practice guidelines of the American Society of Clinical Oncology. J Clin Oncol 2001;19:1539.

13. Overgaard M, Hansen PS, Overgaard J, et al. Postoperative radiotherapy in high-risk premenopausal women with breast cancer who receive adjuvant chemotherapy. N Engl J Med 1997;337:949.
14. Ragaz K, Jackson SM, Le N, et al. Adjuvant radiotherapy and chemotherapy in node-positive premenopausal women with breast cancer. N Engl J Med 1997;337:956.
15. Buchholz TA, Kronowitz SJ, Kuerer HM. Immediate breast reconstruction after skin-sparing mastectomy for treatment of advanced breast cancer: radiation oncology considerations. Ann Surg Oncol 2002;9:820.
16. Strom E. Radiation therapy for early and advanced breast disease. In: Hunt KK, Robb GL, Strom EA, Ueno NT, (eds.), *Breast cancer*. New York: Springer-Verlag; 2001:255–285.
17. Kroll SS, Schusterman MA, Reece GP, Miller MJ, Smith B. Breast reconstruction with myocutaneous flaps in previously irradiated patients. Plast Reconstr Surg 1994;93:460.
18. Evans GRD, Schusterman MA, Kroll SS, et al. Reconstruction and the radiated breast: is there a role for implants? Plast Reconstr Surg 1995;96:1111.
19. Spear SL, Onyewu C. Staged breast reconstruction with saline-filled implants in the irradiated breast: recent trends and therapeutic implications. Plast Reconstr Surg 2000;105:930.
20. Williams JK, Bostwick J III, Bried JT, Mackay G, Landry J, Benton J. TRAM flap breast reconstruction after radiation treatment. Ann Surg 1995;221:756.
21. Kraemer O, Andersen M, Siim E. Breast reconstruction and tissue expansion in irradiated versus not irradiated women after mastectomy. Scand J Plast Reconstr Hand Surg 1996;30:201.
22. Williams JK, Carlson GW, Bostwick J III, Bried JT, Mackay G. The effects of radiation treatment after TRAM flap breast reconstruction. Plast Reconstr Surg 1997;100:1153.
23. Rogers NE, Allen RJ. Radiation effects on breast reconstruction with the deep inferior epigastric perforator flap. Plast Reconstr Surg 2002; 109:1919.
24. Spear SL, Ducic I, Low M, et al. The effect of radiation therapy on pedicled TRAM flap breast reconstruction: outcomes and implications. Plast Reconstr Surg 2005;115:84–95.
25. Kronowitz SJ, Robb GR. Breast reconstruction with postmastectomy radiation therapy: current issues. Plast Reconstr Surg 2004;114:950–960.
26. Kronowitz SJ, Hunt KK, Kuerer HM, et al. Delayed-immediate breast reconstruction. Plast Reconstr Surg 2004;113:1617–1628.
27. Taylor W, Horgan K, Dodwell D. Oncological aspects of breast reconstruction. Breast 2005;14:118–126.
28. Kroll SS, Coffey JA, Winn RJ, Schusterman MA. A comparison of factors affecting aesthetic outcomes of TRAM flap breast reconstructions. Plast Reconstr Surg 1995;96:860.
29. Miller MJ, Rock CS, Robb GL. Aesthetic breast reconstruction using a combination of free transverse rectus abdominis musculocutaneous flaps and breast implants. Ann Plast Surg 1996;37:258–264.
30. Kronowitz SJ, Robb GL. Reconstruction and radiation therapy. In: Singletary SE, Robb GL, Hortobagyi GN, (eds.), *Advanced therapy of breast disease, second edition*. Hamilton, Ontario, Canada: BC Decker Inc.; 2004.
31. Ferguson MK. The effect of antineoplastic agents on wound healing. Surg Gynecol Obstet 1982;154:421.
32. Lawrence WT, Talbot TL, Norton JA. Preoperative or postoperative doxorubicin hydrochloride: which is better for wound healing? Surgery 1986;100:9.

33. Yule GJ, Concannon MJ, Croll GH, Puckett CL. Is there liability with chemotherapy following immediate breast reconstruction? Plast Reconstr Surg 1996;97:969.
34. Furey PC, Macgillivray DC, Castiglione CL, Allen L. Wound complications in patients receiving adjuvant chemotherapy after mastectomy and immediate breast reconstruction for breast cancer. J Surg Oncol 1994;55:194.
35. Allweis TM, Boisvert ME, Otero SE, Perry DJ, Dubin NH, Priebat DA. Immediate reconstruction after mastectomy for breast cancer does not prolong the time to starting adjuvant chemotherapy. Am J Surg 2002;183:218.
36. Caffo O, Cazzolli D, Scalet A, et al. Concurrent adjuvant chemotherapy and immediate breast reconstruction with skin expanders after mastectomy for breast cancer. Breast Cancer Res Treat 2000;60:267.
37. Schusterman M, Kroll S, Weldon M. Immediate breast reconstruction: why the free TRAM over the conventional TRAM flap? Plast Reconstr Surg 1992;90:255.
38. Drake D, Oishi S. Wound healing considerations in chemotherapy and radiation therapy. Clin Plast Surg 1995;22:31.
39. Ariyan S, Kraft RL, Goldberg NH. An experimental model to determine the effects of adjuvant therapy on the incidence of postoperative wound infections II: evaluating preoperative chemotherapy. Plast Reconstr Surg 1990;65:338.
40. Springfield D. Surgical wound healing. In: Verweij J, Pinedo HM, Suit HD, (eds.), *Multidisciplinary treatment of soft tissue sarcomas*. Boston: Luwer Academic Publishers; 1993:81–98.
41. Deutsch MF, Smith M, Wang B, Ainsle N, Schusterman MA. Immediate breast reconstruction with TRAM flap after neoadjuvant therapy. Ann Plast Surg 1999;42:240.
42. Vandeweyer E, Deraemaecker R. Radiation therapy after immediate breast reconstruction with implants. Plast Reconstr Surg 2000;106:56.
43. Robb GL. Reconstructive surgery. In: Hunt KK, Robb GL, Strom EA, Ueno NT, (eds.), *Breast cancer*. New York: Springer-Verlag; 2001:255–285.
44. Hartrampf CR, Bennett GK. Autogenous tissue reconstruction in the mastectomy patient. Ann Surg 1987;205:508.
45. Rosato RM, Dowden RV. Radiation therapy as a cause of capsular contracture. Ann Plast Surg 1994;323:342.

4

Breast Reconstruction

Autogenous Tissue

Joseph M. Serletti

Introduction

Oncologic reconstruction of head and neck cancers, breast cancers, and trunk and extremity cancers has become routine in most academic and larger community medical centers. Reconstruction of many of these oncologic defects can be performed using either autogenous tissue or alloplastic materials. Although there are usually clear indications for the use of either of these basic methods, autogenous reconstructions are usually preferred. Autogenous tissue has the advantage of "replacing like with like," creating a more natural reconstructive result with long-term predictability. Autogenous reconstructions are less likely to result in late infectious sequellae including wound infection, implant exposure, and implant failure as can be seen in alloplastic reconstructions. For breast reconstruction, two primary methods of reconstruction exist: implant reconstruction and autogenous reconstruction. Although there are relative contraindications for each of these methods in selected patients, most patients are candidates for either method.

Patients presenting to the plastic surgeon for breast reconstruction are frequently well informed about their options for breast reconstruction. The internet, patient support groups, and numerous lay books have provided easy access to an abundant amount of information regarding breast cancer treatments and breast reconstruction. Upon presenting to the plastic surgeon, many patients begin by saying they do not want an implant reconstruction. Although this may be an appropriate decision for some patients, many others are misinformed about implants and the plastic surgeon must spend additional time with these patients, properly informing them about the safety and limitations of implant reconstructions.

Both silicone gel and saline implants remain available for breast reconstruction. Thus far, no study has been able to document a cause and effect relationship between silicone or saline implants and a systemic illness *(1–3)*. Why then have implant reconstructions become less popular? The limitations of implant reconstructions are related to the aesthetic results, capsular contracture, and implant failure *(4–7)*. In the unilateral implant breast reconstruction, it is very difficult to match the ptosis and pliability of the natural breast. Without brassiere support, there is usually a vertical discrepancy between the native and reconstructed breast mound, with the native breast more inferiorly positioned. Even in the absence of capsular contracture, the implant breast reconstruction will be firmer and less mobile as compared to the native breast. Over time, all implants will eventually leak as a result of degradation of the silicone bladder. Particularly for younger patients with implant reconstructions, one or more implant exchanges may need to occur over their lifetime *(8)*.

The breast is composed of thin skin surrounding mostly adipose tissue. Throughout the adipose tissue is a network of breast glandular tissue. Autogenous breast reconstructions typically use flaps of skin and adipose tissue, essentially replacing the breast contents with "like" tissue. Autogenous breast reconstructions, therefore, can create a ptotic, soft, pliable, and essentially symmetric breast mound that more significantly mimics the contralateral native breast mound as compared to implant reconstructions. Because of the limitations with implant reconstructions and the more natural results obtained with autogenous reconstructions, many patients are selecting an autogenous method despite these being typically longer, more complex surgical procedures. After 2 or more years following autogenous reconstruction, the early and intermediate postoperative changes and scarring have matured. Not infrequently, some level of sensation occurs in these reconstructed breast mounds *(9,10)*. At this point, many patients view their reconstructed breast mound as a natural part of their body. The reconstructed breast does not tend to remain a constant reminder of the patient's history of breast cancer *(11)*. The same cannot easily be said about implant reconstructions, which have a greater tendency to serve as a permanent reminder of the patient's experience with breast cancer. This difference serves as another compelling advantage of autogenous breast reconstruction.

History of Autogenous Reconstruction

Autogenous breast reconstruction had its beginnings in the early 1900s using the latissimus myocutaneous flap as described by Tansini. This method fell from favor and was not recognized again until the 1970s. During the 1940s and 1950s, most breast reconstructions were preformed using breast-sharing procedures. A portion of the remaining native breast was moved to the mastectomy site in a series of tubed transfers. This method required multiple operative procedures over a course of months to achieve the final result. Thoracoepigastric tube flaps were similarly used to create an autogenous breast reconstruction, again in a series of operative steps. In the 1960s, Cronin and Gerow introduced the silicone gel implant, and in 1982 Radovan introduced the tissue expander concept. These two devices allowed for breast mound reconstruction in fewer steps and avoided donor site considerations. The use and relative ease of these devices also helped establish both delayed and immediate breast reconstruction as routine surgical procedures. The latissimus dorsi myocutaneous flap was re-introduced during the late 1970s as a method of autogenous breast reconstruction alone or used in combination with an implant. A monumental contribution to autogenous breast reconstruction was Hartrampf's introduction of the pedicled transverse rectus abdominis myocutaneous flap (TRAM) in 1982. This technique remains the most common method of autogenous breast reconstruction today. Alterations in the technique for transferring this redundant lower abdominal tissue have occurred and include the free TRAM flap, the deep inferior epigastric perforator (DIEP) flap, and the superficial inferior epigastric (SIE) flap. These alterations have been made to improve the blood supply to the transferred tissue and to limit the abdominal wall donor defect. Other free autogenous choices include the gluteal flap, the superior gluteal artery perforator flap (superior gluteal artery perforator), the lateral thigh flap, and the Ruben's flap. These other choices are typically used in patients who have had a TRAM flap and develop a contralateral breast cancer or in patients who desire an autogenous breast reconstruction but have inadequate abdominal tissue.

The Latissimus Dorsi Myocutaneous Flap

The latissimus dorsi myocutaneous flap was first introduced for coverage of mastectomy defects by Tansini in 1906. Although this technique had a brief period of popularity, it was essentially lost until the 1970s. With the advent of myocutaneous flaps, the latissimus dorsi typically used in combination with a breast implant became a popular method of breast reconstruction. Prior to the use of tissue expansion, the latissimus dorsi skin island provided for the missing breast skin and the underlying volume of the breast was reconstructed with an implant. Using the latissimus dorsi flap in this way allowed for single-stage immediate and delayed breast reconstruction.

The latissimus dorsi muscle is a broad, thin muscle that originates from the iliac crest, lumbar vertebrae, and lower thoracic vertebrae and inserts on the inter-tubercular groove of the humerus. The primary blood supply is the thoracodorsal system, which is a terminal branch of the subscapular vessels. The motor nerve to the muscle is the thoracodorsal nerve. This muscle's functions include shoulder extension, adduction, medial rotation of the arm, and downward and backward movement of the shoulder. Most of these functions are provided by other muscles, and loss of this muscle is usually unnoticed by most patients. A skin island can be designed over almost any portion of the muscle; however, any skin overlying the most inferior portions of the muscle can be problematic. For breast reconstruction, the skin island is usually placed on a transverse orientation in the more superior portion of the muscle. This allows for the donor scar to be potentially hidden by an overlying back of a brassiere or the back of a two-piece bathing suit. Skin markings over the breast site and the latissimus donor site are usually made preoperatively with the patient in the standing position.

In both immediate and delayed reconstruction, surgery may begin with the patient in either the supine or decubitus position. In delayed reconstruction, the breast skin is elevated to redefine the perimeter of the breast pocket. The flap's skin island is incised and skin flaps are elevated to expose the needed boundaries of the latissimus muscle. The back skin is elevated laterally so as to create a subcutaneous tunnel between the latissimus dissection and the mastectomy defect. In most patients, the thoracodorsal vessels do not need to be dissected, and the insertion is left intact. Some surgeons prefer to divide the motor nerve so as to avoid potential motion of the breast reconstruction with shoulder movement. In delayed reconstructions, there remains the potential for prior injury to the thoradorsal vessels from the axillary dissection. Despite division of the thoracodorsal vessels, the latissimus is believed to remain reliable through retrograde flow through its serratus branches. In delayed reconstructive patients, the latissimus muscle should be examined preoperatively. Absence of motor activity within the muscle should raise suspicion about the patency of the thoracodorsal vessels. Flap viability should be assured in these patients during surgery; questionable viability may require microsurgerical intervention.

In radical mastectomy defects, the entire muscle is usually harvested and used for reconstruction of the missing pectoralis muscle. The insertion of the latissimus is usually divided and re-established anteriorly to create an anterior axillary fold. When implants are used in combination with this flap, the implant is placed underneath the pectoralis muscle and latissimus muscle. In patients with smaller contralateral breast volume, a total autogenous latissimus reconstruction can be performed, obviating the need for an implant.

The Pedicled TRAM Flap

The pedicled TRAM flap was introduced by Hartrampf in 1982. The lower abdominal skin island used in this flap remains the most common method of autogenous breast reconstruction, whether transferred as a pedicled TRAM flap, a free TRAM flap, a DIEP flap, or an SIE flap. When considering all methods of breast reconstruction, both alloplastic and autogenous, most surgeons agree that the TRAM flap is unmatched for its ability to create a soft, pliable, and natural breast mound with excellent potential for symmetry to an intact opposite breast.

The pedicled TRAM flap skin island receives its blood supply from perforators arising from the rectus abdominis muscle. The rectus abdominis muscle originates on the pubic symphysis and crest and inserts on the fifth, sixth, and seventh costal cartilages. This muscle is an intimate part of the abdominal wall and flexes the vertebral column. The motor supply to this muscle is the lower six or seven segmental intercostal nerves. This muscle has a dual blood supply. The superior muscle is supplied by the superior epigastric vessels, which are terminal branches of the internal mammary vessels. The inferior muscle is supplied by the inferior epigastric vessels, which originate from the external iliac vessels. These two systems anastomose with each other through choke vessels within the center of the muscle. The entire muscle can, therefore, be elevated on either blood supply. The TRAM skin island in the pedicled TRAM flap is based upon the superior epigastric vessels as it is transferred to the chest defect.

Whether used in immediate or delayed reconstruction, preoperative markings on both the chest and abdomen are made on the patient in the standing position. The abdominal skin island is placed in the lower abdomen and can generally follow native skin creases at the umbilicus and suprapubic region. The upper portion of the skin island is usually placed just above the umbilicus to capture some of the larger perforators exiting from the muscle and the epigastric vasculature. The lower portion of the skin island is placed so as to allow primary closure of the typical abdominoplasty defect. The skin island is typically viewed with four separate zones or quadrants based on its attachment to one rectus muscle. The zone overlying the muscle directly and the adjacent quadrants are generally reliable. The zone furthest from the muscle is usually unreliable and is discarded before insetting a pedicled TRAM flap.

The pedicled TRAM flap is usually begun with elevation of the skin just superior to the TRAM skin island, exposing the upper rectus muscles. A subcutaneous skin bridge is created between the abdominal dissection and the mastectomy defect. This bridge is kept as medial as possible to maintain a significant portion of the inframammary fold but large enough to allow passage of the TRAM skin island. The skin island can be pedicled on one rectus abdominis muscle or both muscles. In preparing the skin island for transfer, all attachements except those of the skin island to the rectus muscle(s) are divided. Whether designed as a unipedicle or bipedicle flap, some surgeons harvest the entire muscle(s), whereas others preserve a lateral and medial band of muscle, harvesting only the central rectus muscle. The early experiences with the pedicled TRAM flap included complications such as abdominal wall laxity/hernia, fat necrosis, and partial flap loss, particularly seen in patients who smoked, were obese, or had other significant medical comorbidities. In such high-risk patients, surgeons have altered their technique for the pedicled TRAM flap so as to augment the blood supply to the skin island. These alterations have included a bipedicle blood supply, thus harvesting both rectus muscles with the flap perfused by both superior epigastric vessels. The pedicled TRAM flap can also be "supercharged" by dissecting a length of the inferior epigastric vessels and anastomosing them to the thoracodorsal vessels, thus employing both sources of the rectus abdominis' blood supply. Muscle sparing techiques have been employed to perserve some muscle and fascia to help improve abdominal donor site results. Onlay and inlay mesh are also used to reinforce the abdominal wall closure. Once the flap is transferred to the chest, the abdominal wall defect is closed. The lower abdominal skin defect is closed by mobilizing the upper abdominal skin flap into the lower skin defect. The previously separated umbilicus is re-inset into the anterior abdominal skin. After completing the abdominal site closure, the patient is placed in the sitting position and the TRAM skin island is trimmed and contoured to match the opposite breast.

The Free TRAM Flap

The rectus abdominis muscle has a dual dominant blood supply, the superior epigastric vessels and the inferior epigastric vessels. The pedicled TRAM flap is based upon the superior epigastric vessels and the free TRAM flap is based on the inferior epigastric vessels. The overlying skin and adipose tissue within the transverse skin island of the TRAM flap receives its blood supply from perforating vessels from the rectus abdominis muscle. These vessels exit from the muscle and perforate the anterior rectus fascia to supply the fat and dermal-subdermal plexus. The skin island in the TRAM flap is positioned over the lower portion of the rectus muscle, actually closer to the inferior epigastric blood supply. This flap design provides for more direct and improved blood supply to the TRAM skin island and represents one of the main advantages of the free TRAM flap over the pedicled flap *(12–14)*.

Prior to beginning surgery, the patient is marked in the standing position. The TRAM skin island and the inframammary fold are marked bilaterally. The entire chest and abdomen are prepped including the contralateral breast whether for an immediate or delayed reconstruction. The upper edge of the TRAM skin island is incised and an upper abdominal flap is raised to the xiphoid and the costal margins. This upper skin flap can be draped over the TRAM skin island so as to ensure an acceptable abdominal closure. The lower portion of the skin island is then incised. A decision has usually been made preoperatively whether to use an ipsilateral or contralateral free flap. This is based upon the shape of the contralateral breast. The lateral portion of the skin island closest to the selected muscle is elevated to the first row of lateral perforators and the fascia is incised. A muscle splitting dissection is performed, and the inferior epigastric vessels are identified and dissected to the external iliac vessels. There is usually a single inferior epigastric vein at this level or a large vein with a smaller counterpart entering the external iliac vein. The opposite side of the skin island is elevated to the first row of medial perforators exiting from the selected muscle. This separates the skin island from the vasculature of the opposite rectus. The anterior rectus fascia is incised here and a medial muscle splitting dissection is performed. The flap is now ready for division and transfer. Prior to doing this, the recipient vessel site has been prepared and the adequacy of their inflow and outflow assessed. Once harvested, there remains a fascial defect in the lower abdominal wall. This is typically repaired by direct closure and onlay mesh or exact repair of the fascial defect with an inlay of mesh. The abdominal donor site is closed similar to that in an aesthetic abdominoplasty. The patient is usually placed in the fully upright position for inset of the free flap. At the end of the procedure, a surface arterial doppler signal is identified or an implantable venous doppler probe is placed. The patient is placed in a postoperative clinical setting that allows frequent flap checks during the first 24 to 48 hours.

Because of the indirect blood supply in a pedicled TRAM, patient selection for this technique has generally followed strict guidelines. Patients with a history of smoking, hypertension, obesity, chronic obstructive pulmonary disease (COPD), previous abdominal surgery, and even diabetes have been considered high-risk patients for the pedicled TRAM flap *(15,16)*. The improved blood supply and more limited donor site defect in the free TRAM technique has allowed this type of breast reconstruction in these higher-risk patients with acceptable complication rates *(5–7)*. Insetting of the free TRAM flap is easier and less restrictive as compared to the pedicled flap. Another advantage of the free TRAM flap over other choices for free flap breast reconstruction is the quality of the soft tissue. The adipose tissue and skin in the free TRAM flap more closely mimics breast skin and fat producing, in general, the most natural reconstructive results.

The DIEP Flap

Criticisms of both the pedicled and free TRAM flap have mostly centered on the abdominal wall donor site *(17)*. Initially, the entire lower portion of the rectus muscle was harvested with the free flap. This was followed by the muscle splitting approach described previously, where both a lateral and medial strip of muscle and anterior rectus fascia are preserved. The DIEP flap uses the same skin island as in the TRAM flap, but preserves all of the rectus muscle and anterior rectus fascia. The skin island in the DIEP flap is based on one or more of the perforating vessels and their connection to the inferior epigastric vasculature.

Prior to surgery, the major perforators on each side of the skin island are identified with a hand-held doppler *(18)*. Upon selecting a side (right or left), the lateral edge of the ipsilateral part of the skin island is elevated off of the fascia. Using loupe magnification and atraumatic technique, an acceptably large perforator(s) is identified. The anterior rectus fascia is incised above the perforator for a short distance and below it to just above the inguinal region. The fascia is reflected off of the muscle in a lateral direction. The muscle is split for a short distance around the perforator, identifying its connection to the inferior epigastric system. The lateral edge of the muscle is elevated off of the posterior rectus sheath for further identification and dissection of the inferior epigastric vessels. Care is taken to maintain all of the intercostal motor nerve supply to the rectus muscle. After completion of flap dissection, the inferior epigastric vessels are divided proximally and passed through the opening in the muscle at the level of the perforator. The flap is separated from its remaining attachments to the abdominal wall and passed to the chest for anastomosis and inset. The incision in the anterior rectus fascia is closed directly without the need for mesh and the entire muscle with its nerve supply has been preserved. Proponents for this technique suggest that there is less postoperative pain, shorter hospitalization, more prompt recovery, and little or no functional deficit in the abdominal donor site. Because of this flap relying on one or two perforators, it has been recommended to avoid this technique in smokers and obese patients *(19)*.

The SIE Flap

More recently, the SIE blood supply to the typical TRAM skin island has been identified as yet another free flap method of transferring the excess lower abdominal tissue to the chest for breast reconstruction. The SIE vessels arise from the common femorals and course into the lower abdominal soft tissue, usually just medial to the iliac crest. These vessels arise off of the femorals either independently of the superificial iliac circumflex vessels or as a shared originating vessel. The SIEs are identified during the dissection of the lower incision of the typical transverse lower abdominal skin island. They are usually found just medial to the iliac crest and are either just below or just above scarpa's fascia. The SIE vessels are either absent or too small to use as a free flap transfer of the abdominal tissue in the majority of patients. Approximately 20–30% of the time, they are large enough to use for free tissue transfer and should be strongly considered in this setting. This pedicle only reliably perfuses the ipsilateral half of the lower abdominal skin island. These vessels are smaller in caliber than the inferior epigastrics and generally do require the operating microscope in order to reliably perform the anastomoses. When this flap is harvested, there is no fascial incision or any muscle dissection. Whereas the abdominal donor site advantages of the DIEP flap over the fTRAM flap remain questionable, there is essentially no abdominal wall morbidity when the SIE flap is used. Smokers, large breast reconstructions, and patient who are planned for postoperative radiotherapy are considered contraindications for using this flap.

The Superior and Inferior Free Gluteal Flap

The free superior and inferior gluteal myocutaneous flap is based upon the gluteus maximus muscle supplied by either the superior gluteal or inferior gluteal vasculature and its overlying skin. With the patient in the decubitus or prone position, a line is drawn from the posterior superior iliac spine to the top of the greater trochanter. The superior gluteal pedicle is located near the junction of the superior and middle one-thirds of that line. The skin island can be centered along this oblique line or may be rotated to a more horizontal position overlying the upper portion of the gluteus maximus muscle. With the inferior gluteal flap, the pedicle is 4–5 cm inferior to the location of the superior gluteal vessels. The skin island can similarly be oriented transversely or obliquely about this point. The width of either skin island can be up to 13 cm and the length can vary between 10 and 30 cm. While the most limiting parameter is skin paddle width, an abundant amount of adipose tissue can be taken both above and below the margins of this skin island, allowing for reconstruction of a large breast. Prior to positioning the patient for flap harvest, the vertical and horizontal dimensions of the remaining breast are recorded and used for design of the gluteal flap. The superior and inferior edges of the skin island are incised first and skin flaps are raised, leaving an appropriate amount of adipose tissue attached to the muscle. This fat will be part of the flap used for breast reconstruction. With the superior gluteal flap, the superior edge of the gluteus maximus is identified and elevated off of the gluteus medius. Dissection then follows to the lateral margin of the muscle as it heads toward the greater trochanter. The lateral muscle here is incised. The upper portion of the medial gluteus maximus muscle can also be incised, allowing for improved visualization of the deep surface of the muscle. The superior gluteal vessels are identified on this deep surface and followed to their origin approximately 5 cm lateral to the sacral edge, between the gluteus medius and the piriformis. It is imperative that the vessels here are carefully dissected, as they are fragile and the space for dissection is quite limited despite using self-retaining retractors. A pedicle length of 2–3 cm is typically obtained. The lower edge of the flap with its attached muscle is incised and the gluteus maximus muscle is split at that level. The vessels are divided, as is the remaining soft tissue attachments to the flap. With the inferior gluteal flap, the lower edge of the gluteus muscle is identified laterally. This lateral muscle is incised along its attachment to the greater trochanter and the gluteus muscle along the superior edge of the skin island is split. The skin island and attached gluteus muscle are reflected medially, exposing the sciatic nerve and the inferior gluteal vasculature. During this flap dissection, the posterior cutaneous nerve of the thigh is sacrificed. The inferior gluteal vessels can be dissected just underneath the piriformis muscle, obtaining a pedicle length of 4–6 cm. While the donor site is being closed, the superior or inferior flap is taken to the side table for further dissection of the pedicle from the muscle. This can yield an additional 1–2 cm of length. The patient is returned to the full supine position for flap anastomosis and inset. Because of the short pedicle length, the internal mammary vessels are preferred, allowing for medial placement of this tissue. Some surgeons have regularly used vein grafts with this flap so as to overcome the difficulties with the short pedicle *(20–22)*. It is useful to harvest the smallest amount of muscle needed to capture either the superior or inferior gluteal blood supply. This helps to overcome some of the pedicle length limitations and avoids excessive bulk from the muscle when insetting the flap.

Patients selected for this technique have insufficient abdominal tissue, or have had a prior abdominoplasty. This technique is also used following a unilateral TRAM reconstruction when a secondary contralateral mastectomy and reconstruction are being performed. A significant advantage of this technique is the more rapid recovery and less postoperative discomfort as compared to the TRAM flap. The adipose tissue in the gluteal flap is more septated and less pliable than in both the native breast and the TRAM flap, which makes insetting more challenging and the final result somewhat firmer than a natural breast. Despite these limitations, the gluteal flap remains an excellent and reliable method for autogenous breast reconstruction.

The SGAP and Inferior Gluteal Artery Perforator (IGAP) Flap

The SGAP or IGAP flap uses the skin island of the gluteal flap based on one or more perforators from either the superior or inferior gluteal vasculature. As with the DIEP flap, all of the gluteus maximus muscle is preserved. Using a hand-held doppler, the location of the superior or inferior gluteal vessels is identified on the skin using the line drawn from the posterior superior iliac spine to the greater trochanter as described previously. One or more perforators from either system to the skin can be identified just lateral to the position of the gluteal vessels. A transverse or slightly oblique skin paddle is designed to incorporate the perforators and the gluteal vessels. The upper and lower edges of the skin paddle are prepared just as in the gluteal flap. Beginning at the lateral edge of the skin island, a subfascial dissection is performed until an acceptable perforator is identified. The muscle fibers are split and the perforator is dissected away from its muscle attachments to where it joins a major muscle branch of the gluteal vessels. This major muscle branch is further dissected to the proximal portion of the main vessel and divided. All other attachments of the skin island to the muscle are divided and the flap is passed to the chest for anastomosis and inset.

The advantages of this flap include the considerably longer pedicle length obtained with this dissection. A pedicle length of 6 cm or more can be achieved, which makes performing the anastomosis more straightforward than with the gluteal mycutaneous flap. Without the bulk of the muscle, insetting the flap is easier and the intraoperative result more closely mimics the matured postoperative result of a standard gluteal flap. Preserving all of the gluteus maximus muscle has significant functional considerations and leaves a less depressed contour deformity compared to the gluteal flap. The main disadvantage is that this flap along with the DIEP flap are technically more demanding than their myocutaneous counterparts *(23)*.

Recipient Vessel Sites for Free Flap Breast Reconstruction

The two most common recipient vessel sites in free tissue reconstruction of the breast are the thoracodorsal vessels and the internal mammary vessels. In immediate breast reconstruction, the thoracodorsal vessels are either fully or partially exposed if a modified radical mastectomy has been performed. Only a short amount of surgical time is usually required for full preparation of these vessels in this setting. The thoracodorsal vessels are usually chosen as long as the autogenous flap for reconstruction has a sufficiently long donor pedicle. This combination provides enough vessel length to allow for satisfactory medial placement of the reconstructed breast mound. The thoracodorsal artery and vein are dissected free from the take-off of the scapular circumflex vessels to the vessels to the serratus. The thoracodorsal vessels are also separated from the nerve, all other surrounding attachments, and each other for one-half their length. This dissection allows for a long length of recipient vessels, which can be positioned more superficially for easier anastomosis. The free flap is not inset at this point but rather temporarily secured, so as to allow for an unencumbered positioning and view of both recipient and donor vessels during the anastomoses. End-to-end anastomoses are performed using either interrupted 8-O or 9-O nylon sutures for both the artery and vein, or sutures for the artery and a coupler for the vein. In the delayed breast reconstructive setting, some surgeons choose the thoracodorsal recipient vessels because of their familiarity with flap insetting in immediate reconstruction and the proven efficacy of these vessels in the delayed setting.

For many surgeons, the internal mammary vessels are the recipient vessels of choice in delayed free flap breast reconstruction *(24,25)*. This recipient site has the advantage of avoiding surgery in the previously operated axilla. Some surgeons use this recipient site primarily in immediate reconstruction as well because it allows more medial positioning of the flap for improved symmetry and aesthetics. The internal mammary vessels have also been used preferentially in mastectomy alone or when combined with sentinel node biopsy. There is limited axillary dissection with sentinel node biospy such that considerable further dissection would be required for using the thoracodorsal vessels. The internal mammary vessels are first approached by separating the fibers of the pectoralis muscle overlying the third costal cartilage. The perichondrium is incised and separated off of the cartilage first on the anterior surface and extending to its posterior surface. The costal cartilage is then removed using a rongeur. The deep surface of the perichondrium is incised to expose the internal mammary vessels. The internal mammary vein tends to be larger on the right side as compared to the left. Previous descriptions for approaching this site used the fifth costal cartilage; however, the size of the internal mammary vein was not routinely reliable for free tissue transfer at this location. Although the third cartilage is currently recommended, the second cartilage can be similarly removed for access to a greater diameter recipient vein. Once fully dissected, the internal mammary artery and vein are divided distally so as to perform end-to-end anastomoses. The free flap is temporarily positioned to allow easy performance of the anastomoses.

Immediate Versus Delayed Autogenous Breast Reconstruction

Free flap breast reconstruction can occur at the time that the mastectomy is performed; this is referred to as an immediate breast reconstruction. A delayed reconstruction can occur any time following the mastectomy. A delayed reconstruction is usually not performed sooner than 6 months following mastectomy because of the immature scarring and scar contracture seen in the early months following surgery. There is no temporal limit beyond this that a delayed reconstruction cannot be performed, with some patients having a delayed reconstruction 20 or more years following mastectomy.

In performing a delayed autogenous breast reconstruction, the plastic surgeon needs to consider the quality of the chest wall skin and the available recipient vessel sites if a free flap is planned. Some patients for delayed reconstruction will have had chest wall irradiation. In beginning a delayed autogenous reconstruction, the mastectomy scar is excised and the mastectomy defect is recreated by elevating the prior mastectomy flaps. This is done to the prior perimeter of the breast, which can be more easily identified using the opposite native breast as a guide. Thin, atrophic breast flap skin should be removed and replaced by the skin of the flap. In particular, radiated skin should be removed because of its impaired vascularity and poor compliance. Even in the non-irradiated mastectomy skin, sufficient contracture may have occurred to limit the ptosis and inset of the flap. When that happens, the contracting mastectomy flap skin is either resected and/or radially incised to allow full volumetric creation of the prior mastectomy defect.

Most surgeons agree that with immediate free flap breast reconstruction, the aesthetic results and technical ease of the procedure are improved as compared to performing delayed reconstructions. There is no scar contracture to overcome. With most experienced general surgeons, a well-defined mastectomy defect is created such that filling that defect with the flap mimics the borders of the contralateral native breast. Most centers active in immediate autogenous breast reconstruction have their general surgeons using skin sparing mastectomies. A skin sparing mastectomy removes the nipple-areola complex with usually a lateral extension towards the axilla. Skin sparing mastectomies have allowed for satisfactory local control of the breast cancer while preserving the natural skin brassiere of the breast *(26–28)*. By preserving this natural skin brassiere, the inset of the flap is more straightforward, leading to more reliable symmetry with the opposite breast. The final decision with regard to local tumor control and the pattern for skin excision with the mastectomy, however, is always left to the judgement of the oncologic general surgeon.

Conclusion

Autogenous breast reconstruction allows for the creation of a generally soft, pliable, and ptotic breast mound with unmatched ability to mimic an intact native breast. Autogenous reconstruction can be achieved in most patients despite age or the presence of significant medical comorbidities. Flap selection and other issues related to the technical considerations of autogenous reconstruction should be based on patient needs and the surgeon's experience. With this in mind, autogenous reconstruction can be successfully achieved in the broad spectrum of patients with high patient satisfaction and low incidence of complications.

References

1. Buncke HJ, Buncke CM, Schulz WP. Experimental digital amputation and replantation. Plast Reconstr Surg 1965;36:62.
2. Chen ZW, Chen YC, Pao YS. Salvage of the forearm following complete traumatic amputation. Clin Med J 1963;82:632.
3. Kleinert HE, Kardan ML, Romero JL. Small blood vessel anastomosis for salvage of severely injured upper extremity. J Bone Joint Surg 1963;45:788.
4. Daniel RK, Taylor GI. Distant transfer of an island flap by microvascular anastomosis. Plast Reconstr Surg 1973;52:111–117.
5. McLean DH, Buncke HJ. Autotransplantation of omentum to scalp defect with microsurgical revascularization. Plast Reconstr Surg 1982;49:268–274.
6. Kaplan EL, Buncke HJ, Murray DE. Distant transfer of cutaneous island flaps in humans by microvascular anastomosis. Plast Reconstr Surg 1973;52:301–305.
7. Glicksman A, Ferder M, Casale P, Posner J, Kim R, Strauch B. 1457 years of microsurgical experience. Plast Reconstr Surg 1997;100:355–363.
8. Khouri RK, Benes CO, Ingram D, et al. Outcome date from a prospective survey of 486 microvascular free flaps. Proceedings of the 75th ASPS Meeting, Hilton Head, SC, May 5–8, 1996.
9. Kroll SS, Schusterman MA, Reece GP, et al. Choice of flaps and incidence of free flap success. Plast Reconst Surg 1996;98:459–463.

10. Holmstrom H. The free abdominoplasty flap and its use in breast reconstruction: An experimental study and clinical case report. Scan J Plast Reconstr Surg 1979;13:423–437.
11. Friedman Rj, Argenta LC, Anderson R. Deep inferior epigastric free flap for breast reconstruction after radical mastectomy. Plast Reconstr Surg 1985;76:455–460.
12. Grotting JC, Urist MM, Maddox WA, Vasconez LO. Conventional TRAM flap versus free microsurgical TRAM flap for immediate breast reconstruction. Plast Reconstr Surg 1989;83:828–841.
13. Serletti JM, Deuber MA, Guidera PM, Reading G. Comparison of the operating microscope and loupes for free microvascular tissue transfer. Plast Reconstr Surg 1995;95:27–76.
14. Arnez ZM, Khan U, Pogurelec D, Planinseh F. Rational selection of flaps from the abdomen in breast reconstruction to reduce donor site morbidity. Br J Plast Surg 1999;52:351–354.
15. Hartrampf CR, Bennett GK. Autogenous tissue reconstruction in the mastectomy patient: a critical review of 300 patients. Ann Surg 1987;205:508–512.
16. Scheflan M, Dinner MI. The transverse abdominal island flap: I. Indications, contraindications, results, and complications. Ann Plast Surg 1983;10:24–35.
17. Hochberg M, Perlmutter D, Medsger T, et al. Lack of association between augmentation mammoplasty and systemic sclerosis (scleroderma). Arthritis Rheum 1996;39:1125–1131.
18. Lewin S, Miller T. A review of epidemiologic studies analyzing the relationship between breast implants and connective tissue disease. Plast Recon Surg 1997;100:1309–1313.
19. Karlson EW, Hankinson SE, Liang MH, et al. Association of silicone breast implants with immunologic abnormalities: a prospective study. Am J Med 1995;106:11–19.
20. Bailey MN, Smith JW, Caras L, et al. Immediate breast reconstruction: reducing the risks. Plast Reconstr Surg 1989;83:845–851.
21. Spear SL, Onyewu C. Staged breast reconstruction with silicone-filled implants in the irradiated breast: recent trends and therapeutic implications. Plast Reconstr Surg 2000;105:930–942.
22. Collis N, Sharpe DT. Breast reconstruction by tissue expansion: a retrospective technical review of 197 two-staged delayed reconstructions following mastectomy for malignant breast disease in 189 patients. Br J Plast Surg 2000;53:37–41.
23. Yeh KA, Lyle C, Wei JP, Sherry R. Immediate breast reconstruction in breast cancer: morbidity and outcome. Am Surg 1998;64:1195–1199.
24. Rohrich RJ, Adams WP, Beran SJ, et al. An analysis of silicone gel-filled breast implants: diagnosis and failure rates. Plast Reconstr Surg 1998;102:2304–2308.
25. Place MJ, Song T, Hardesty RA, Henricks DL. Sensory reinnervation of autologous tissue TRAM flaps after breast reconstruction. Ann Plast Surg 1997;38:19–22.
26. Lieu S, Hunt J, Penning MD. Sensory recovery following free TRAM flap breast reconstruction. Br J Plast Surg 1996;49:210–213.
27. Cederna PS, Yates WR, Chang P, et al. Postmastectomy reconstruction: Comparative analysis of the psychosocial functional, and cosmetic effects of transverse rectus abdominus flap versus breast implant reconstruction. Ann Plast Surg 1995;35:458–468.
28. Serletti JM, Moran SL, Orlando GS, Fox I. Thoracodorsal vessels as recipient vessels for the free TRAM in delayed breast reconstruction. Plast Reconstr Surg 1999;104:1649–1655.

5

Breast Reconstruction

Implant and Nipple Reconstruction

Joseph J. Disa and Colleen M. McCarthy

Introduction

Breast reconstruction following mastectomy has been shown to have a positive effect on the psychological well being of women with breast cancer. Nearly 65,000 women in the United States alone had breast reconstruction last year, a 130% increase from just more than a decade ago *(1)*.

Recent refinements in surgical technique and improvements in prosthetic technologies have continued to improve reconstructive outcomes. Both the increased use of skin-sparing mastectomies and the introduction of novel implant technologies have played a role in the advancement of post-mastectomy breast reconstruction. Along with continuing progress in reconstruction of the breast, new concepts in nipple-areola reconstruction have developed, limiting or eliminating pain with this procedure. Although some techniques have been discredited to historical significance only, others such as the use of commercially available soft-tissue fillers are evolving to become accepted adjuncts to traditional reconstructive techniques. And so, as the treatment of breast cancer continues to evolve, so does the practice of breast reconstruction.

The following is an overview of current implant-based breast reconstruction and nipple-areolar reconstructive techniques. Indications, contraindications, advantages, and disadvantages of both prosthetic breast reconstruction and nipple reconstruction will be discussed.

Reconstructive Options

Contemporary techniques provide numerous options for postmastectomy reconstruction. These options include: single-stage reconstruction with a standard or adjustable implant, tissue expansion followed by placement of a permanent implant, combined autologous tissue/implant reconstruction, or autogenous tissue reconstruction alone.

Procedure selection is based on a range of patient variables, including: location and type of breast cancer, availability of local, regional, and distant donor tissue, size and shape of the desired breast(s), surgical risk, and most importantly, patient preference. For many, the relative simplicity, rapid recovery, and elimination of donor-site morbidity associated with implant-based breast reconstruction is appealing. Individualized selection of a reconstructive technique for each patient remains the key to success.

Implant Reconstruction

The overriding goal of postmastectomy breast reconstruction is to recreate a breast that looks and feels like the removed breast. Thus, the ideal reconstructive technique will fashion a breast mound with a natural contour, natural consistency, and minimal scarring. Symmetry, with respect to the size and shape of the contralateral breast, is the objective. In spite of ideals, a good reconstruction is one that provides symmetry in clothing, as it may never be possible to achieve exact symmetry with reconstruction.

Implant reconstruction has the distinct advantage of combining a lesser operative procedure with the capability of achieving excellent results. Tissue expansion provides donor tissue with similar qualities of skin texture, color, and sensation compared to the contralateral breast. Donor-site morbidity is eliminated with use of a prosthetic device; and by using the patient's mastectomy incision (scar) to place the prosthesis, no new or additional scars are introduced.

Immediate, single-stage breast reconstruction with a standard implant is best suited to the occasional patient with adequate skin at the mastectomy site and small, non-ptotic breasts. Selection criteria for single-stage, adjustable implant reconstruction is similar; yet, it is the preferred technique when the ability to adjust the volume of the device postoperatively is desired. In small-breasted women in whom the skin deficiency is minimal, the implant can be partially filled at the time of reconstruction and gradually inflated to the desired volume post-operatively. Disadvantages of this technique include the placement of a remote port, the need for its subsequent removal and the inability to improve the result at a planned second operation.

Although satisfactory results can be obtained with single-stage reconstruction, in the vast majority of patients, a far more reliable approach involves two-stage expander/implant reconstruction. Tissue expansion is used when there is insufficient tissue after mastectomy to create the desired size and shape of a breast in a single stage.

A tissue expander is placed under the skin and muscles of the chest wall at the primary procedure (Figure 5.1). Anatomic expanders are used to preferentially expand the lower one-half of the breast, facilitating creation of breast ptosis.

Post-operatively, tissue expansion is performed over a period of weeks or months, the soft tissues stretched until the desired breast volume is achieved (Figure 5.2).

Exchange of the temporary expander for a permanent implant occurs at a subsequent operation. At the second procedure, access to the implant

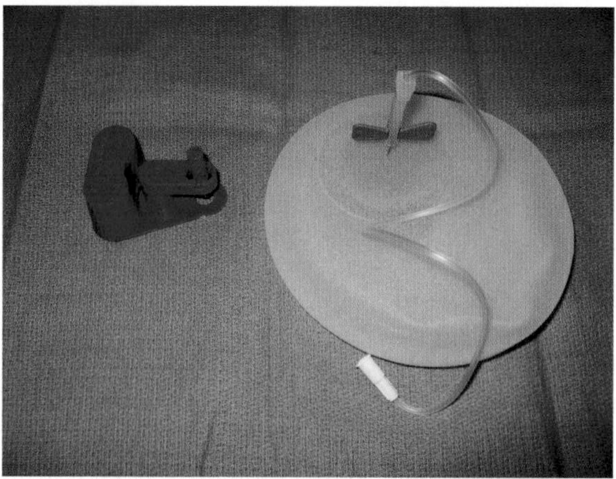

Figure 5.1. Textured surface, integrated valve, biodimensional shaped tissue expander with Magnasite® (Inamed Aesthetics, Santa Barbara, California) fill port locating device.

pocket enables adjustments to improve the final breast form. A capsulotomy is often performed at this second stage. By releasing the surrounding scar capsule, breast projection and breast ptosis are increased. Similarly, precise positioning of the inframammary fold can be addressed.

Re-evaluation of the height and width of the natural breast facilitates the appropriate selection of a permanent implant. Currently, both saline and silicone gel implants are available for use in breast reconstruction (Figure 5.3). Although the stigma surrounding the use of silicone filled implants still exists, issues of silicone safety have been carefully investigated. To date, there is no definitive evidence linking breast implants to cancer, immunologic diseases, neurologic problems, or other systemic diseases. The use of silicone gel implants generally allows for a softer, more natural-looking breast.

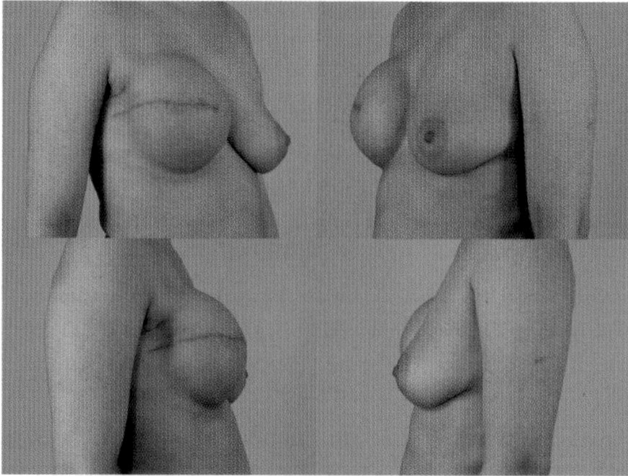

Figure 5.2. Unilateral, right breast reconstruction with tissue expander. The expander is intentionally overfilled to maximize projection and inferior pole skin.

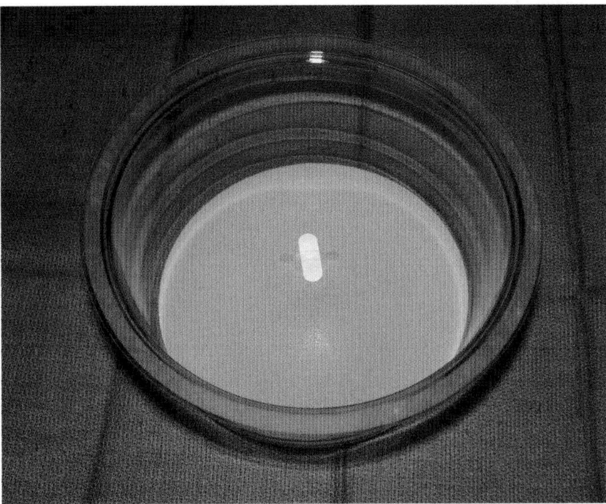

Figure 5.3. Permanent saline implant.

Alternatively, the use of saline-filled implants allows for minor volume adjustments to be made at the time of implant placement. And although saline-filled implants may offer the greatest piece of mind for some patients in terms of safety, implant palpability and rippling is more likely (Figures 5.4 and 5.5).

Combined Autogenous Tissue/Implant Reconstruction

Nearly every patient who undergoes a mastectomy is a candidate for some form of implant-based reconstruction. Implant reconstruction alone is contraindicated, however, in the presence of an inadequate skin envelope. A large skin excision at the time of mastectomy, owing to previous biopsies or locally advanced disease, may preclude primary coverage of a prosthetic device.

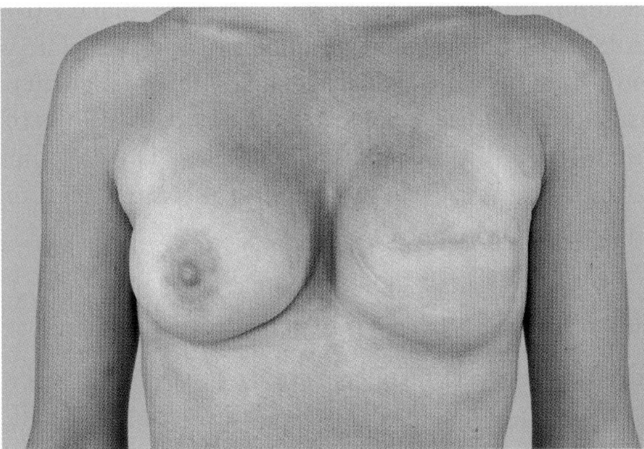

Figure 5.4. Unilateral, left breast reconstruction with saline implant. Photo taken prior to planned nipple-areola reconstruction.

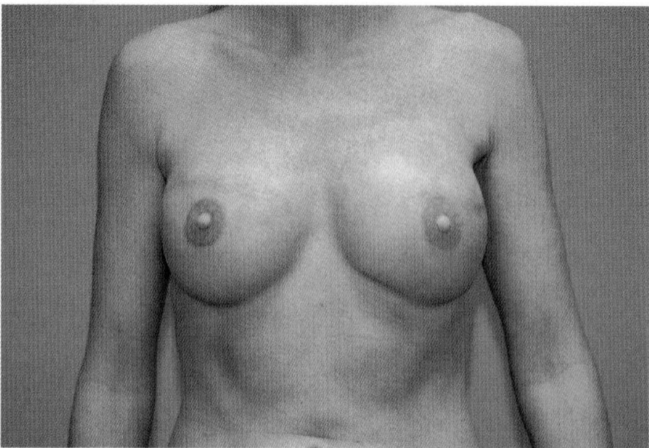

Figure 5.5. Bilateral breast reconstruction with silicone gel implants after nipple-areola reconstruction.

Similarly, previous chest wall irradiation and/or post-mastectomy radiotherapy are considered by many to be a relative contraindication for implant-based breast reconstruction *(2,3)* (*see* Adjuvant Therapy).

In patients with thin, contracted, or previously irradiated skin, the ipsilateral latissimus dorsi myocutaneous flap can provide additional skin, soft tissue, and muscle, obviating the need for or facilitating the process of tissue expansion. The skin island is designed under the bra line or along the lateral margin of the muscle, and the flap is tunneled anteriorly into the mastectomy defect. Although the latissimus dorsi myocutaneous flap is extremely reliable, the tissue bulk is usually inadequate. Thus, a permanent implant is often placed beneath the flap to provide adequate volume.

The latissimus dorsi flap is advantageous in that it can provide additional vascularized skin and muscle to the breast mound in a single operative procedure. Its disadvantages include the creation of new chest scars, a back donor scar, and the fact that the transfer of autogenous tissue does not, in this setting, eliminate the need for an implant.

In cases where large amounts of new skin are required at the mastectomy site, a temporary tissue expander can be placed to enlarge the latissimus dorsi skin island following inset of the flap. The combination of a latissimus dorsi flap and tissue expansion may be particularly appropriate in cases in which the remaining mastectomy skin is of insufficient quality or quantity to tolerate tissue expansion. This is typically the case in the insetting of delayed reconstruction after mastectomy and post-operative radiation therapy (Figure 5.6).

Complications

Prosthetic breast reconstruction is a relatively simple technique that is generally well tolerated. Complications are generally centered on the breast, with minimal systemic health implications and minimal overall patient morbidity. Thus, implant reconstruction can often be performed on patients who might not be suitable candidates for the more complex

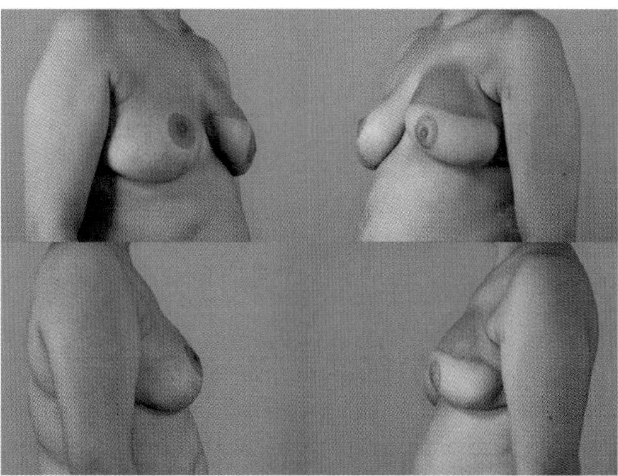

Figure 5.6. Unilateral, left latissimus-dorsi flap reconstruction. Note radiation-induced skin changes native skin flaps. Right vertical scar pattern reduction mammoplasty.

surgical procedure required for breast reconstruction with autogenous tissue.

Initial reports of tissue expander/implant reconstruction using smooth-surface expanders with remote ports demonstrated high rates of complications. Expander extrusions, port complications, and capsular contractures were common. The subsequent change in technology to textured-surface expanders with integrated valves has generally improved complication rates *(4)*. Despite these technologic advances, peri-operative complications including hematoma, seroma, infection, skin flap necrosis, and implant exposure/extrusion do occur.

Late complications include device malfunction and capsular contracture. Although capsular contracture occurs to some extent around all implants; in some, the degree of contracture will increase in severity over time *(5)*. A pathologic capsular contracture, implant deflation, and/or rupture may require revisional surgery years following completion of reconstruction.

Advantages/Disadvantages

Although implant techniques are technically easier than autologous reconstruction, with shorter hospitalization and a quicker recover, they do provide additional reconstructive challenges.

Patients who undergo tissue expander/implant breast reconstruction will experience varying degrees of discomfort and chest wall asymmetry during the expansion phase. In addition, patients must make more frequent office visits for percutaneous expansion.

The breast mound achieved with implant reconstruction is generally more rounded, less ptotic, and will often require a contralateral matching procedure in order to achieve symmetry. Recent advances in prosthesis design have resulted in anatomically shaped, textured devices that provide significant improvements in overall breast shape. These devices limit the upper pole fullness that results from the use of round devices, while at the same time lowering the point of maximal projection to a more anatomic location. For a patient with large, ptotic breasts, however, it remains difficult to achieve symmetry if a contralateral breast procedure is not desired.

Timing of Reconstruction

Immediate post-mastectomy reconstruction is currently considered the standard of care in breast reconstruction. Numerous studies have demonstrated that reconstruction performed concurrently with mastectomy is an oncologically safe option for women with breast cancer. Immediate reconstruction is assumed to be advantageous when compared with delayed procedures on the basis of improved cost-effectiveness and reduced inconvenience for the patient. Moreover, studies have shown that women who undergo immediate reconstruction have less psychological distress about the loss of a breast and have a better overall quality of life *(6)*.

Technically, reconstruction is facilitated in the immediate setting because of the pliability of the native skin envelope and the delineation of the natural inframammary fold. The increasing use of post-operative radiotherapy for earlier-staged breast cancers has, however, challenged this thinking. Adjuvant radiotherapy has been shown to increase the risk of post-operative complications *(7,8)*. Based on this data, whether or not to perform immediate, implant-based reconstruction for patients in whom radiation therapy is planned remains controversial (*see* Adjuvant Therapy and Implant Reconstruction).

Similarly, for those who may be unwilling to decide about reconstruction while adjusting to their cancer diagnosis, delayed breast reconstruction remains an option.

Skin-Sparing Mastectomy

Mastectomy techniques have changed dramatically in the past 50 years. Today, it is understood that the skin envelope of the breast can safely be preserved in the absence of direct tumor invasion. Several long-term studies have shown equivalent local recurrence rates and disease-free survival for patient cohorts undergoing skin-sparing mastectomy or conventional mastectomy *(9,10)*.

A skin-sparing mastectomy includes resection of the breast tissue, the nipple-areola complex (NAC), and often the previous biopsy scar. In many cases, this can be achieved by performing the mastectomy through an elliptical incision that encompasses both the NAC and the adjacent biopsy scar. Alternatively, if the diagnosis of cancer has been made by fine-needle aspiration or needle-core biopsy, the mastectomy can be accomplished through a periareolar incision in the breast.

The largely intact, mammary skin envelope preserves the contour of the native breast, once the immediate breast volume is restored with a prosthesis. Restoration of breast symmetry is thus facilitated. The resulting peri-areolar scars are often well hidden after nipple reconstruction and areolar tattooing are completed.

Adjuvant Therapy and Implant Reconstruction

Earlier breast cancers are being increasingly treated with adjuvant chemotherapy and radiotherapy in an attempt to increase survival. Multiple reports have demonstrated that patients who undergo immediate breast reconstruction are not predisposed to delays in administration of adjuvant chemotherapy compared with patients undergo mastectomy alone. In addition, the administration of either pre- or post-operative chemotherapy does not increase the risk of peri-operative complications *(11–13)*.

The possible implications of radiotherapy on implant-based breast reconstruction are, however, both profound and controversial. Not only is tissue expansion difficult in the previously irradiated tissues, but the risks of infection, expander exposure, and subsequent extrusion are increased. For these reasons, it is generally agreed that either autologous tissue reconstruction alone or combined autologous tissue/implant reconstruction is preferable in patients who have a history of previous chest wall irradiation. Recent reports have also demonstrated that patients who received post-operative radiotherapy had a significantly higher incidence of capsular contracture than controls.

The increasing use of post-mastectomy radiation and chemotherapy in patients with early-stage breast cancer necessitates increased communication between the medical oncologist, radiation oncologist, breast surgeon, and plastic surgeon during treatment planning. Paramount to a successful outcome is a frank discussion between the plastic surgeon and the patient about the potential risks of adjuvant radiotherapy on immediate reconstruction versus the additional surgery required for delayed reconstruction. There is no single "standard of care" in the setting of adjuvant radiotherapy and each case must be individualized.

Nipple-Areola Reconstruction

Although the creation of a breast mound restores the contour of the native breast, reconstruction of the NAC represents the completion of the restorative process. Not only can recreation of the NAC improve the overall aesthetic result, it can improve patient acceptance and integration of the reconstructed breast. In a recent study investigating patient satisfaction following breast reconstruction, a highly significant correlation was seen between the level of satisfaction and the presence of the nipple-areola complex *(14)*. There are patients, however, who choose to minimize their exposure to surgery and thus will elect not to proceed with nipple reconstruction.

Reconstruction of the size, shape, and color of the NAC are attainable goals. Contemporary reconstructive techniques do not, however, allow for functional restoration of sensation and/or erectile ability. Multiple techniques have been described for reconstruction of the nipple, including: local flaps, composite grafts, and nipple-sharing techniques where the opposite nipple is used as a donor site. A number of techniques are also available for reconstruction of the areola, including: areolar tattooing alone, skin grafting from a distant donor site, or a combination of both. These procedures, when performed in conjunction with tattooing of the entire nipple-areolar reconstruction, can create an aesthetically pleasing NAC.

Timing

The reconstructed nipple must appear centered on its reconstructed breast mound, yet symmetrical both in and out of clothing with respect to the contralateral nipple. Often a compromise here must be sought. When breast mounds themselves are inherently asymmetrical, as often occurs after prosthetic reconstruction, the goal of symmetry is more challenging. Nipple reconstruction is therefore often delayed for 3–6 months following reconstruction of the breast mound. The optimal nipple-areolar position can then be determined once the post-operative swelling has resolved and the reconstructed breast has achieved its final shape. Determining the ultimate position of the NAC is a critical step in the reconstructive process, as secondary corrections of nipple asymmetry are difficult to perform.

Relevant Anatomy

Nipple-areola anatomy is remarkably variable in dimension, texture, and color across ethnic groups. In fact, in most women the two NACs exhibit varying degrees of asymmetry. Typically, the nipple lies opposite or just above the inframammary fold overlying the fourth intercostal space. The average distance from the sternal notch to the nipple varies from 17–22 cm, but may be more or less depending on the patient's stature and the degree of breast ptosis. In general, an aesthetically balanced breast will have an areola diameter of 4–5 cm, with the nipple diameter and projection or height equal to one-quarter to one-third of the areolar diameter *(15)*.

Nipple Reconstruction

The most challenging aspect of nipple reconstruction is the creation of a three-dimensional projecting structure with texture, dimensions, and contour similar to the contralateral nipple. Nipple reconstruction enhances the realism of breast reconstruction, and the more projecting and three-dimensional the structure, the more lifelike the reconstruction. Various options have included nipple sharing, nipple tattooing, grafting of autogenous tissues, introduction of soft tissue fillers, and local flaps.

Nipple sharing

The most realistic nipple is one produced by grafting part of the contralateral, normal nipple to the reconstructed breast mound. This technique creates a nipple with a perfect color and texture match and can be combined with areolar tattooing with or without skin grafting. A relatively projecting donor nipple is required, however, in order to be effective without eliminating projection at the donor site. In addition, because the structure of the contralateral nipple is altered, nipple sharing may potentially harm the only erogenous structure left on the woman's chest.

Nipple tattooing

In patients who neither wish nor are candidates for local flap reconstruction, nipple tattooing remains an option. Intradermal tattooing restores the appearance of a nipple by employing a strictly optical effect. Restoration of the structural support and/or the texture typical of a natural NAC is not achieved by tattooing alone. Thus, tattooing is best employed as a stage of the combined approach toward nipple reconstruction, whether performed prior to or after elevation of the nipple structure (*see* Areolar Reconstruction).

Grafting and soft-tissue fillers

Many techniques have been used previously to obtain and maintain nipple projection, including dermal, fat, auricular, and/or rib grafting. These reconstructive methods add a layer of complexity to a seemingly simple problem, and increase the potential for further donor site morbidity. In cases of secondary treatment of failed nipple reconstructions, various treatment options are available, including inserting banked or immediate autologous grafts under a new skin flap to improve structural support and projection.

More recently, augmenting the projection of a collapsed nipple has been performed by inserting rolled dermal tissue or commercially available, processed dermis (Alloderm). Others have advocated the use of injectable, semi-permanent soft-tissue fillers such as calcium hydroxylapatite as a way to augment projection *(16,17)*. Further evaluation of the long-term outcomes following these novel techniques is on-going.

Local flaps

For the majority of patients in whom nipple sharing is not feasible or desired, local flaps with or without skin grafting are our preferred methods of reconstruction. Multiple local flap techniques have been described to reconstruct the nipple, each with its own advantages and disadvantages. These include: the skate flap, C-V flap, bell flap, double opposing tab flap, star flap, and twin flap. Although each technique has is advantages and disadvantages, the skate flap has proven to be a reliable workhorse and is thus our local flap of choice. The skate flap uses local cutaneous flaps to recreate a three-dimensional nipple, leaving behind a split-thickness donor defect that requires immediate skin grafting. If a patient neither wishes nor is a candidate for skin grafting of the areola, however, then a C-V flap is our preferred method of reconstruction. In using the C-V flap reconstruction, local flaps are designed so that the donor sites may be closed primarily.

The "skate flap": a technical approach

A 38-mm cookie cutter is used to create a perfect circle for the areola, and a 1-cm nipple diameter is selected. Positioning is confirmed by performing sternal notch-nipple measurements (Figure 5.7).

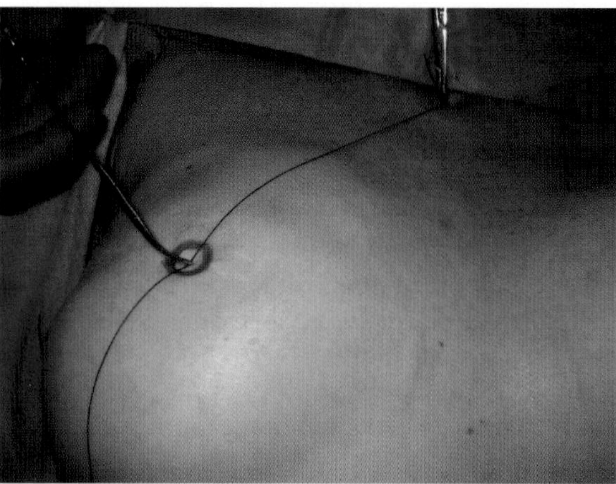

Figure 5.7. Symmetry of nipple position is confirmed through measurement of the sternal notch-nipple distance.

Positioning of the reconstructed nipple should be performed so that the nipple is located adjacent to the mastectomy scar whenever possible. The nipple reconstruction can be oriented superiorly or inferiorly, depending on the position of the mastectomy scar and the selected nipple position. In this case, the pedicle for the nipple complex will be superior, as indicated by the vertical limbs in the patient markings (Figure 5.8).

The superior skate flap nipple reconstruction is begun by drawing a line across the proposed nipple base, and the skin above this line is de-epithelialized. This line should be directly on the mastectomy scar whenever possible. Conversely, if the nipple reconstruction is oriented

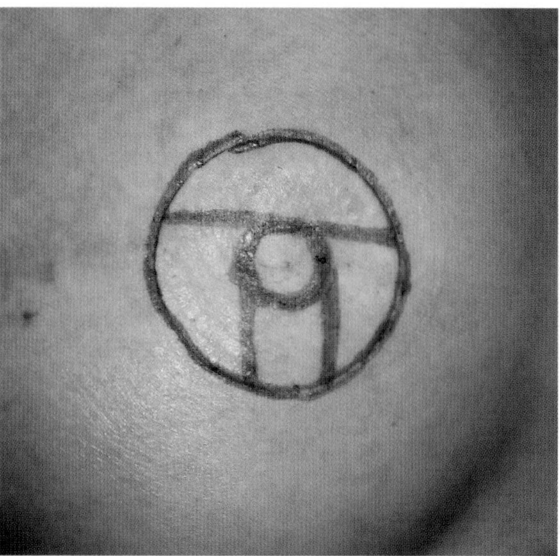

Figure 5.8. The skate-flap is marked on the breast mound. A 3.8-cm areola is marked around a 1-cm nipple base. The nipple flaps are oriented inferiorly.

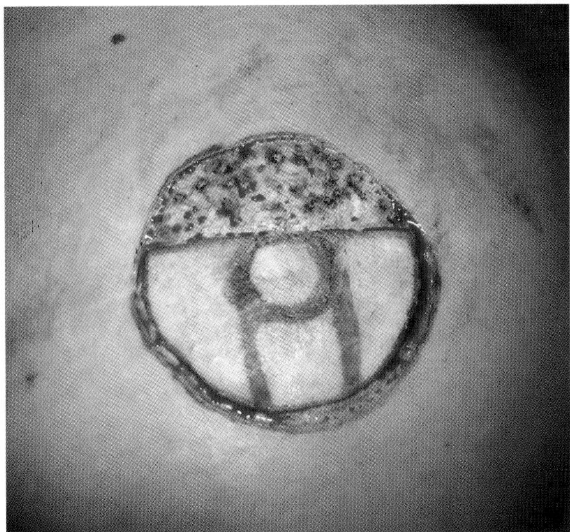

Figure 5.9. The areola is incised circumferentially and the superior portion is de-epithelialized.

inferiorly, the line is drawn across the bottom of the proposed nipple, and the skin below the line is de-epithelialized. If the mastectomy scar crosses the area, the flap is drawn so that the wings and body of the skate are designed away from the scar (Figure 5.9).

The lateral wings of the skate flap are raised in the deep dermal level, extending only to the previously drawn vertical lines. These lines demarcate the outer edge of the proposed nipple. The forceps are holding the raised lateral wings of the skate flap. Note that the central portion of the skate flap remains adherent (Figure 5.10).

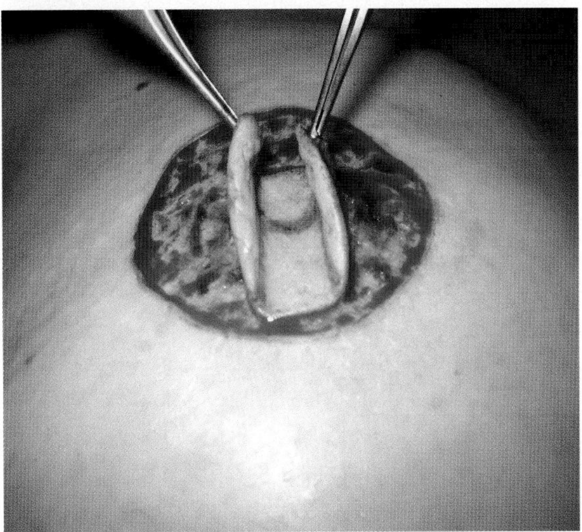

Figure 5.10. The split-thickness, lateral flaps are elevated peripherally to centrally until the outer limits of the proposed nipple base.

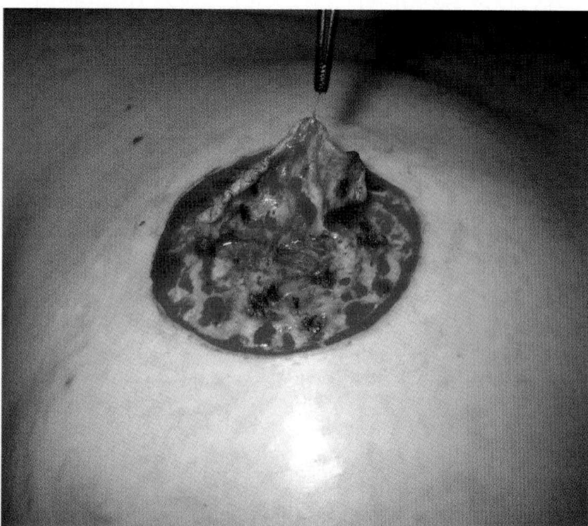

Figure 5.11. The central portion of the flap is elevated and includes a layer of subcutaneous fat attached to the inferior flap centrally to provide bulk.

The central portion of the skate flap (between the two vertically drawn lines) is undermined at the level of the subcutaneous fat, deep to the dermis, until the flap can be raised in a perpendicular plane from the planned areola. The subcutaneous fat is included with the central portion of the flap to provide bulk to the nipple reconstruction (Figure 5.11).

The lateral wings of the skate flap are then folded around the central portion and sutured to one another with interrupted chromic sutures (Figure 5.12).

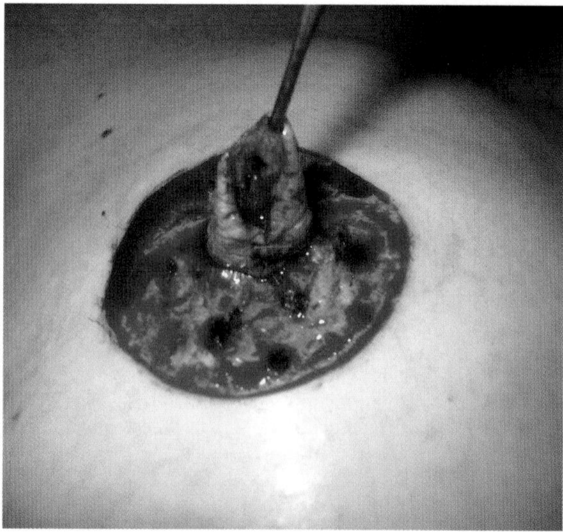

Figure 5.12. The nipple cylinder is formed by wrapping the lateral flaps centrally.

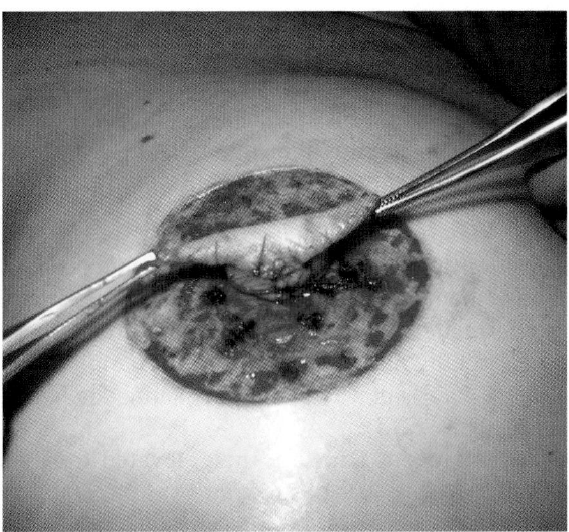

Figure 5.13. The lateral flaps will be trimmed to match the size of the underlying nipple cylinder.

The excess tissue at the top of the skate flap is trimmed on either side, and the newly created nipple cylinder is closed with chromic sutures (Figure 5.13).

A full-thickness skin graft is sutured onto the areolar bed with absorbable sutures, over the newly created nipple cylinder. A 1-cm hole is made in the center of the skin graft to allow the nipple to be delivered, and the skin graft is sutured to the nipple base (Figure 5.14).

The reconstructed nipple should be protected in the post-operative period. The dressing should provide some compression to the skin graft

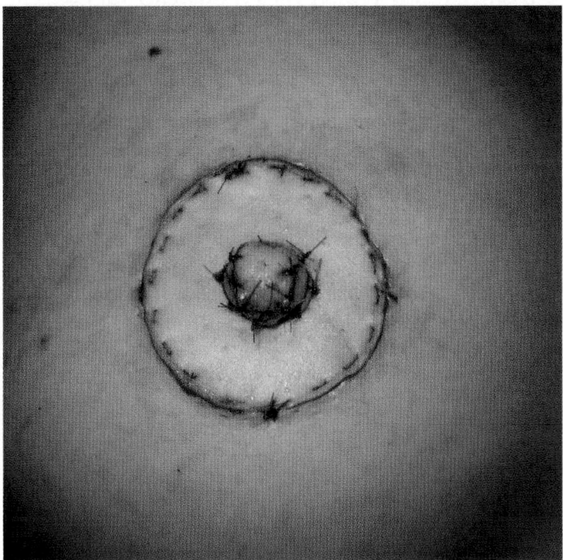

Figure 5.14. A full-thickness graft is used to reconstruct the areola.

and thus firmly maintain the position of the skin graft against the underlying bed. It should prevent any accumulation of hematoma/seroma under the graft or a sheering motion between the graft and the bed, thus ensuring rapid revascularization of the graft. Finally, it should provide a moist environment to promote rapid wound healing and should serve to protect the wound from outer physical trauma.

The C-V flap: a technical approach

The nipple position is marked on the breast mound (*see* "The Skate Flap"). The base diameter of the nipple will be determined using the width of the contralateral, normal nipple. Two triangular "V-shaped" flaps extending laterally and medially from the nipple base are drawn. The width of the V-flaps will be equal to the planned height of the reconstructed nipple (Figure 5.15)

Full-thickness, cutaneous flaps are then elevated from peripheral to central direction, leaving a core of subcutaneous fat attached to the base centrally (Figure 5.16).

The central core of subcutaneous tissue is then released opposite of the nipple base, which allows vertical rotation of the elevated skin flaps (Figure 5.17).

The distal-most ends of the elevated flaps are then wrapped around the central core and sutured to each other. The "cap" of the nipple is closed over the top of the nipple and sutured in place. The triangular flap donor sites are closed primarily (Figures 5.18–5.20).

Complications

Possible complications of nipple reconstruction include partial and total loss of the nipple, epidermolysis, and loss of nipple projection. Avoidance of smoking, accurate dissection, and the creation of a nipple that is initially 20–30% larger than the contralateral side minimize the chances of complications. Despite these precautions, loss of nipple projection is a common occurrence a few years post-reconstruction (*see* Nipple Reconstruction Using Grafting and Soft-Tissue Fillers).

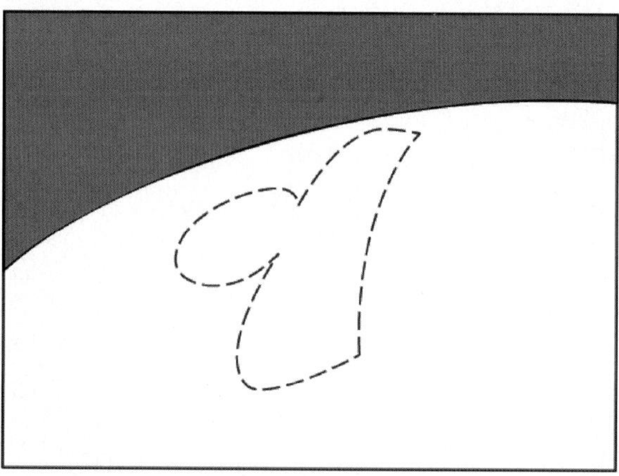

Figure 5.15. The C-V flap is designed over the breast mound. The flap will be superiorly based.

Figure 5.16. The full-thickness lateral flaps are elevated peripherally to centrally until the outer limits of the proposed nipple base.

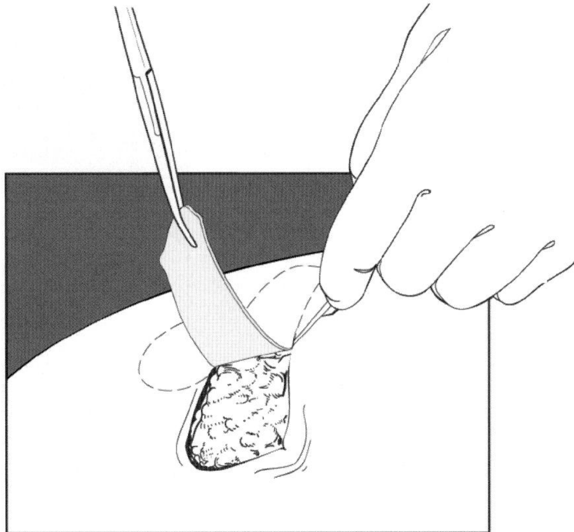

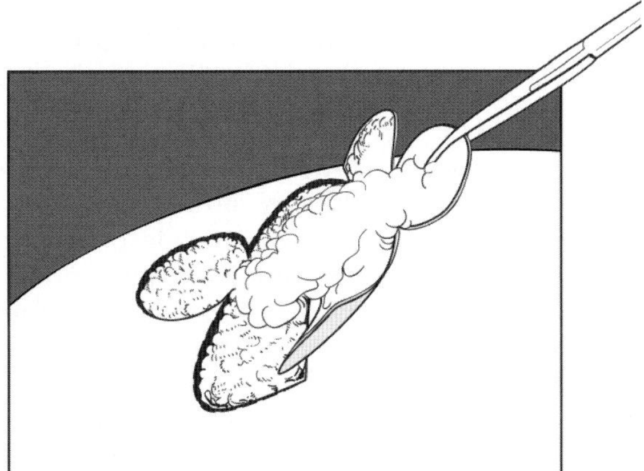

Figure 5.17. The central portion of the flap is elevated and includes a layer of subcutaneous fat attached to the flap centrally to provide bulk.

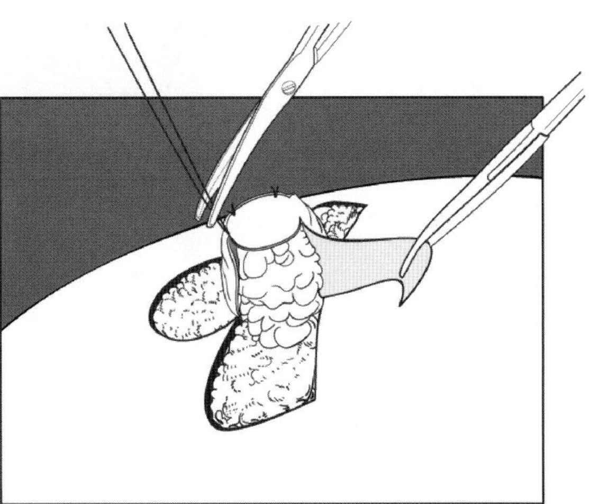

Figure 5.18. The nipple cylinder is formed by wrapping the lateral flaps centrally. The central flap forms the roof of the cylinder.

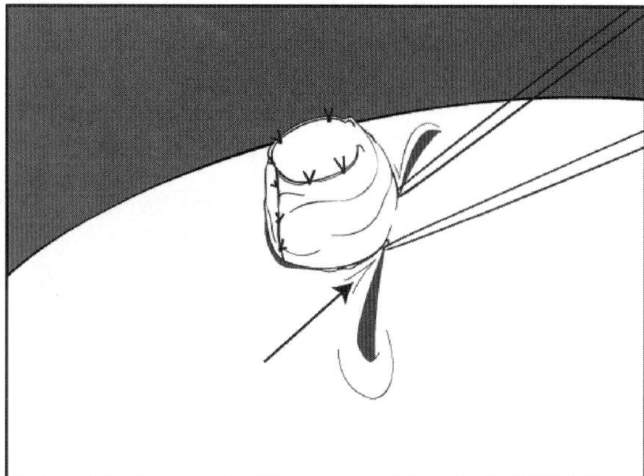

Figure 5.19. The donor site defect is closed primarily.

Areola Reconstruction

Areolar reconstruction can be accomplished by intradermal tattooing alone. Colorization of a reconstructed nipple may be performed in conjunction with areolar tattooing. Intradermal tattooing should be staged, however, following local flap or composite grafting for nipple reconstruction.

Primary intradermal tattooing

Primary intradermal tattooing for areolar reconstruction is a safe and effective method of reconstruction. The procedure is simple, easy to perform, and requires no significant recovery time. There is no donor site morbidity and the risk of major complications is low.

Reconstruction of the areola by tattooing allows a great degree of control over size and color match with the contralateral side; however, results are usually less than satisfactory when used in the absence of three-dimensional reconstruction of the nipple. Many tattoo pigments are available, allowing precise color matching with the contralateral

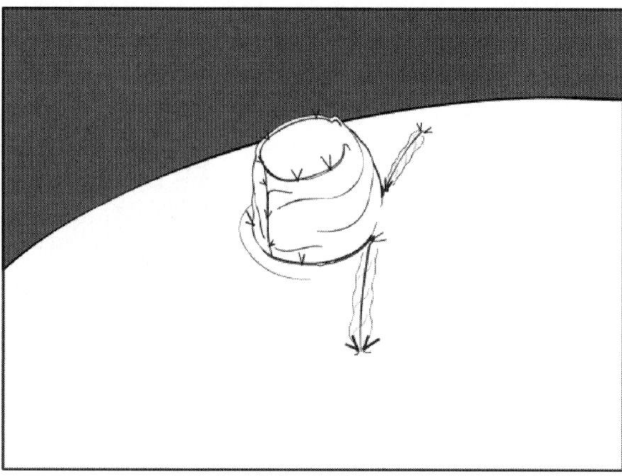

Figure 5.20. The reconstructed nipple.

areola. One or more applications may be necessary to obtain the desired result. Feathering of pigment across the junction between the skin-graft and breast mound may effectively conceal suture lines.

Skin-grafting

Simple tattooing alone provides pigmentation only in the region of the areola, without the appropriate areolar texture. Skin grafting used in combination with areolar tattooing can both recreate the areolar pigment and provide a slightly irregular texture that is distinctly different from the surrounding breast skin.

Split-thickness skin grafts may be harvested from the groin, the axilla, the lower abdomen, or other sites of previously existing scars. Groin skin is appropriately pigmented and provides a more realistic contrast with native breast skin than does axillary skin, which tends to have a very white color in Caucasian patients. Although the donor site can be concealed in the bikini line, it is often associated with more peri-operative discomfort. Axillary skin has the advantage of being within the operative field and can usually be harvest from the axillary dog-ear deformity that so often accompanies mastectomy scars, particular in large-breasted women.

Conclusion

For patients who undergo mastectomy for the treatment of breast cancer, the preservation of a normal breast form through breast reconstruction is important to their physical and mental quality of life. Prosthetic breast reconstruction has the capability of producing excellent results in the properly selected patient. Complete breast reconstruction includes the restoration of a NAC that is symmetric with respect to the contralateral nipple. Aesthetic qualities such as nipple position, size, color, projection, and position are important determinants of the overall aesthetics of a reconstruction, qualifying a soft-tissue mound as the new breast.

Although the overriding goal of reconstructive breast surgery is to satisfy the patient with respect to her own self-image and expectations for the aesthetic result, individualized selection of a reconstructive technique for each patient remains a predominant factor in achieving a reconstructive success.

References

1. American Society of Plastic Surgeons. www.plasticsurgery.org. Date accessed: 7/30/07.
2. Krueger EA, Wilkins EG, Strawderman M, et al. Complications and patient satisfaction following expander/implant breast reconstruction with and without radiotherapy. Int J Radiat Oncol Biol Phys 2001;49:713–721.
3. Evans GR, Schusterman MA, Kroll SS, et al. Reconstruction and the radiated breast: is there a role for implants? Plast Reconstr Surg 1995;96:1111–1115.
4. Maxwell GP, Falcone PA. Eighty-four consecutive breast reconstructions using a textured silicone tissue expander. Plast Reconstr Surg 1992;89:1022–1034.

5. Spear SL, Baker JL Jr. Classification of capsular contracture after prosthetic breast reconstruction. Plast Reconstr Surg 1995;96:1119–1123.
6. Al Ghazal SK, Sully L, Fallowfield L, Blamey RW. The psychological impact of immediate rather than delayed breast reconstruction. Eur J Surg Oncol 2000;26:17–19.
7. Spear SL, Onyewu C. Staged breast reconstruction with saline-filled implants in the irradiated breast: recent trends and therapeutic implications. Plast Reconstr Surg 2000;105:930–942.
8. Cordeiro PG, Pusic AL, Disa JJ, McCormick B, VanZee K. Irradiation after immediate tissue expander/implant breast reconstruction: outcomes, complications, aesthetic results, and satisfaction among 156 patients. Plast Reconstr Surg 2004;113:877–881.
9. Singletary SE, Robb GL. Oncologic safety of skin-sparing mastectomy. Ann Surg Oncol 2003;10:95–97.
10. Carlson GW, Losken A, Moore B, et al. Results of immediate breast reconstruction after skin-sparing mastectomy. Ann Plast Surg 2001;46:222–228.
11. Nahabedian MY, Tsangaris T, Momen B, Manson PN. Infectious complications following breast reconstruction with expanders and implants. Plast Reconstr Surg 2003;112:467–476.
12. Vandeweyer E, Deraemaecker R, Nogaret JM, Hertens D. Immediate breast reconstruction with implants and adjuvant chemotherapy: a good option? Acta Chir Belg 2003;103:98–101.
13. Wilson CR, Brown IM, Weiller-Mithoff E, George WD, Doughty JC. Immediate breast reconstruction does not lead to a delay in the delivery of adjuvant chemotherapy. Eur J Surg Oncol 2004;30:624–627.
14. Shaikh-Naidu N, Preminger B, Rogers K, Messina P, Gayle L. Determinants of aesthetic satisfaction following TRAM and implant breast reconstruction. Ann Plast Surg 2004;52:465–470.
15. King T, Borgen P. *Atlas of procedures in breast cancer surgery.* New York: Taylor & Francis; 2000.
16. Panettiere P, Marchetti L, Accorsi D. Filler injection enhances the projection of the reconstructed nipple: an original easy technique. Aesthetic Plast Surg 2005;29(4):287–294.
17. Evans K, Rasko Y, Lenert J, Olding M. The use of calcium hydroxylapatite for nipple projection after failed nipple-areolar reconstruction: early results. Ann Plast Surg 2005;55(1):25–29.
18. Farhadi J, Makxveytyte GK, Schaefer D, Pierer G, Scheufler O. Reconstruction of the nipple-areolar complex: an update. J Plast Reconstr Aesthet Surg 2006;59(1):40–53.

6

Skin Cancer and Reconstruction

John Y.S. Kim

Introduction

Skin cancer is by far the most common cancer, with more than 1 million new cases diagnosed in the United States alone *(1)*. This represents approximately 40% of all cancers. Typically, skin cancer is divided into melanoma and non-melanoma skin cancer (NMSC). The distinction between melanoma and NMSC is especially relevant from a treatment and outcomes perspective, because melanoma, though only representing 6% of new skin cancers, represents the majority of mortality associated with skin cancer (74%).

The overall incidence of skin cancers is increasing, and this is attributed to a complex of factors including enhanced surveillance and increased exposure to ultraviolet (UV) radiation (by virtue of changing atmospheric conditions and cultural mores). There is also a preponderance of health care costs that are diverted to treatment of skin cancer; recent economic studies estimated the annual cost of NMSC in the Medicare population at 426 million dollars *(2)* and the cost of cutaneous melanoma treatment at 563 million dollars *(3)*.

The heightened impact of skin cancer has, in turn, generated an increased need for appropriate reconstructive strategies. As with reconstruction for other cancers, the general imperative is to preserve function and form.

Epidemiology

More than 95% of NMSC are comprised of basal cell carcinomas (BCC) and squamous cell carcinomas (SCCA) *(4)*. The ratio of BCC to SCCA is 4:1. The lifetime risk for BCC in the Caucasian population is 33–39% in men and 23–28% in women *(5)*. The age-adjusted incidence in this population (per 100,000) is 475 for men and 250 for women. The lifetime risk of SCCA is 9–14% in men and 4–9% in women with an age-adjusted incidence of 100–150 per 100,000 *(6)*. There is geographic variation, with a doubling of incidence with every 8–10° move towards the equator. For both SCCA and BCC, there is an increase in incidence with age *(7,8)*.

The incidence of melanoma in the United States is estimated to be more than 59,000 for 2005, with male/female ratio of 57:43 *(1)*. The mortality caused by melanoma is expected to be nearly 8000 for 2005. There has been a 3–6% annual increase in melanoma incidence since the 1980s. The lifetime risk for melanoma is approximately is 2% in men and 1% in women.

Pathophysiology

BCC arises from the keratinocytes in the basal cell layer of the epidermis or follicular structures (Figure 6.1) *(9)*. SCCA frequently arises from keratinocytes, particularly in areas exposed to the sun (actinic keratoses is a precursor lesion). Melanoma, in contrast, arises in melanocytes that are of neural crest origin. A host of environmental and genetic factors have been implicated in the multi-factorial pathogenesis of diverse forms of skin cancer *(10)*. UV radiation has been exhaustively studied, and peak carcinogenicity is found in the UVB (280–320 nm) portion of the electromagnetic spectrum *(11,12)*. Typically, photocarcinogenesis stems from DNA base pair mutations in critical cell-cycle regulatory and tumor-suppressor genes such as p53 (NMSC) and p16 (melanoma) *(13,14)*. Other identified environmental factors include ionizing radiation and assorted chemicals such as polycyclic hydrocarbons and arsenic *(15)*. In terms of infectious agents, human papillomavirus (types 6 and 11) have been associated with SCCA. The significance of genetic influences is highlighted by syndromic manifestations of skin cancer such as xeroderma pigmentosum and nevoid basal cell syndrome (Figure 6.2). In

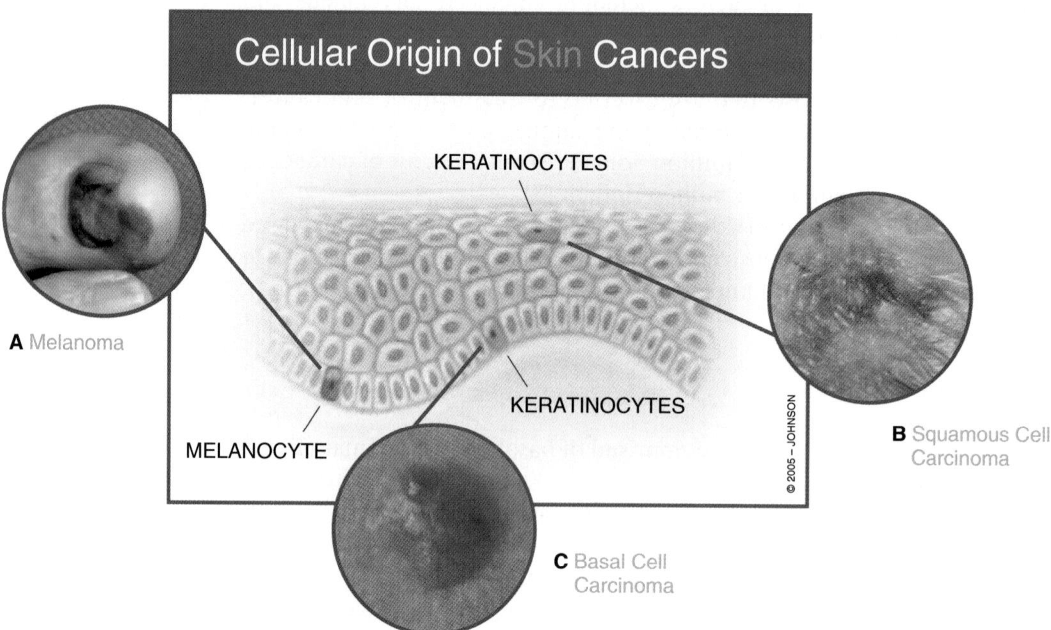

Figure 6.1. Cellular origin of common skin cancers. **(A)** Melanoma arises from melanocytes. **(B)** SCCA and **(C)** BCC originate from keratinocytes.

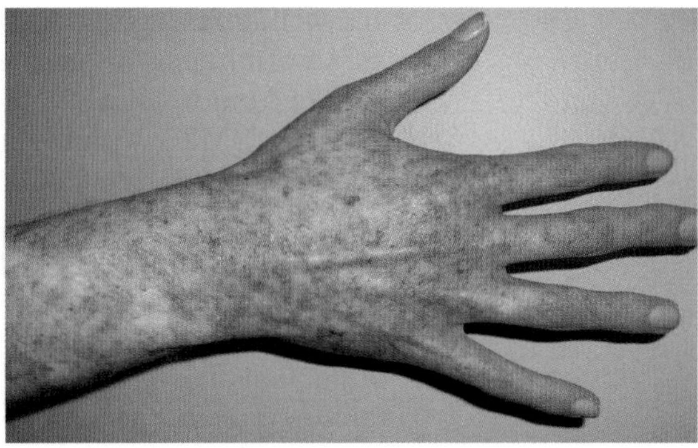

Figure 6.2. Xeroderma pigmentosum of the upper extremity. The patient has had numerous excisions of BCC, SCCA, and melanoma.

turn, as the molecular basis of these genetic disorders becomes known, novel diagnostic techniques such as comparative genomic hybridization are being developed *(16)*.

The largely cultural phenomenon of voluntary sun or direct UV exposure, especially during childhood, has been implicated in an increased overall risk of skin cancer *(17,18)*. Surrogates of skin sensitivity such as Fitzpatrick class I (easily burns without tanning), blue eyes, blonde or red hair, and freckles on the skin increase the relative risk of developing skin cancer by two- to 5-fold. A history of significant sunburn also increases this risk twofold *(19)*.

For melanoma, a history of multiple atypical nevi or more than 100 benign nevi confers an 11-fold increase in risk.

Classification

BCC are divided into nodular, superficial, morpheaform and micronodular, pigmented, and mixed subtypes *(20)*. Nodular and mixed-nodular basal cells are the most common (50–75%) and will typically present as a well-defined solitary nodule or papule with a translucent surface with traversing telangiectasias (Figure 6.1) *(21,22)*. The superficial subtype comprises 10% of BCC and presents as an irregular, erythematous plaque. Infiltrative BCCs such as micronodular and morpheaform are relatively rare, representing 2–5% of BCC. They are generally light-colored, atrophic plaques with ill-defined borders, and can have deeper involvement—all of which serves to make both diagnosis and clearance of margins difficult. Pigmented BCC is a rare subtype, representing 6% of BCCs, and can be confused with melanoma because of the melanin composition.

SCCA can be classified by degree of differentiation and etiology *(23)*. Generally they present as erythematous, ill-defined elevated plaques or more circumscribed nodules with occasional ulceration or cutaneous horn formation (Figure 6.1). In contradistinction to BCC, SCCA are more aggressive and the risk of nodal metastases is 5% at 5 years. There are several variants of SCCA. Bowen's disease is a SCCA *in situ* that has a 10% local invasion rate. Penile lesions are termed erythroplasia of Queyrat. SCCA arising in longstanding wounds, ulcers, or scars is frequently termed Marjolin's ulcers and tend to be more aggressive variants, with a metastases rate approaching 40% *(24,25)*. Verrucous carcinomas are well-differentiated SCCA with a verrucous appearance. Although keratocanthomas are not technically SCCA, they are difficult to differentiate from well-differentiated SCCA *(26)*.

Other NMSC variants that do not fall under the aegis of BCC or SCCA include: dermatofibrosarcoma protuberans, which is a rare cutaneous sarcoma characterized by indolent growth and treated with wide resection with possible adjuvant radiation therapy *(27)*; and Merkel's cell carcinoma—a rare, aggressive cutaneous neoplasm that arises from Merkel cell clusters (cells of possibly neuroendocrine and epithelial origin that may be involved in mechanoreceptor function) *(28,29)*. These tumors resemble violaceous SCCA and have a high rate of local recurrence (44%) and both nodal (55%) and distant (34%) metastases *(30)*.

Melanomas can present as raised or flat pigmented lesions (amelanotic variants do exist however) (Figure 6.1). As described by the "ABCD" diagnostic criteria, these lesions may have **A**symmetry, irregular **B**orders, variegated **C**olor, and an enlarging **D**iameter (>6mm). Melanomas are classified by common clinicopathologic subtypes: (1) superficial spreading (70% incidence); (2) nodular (15–30%); (3) acral lentiginous (2–8% in Caucasians, 29–72% in darker-pigmented patients of African, Hispanic, and Asian descent); and (4) lentigo maligna (4–10%) *(31–33)*. Rare variants include desmoplastic, amelanotic, mucosal, and verrucous melanoma.

Treatment: Surgical

General principles of treatment of both melanoma and NMSC include: biopsy, definitive excision, and reconstruction. Relatively recent modifications of this paradigm include Mohs' micrographic surgery for excision and sentinel lymph node biopsy *(34,35)*. A sound reconstructive strategy is predicated on a clear understanding of the issues involved in oncologic ablation.

Margins

Although margin control is vital to optimal oncologic treatment of skin cancer, there is some variation in the adoption of margin strategies. For NMSC, historically, 2–5mm of margins have been advocated *(36,37)*. For primary BCC and SCCA, 4-mm surgical margins were sufficient to give histologic clearance for 96% of BCC and 97% of SCCA lesions *(38)*. Mohs' micrographic surgery has the benefit that fresh sections are visualized at the time of excision, with the potential that additional margins can be taken as needed. Some general indications for Mohs' surgery of NMSC include: recurrent cancer, aggressive histopathology (morpheaform, sclerosing), large tumors (>20mm), cosmetically sensitive areas, or those anatomic regions prone to higher recurrence (nose, embryonic fusion planes) *(39)*. Mohs' surgery has been reported to have a less than 1% error rate in clearance of margins *(40)*. In contrast, routine frozen section analysis has an 85–91% accuracy rate *(41,42)*.

For melanoma, recommended margins are: 0.5- to 1-cm margins for melanoma *in situ*; 1-cm margin for melanomas 1-mm thick or less; 1- to

2-cm margin for melanomas 1–2 cm thick; and 2-cm margin for melanomas 2-mm thick or greater *(43)*. These guidelines are based on historical comparative studies, such as the World Health Organization trial, the Intergroup Melanoma Study, and the Swedish Melanoma Study Group trials, and have been subject to scrutiny *(44–47)*.

Reconstruction

Timing

The aforementioned issue of margin status is central to the timing of reconstruction. For post-oncologic resection defects that require a flap or skin-graft reconstruction, there should be a reasonable certainty of clearance of tumor. For recurrent, aggressive, or larger NMSCs, the Mohs' surgical technique can accomplish this in the immediate setting. Alternatively, for this same class of advanced, aggressive lesions, if a single-stage resection and reconstruction without Mohs is being considered (and margin status may be in question), routine frozen sections may be helpful. The problem of performing a complex graft and flap reconstruction without margin security is that any *post hoc* positive margin on permanent sections can necessitate a takedown of the reconstruction.

If margin control cannot be sufficiently determined in this scenario, then a delayed reconstruction is a judicious approach after permanent section margin status is confirmed.

The corollary to this issue of uncertain margin status and reconstruction is that for simple, primary, localized, and smaller NMSC, a 4-mm margin is sufficiently accurate (96 and 97% for BCC and SCCA, respectively) that primary closure can proceed without unduly risking a positive permanent margin; which, if it does occur, can normally be handled by re-excision without loss of graft or flap territory.

Although there is no consensus on the utility of Mohs' surgery or frozen section analysis for melanoma, there are studies suggesting its potential benefit vis-a-vis conventional techniques, especially in anatomic regions such as the head and neck where standard margins may be difficult to achieve *(48,49)*.

Techniques

Reconstruction is predicated on the defect itself. There are, of course, the simple facts of the dimensions of the defect; but a variety of host and donor factors must also be taken into consideration during planning: its location; the presence of exposed vital structures; the quality and quantity of neighboring skin (and the secondary effect that moving or altering this may have on critical anatomy); the orientation of the defect relative to relaxed tension lines; the influence of host factors such as diabetes, vascular or immune system impairment, and previous or anticipated local radiation therapy.

To balance this complex of needs are a number of reconstructive techniques (Figure 6.3). A single defect may readily have a number of

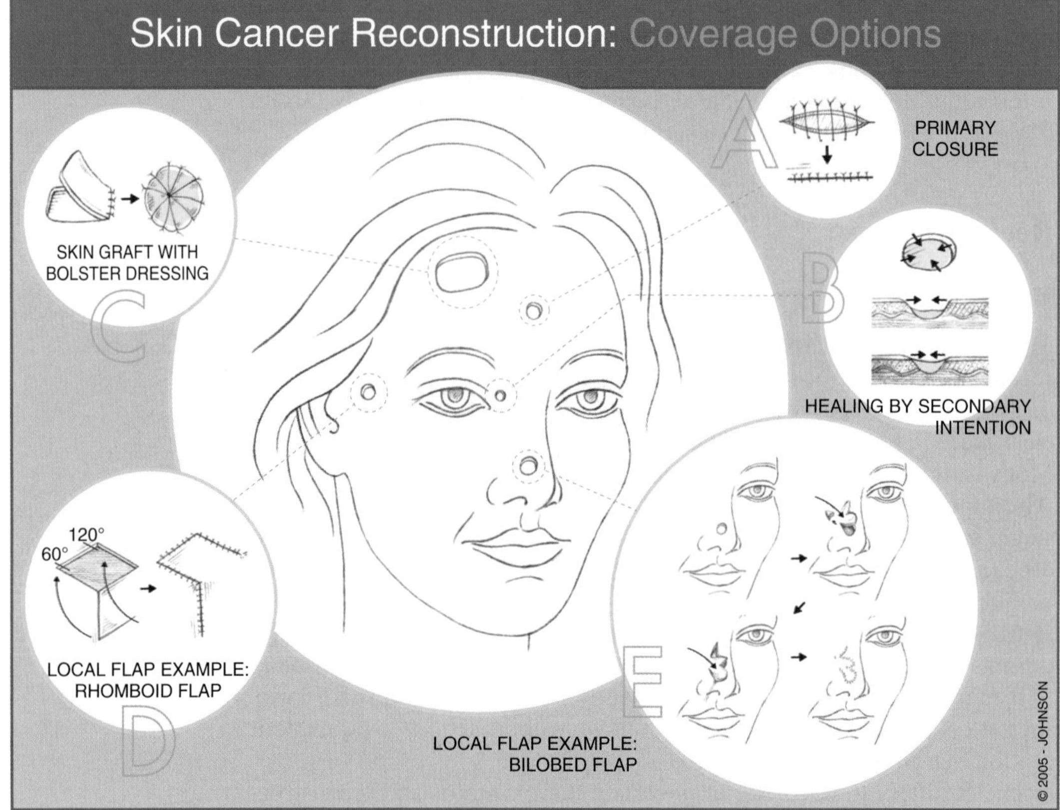

Figure 6.3. Skin cancer reconstruction coverage options: **(A)** Primary closure involves direct suture repair of the defect; **(B)** Healing by secondary intention can be done for smaller lesions in select anatomic zones such as the medial canthal region—re-epithelialization occurs from the periphery; **(C)** Skin grafts can be used for larger defects where local flaps are not suitable; **(D)** local flap example—rhomboid flaps can be useful in the face. Note the approximate 60 and 120° angles; and **(E)** local flap example—bilobed flap is a complex transposition flap that has utility for nasal defects.

suitable reconstructive options. There is, however, a general hierarchy of reconstructive options that progresses from simple closure to complex flap reconstruction.

Primary closure

The simple approximation of the layers of dermis and epidermis that define the wound is termed primary closure. The skin has a topography of tensions, which have been mapped by cadaveric studies. If possible, the defect is oriented along these lines of relaxed skin tension so that there is minimal tension-induced scar widening. If necessary, deeper dermal sutures can be used in conjunction with more superficial epidermal sutures. Eversion of the skin edges is an important technical consideration in primary closure and helps prevent the ensuing scar from becoming depressed. A number of different suture techniques exist including subcuticular, interrupted, and mattress sutures (horizontal, vertical) to facilitate secure closure.

An important corollary to minimizing tension is the judicious undermining of the wound edges. This will help distribute the tension along a greater surface area. Post-operatively, the use of adhesive tapes can provide some external splinting of the wound while the processes of inflammation and wound healing bring the cut edges into more permanent apposition.

Healing by secondary intention

There are both oncologic and reconstructive reasons not to close an ablative defect primarily. If, as discussed previously, there are concerns about the margin status, then the wound may be left open with dressing changes until definitive reconstruction can safely proceed. For smaller defects—and depending on particular anatomic locations such as the medial canthal region—normal wound healing with granulation and re-epithelialization of tissue may be sufficient to close the defect entirely. This type of wound healing is termed healing by secondary intention (Figure 6.3). Alternatively, a combined closure and delayed closure technique is possible, wherein partial closure is performed and the remainder of the wound is allowed to heal by secondary intention. A purse-string type suture employs this very strategy, but this option should be weighed against direct, primary closure.

Skin grafts

When primary closure is not possible because of the magnitude of the defect, a skin graft or flap should be considered. A skin graft is epidermal and varied amounts of dermal tissue taken from another region of the body and engrafted onto a defect (Figure 6.3). The skin graft undergoes a well-defined sequence of healing and incorporation into the wound. During the initial phase, the graft survives by diffusion of nutrients from the recipient bed. Over the next several days, inosculation occurs and vessels from the graft eventually join with and/or get replaced by vessels from the wound bed. The process of neovascularization allows the graft to survive, long-term, through independent proliferation of new growth vessels from the wound into the graft.

Skin grafts are classified by thickness; split-thickness grafts (STSG) are generally 0.012–0.018 inches (0.30–0.45 mm) thick and are routinely harvested with a dermatome. The entire epidermis and the superficial aspect of the dermas is harvested, resulting in a partial-thickness donor site defect, which will heal by re-epithelialization from basal keratinocytes located at the defect edge and within adnexal structures (sweat glands and hair follicles) over several weeks. Full-thickness grafts are harvested by direct excision of the entire thickness of the epidermis and then careful manual thinning of the graft is performed to remove any attached subcutaneous fat, which can act as a barrier to vasculation of the graft. The donor site is usually closed primarily because re-epithelialization is not a facile process over a full-thickness defect. The choice of whether to use a STSG or full-thickness graft for a defect is a matter of clinical judgment and the physical parameters of the oncologic defect. A larger defect often can be reconstructed with a STSG or a flap because of limitations of the donor site surface area for full-thickness skin grafts. A full-thickness graft resists secondary contraction to a greater degree than STSG because of a greater thickness of dermis and is more suitable if a significant degree of durability is needed. For defects of the face, a full-thickness graft is more cosmetically appropriate because its color and texture is superior to a STSG. Moreover, there are distinct differences in color and texture among the candidate donor sites for full-thickness skin grafts and matching the donor site to the context of the donor site is based on individual circumstance. For very large surface area defects of the face, occasionally skin grafts are employed. In this particular case, attention to the aesthetic subunits of the face can be helpful in optimizing outcome—this may mean that excision of small remnants of subunits and full re-surfacing of the entire subunit with the graft may yield a more reasonable appearance than simply grafting the isolated defect itself.

Regardless of the type of graft or donor-recipient site issues, loss of the graft is the major complication the surgeon endeavors to avoid. The most common cause of failure of a graft to take is fluid collections (seroma or hematoma) under the graft, which separate the graft from the recipient wound bed and thereby interrupt the sequence of wound healing and incorporation of the graft described previously. Accordingly, careful hemostasis and debridement of the wound is necessary. This is followed by creating small incisions in the graft or meshing it outright to allow fluid to seep through. A bolster dressing will lend some compressive support to the graft as well.

Skin grafts will undergo contracture according to the relative thickness of the dermal component. STSGs tend to contract more than full-thickness grafts. As the grafts mature, pigmentary changes may occur with STSGs undergoing varying degrees of hyperpigmentation. For the face, where even subtle pigmentation and texture differences may be especially obvious, full-thickness grafts may be superior to STSGs. Reinnervation may occur to a limited extent with potential return to protective sensation in some circumstances.

Flaps

Flaps comprise tissue that can be transferred into defects with its own blood supply as opposed to grafts, which establish a sufficient vasculature from the wound bed once transferred (Table 6.1) *(50,51)*. Flaps can be classified by method of transfer, composition, or characteristic blood supply with overlapping inclusion criteria within these classification schemes. Local flaps are distinguished from free flaps by virtue of the continuity of the vascular supply free flaps are disconnected from the donor site and re-connected to vessels at the recipient site (Figure 6.4).

Random flaps are comprised of skin and subcutaneous tissue without a prominent, defined muscular or septal perforating vessel. These flaps are nourished by multiple, smaller vessels that enter at the base of the flap; consequently, broadening the base of this flap allows the incorpora-

Table 6.1. Classification of Flaps for Reconstruction of Skin Cancer

Vascularity	Composition	Movement and Design
Random	Cutaneous	Local flaps
Axial	Fascial	Advancement
Musculocutaneous	Fasciocutaneous	Transposition
Fasciocutaneous	Adipofascial	Rotation
Free (microvascular approximation)	Muscular	Interpolation
	Musculocutaneous	Distant flaps
		Pedicled
		Free or microvascular

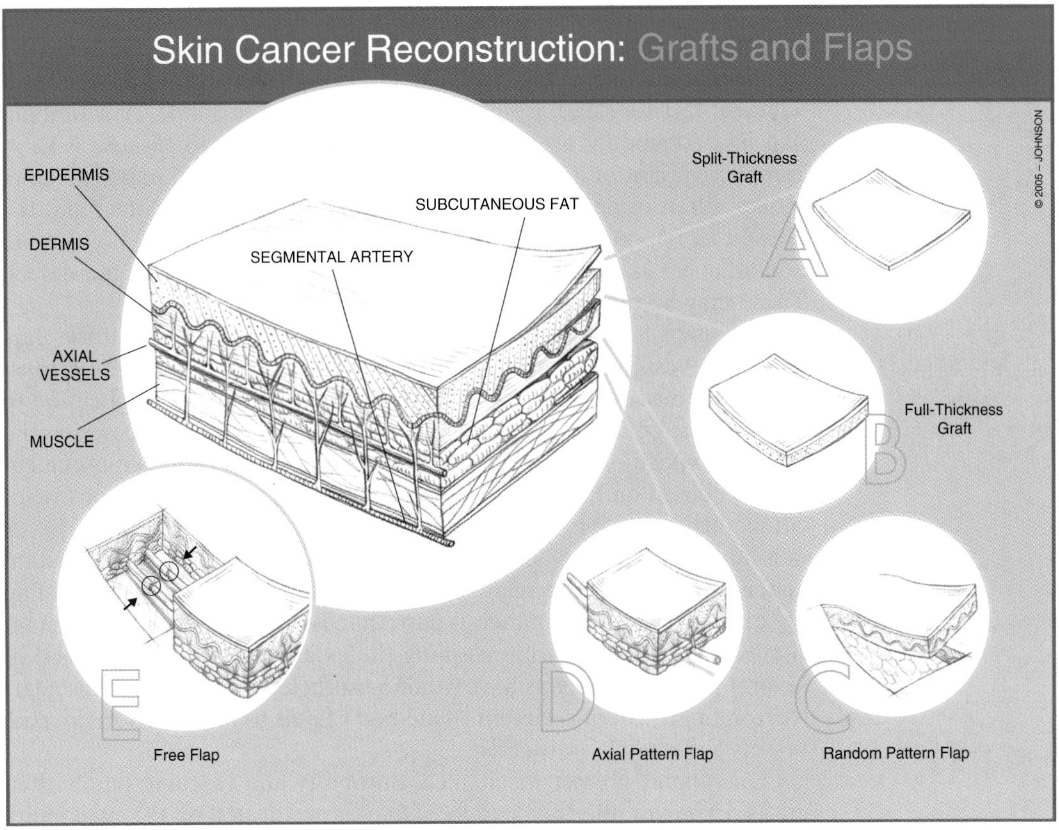

Figure 6.4. Graft and flap types: **(A)** STSG; **(B)** full-thickness graft; **(C)** random flap; **(D)** axial pattern flap with the major feeding vessel coursing through the base of the flap; and **(E)** free flap with microvascular connection of flap vessels to vessels at the recipient site.

tion of a greater density of vessels and can make the distal portions of the flap more robust in terms of vascularity. Random flaps can be categorized by method of movement or design: (1) Advancement flaps simply entail the linear movement of the random flap into the defect without lateral movement of the base (Figure 6.5). Undermining and excision of

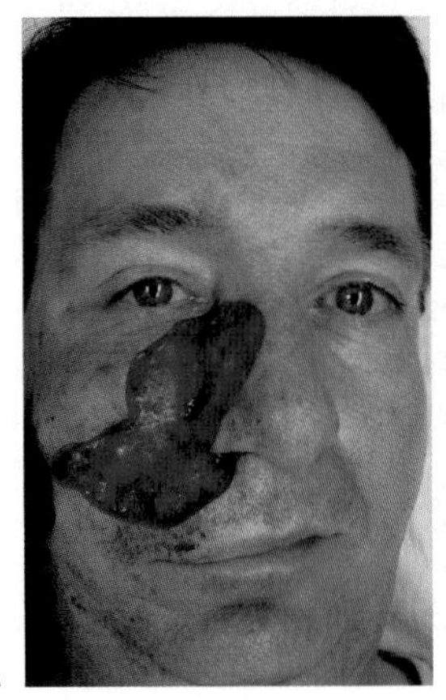

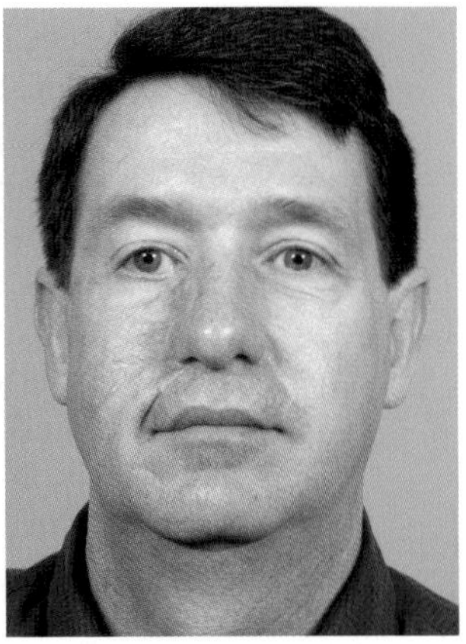

Figure 6.5. Check advancement flap and skin graft coverage of a Moh's defect of the face. **(A)** Pre-operative view and **(B)** 6-month follow-up prior to secondary revision.

small triangles at the base of the flaps can enhance movement. (2) Rotation flaps are generally circular in design and moved into a defect by rotation of the flap at the base. (3) Transposition flaps are moved from adjacent territory and are generally rectangular in shape. A rhomboid flap is a commonly used example of such a local flap (Figure 6.3). A complex variant of a transposition flap is a bilobed flap, in which serial transposition of flaps is used to minimize the donor site defect and the tension of flap motion (Figure 6.3). Interpolation flaps are taken from non-adjacent skin and moved across intervening tissue into the defect. These may be random or axial flaps.

Axial flaps have vessels that are aligned along the length of the flap, and these vessels may have perforators that are direct cutaneous, musculocutaneous, or fasciocutaneous in nature. These terms can be used to describe the course of the vessels, but can also be used to describe the actual composition of the flap. Hence, a flap may be termed musculocutaneous based on its makeup of muscle and skin components or fasciocutaneous based on its makeup of fascia and skin (Table 6.1). A musculocutaneous or fasciocutaneous flap may be local or distant depending on its origin relative to the defect. A groin or forehead flap are examples of fasciocutaneous flaps that can be pedicled from a distant site without necessarily interrupting the axial vessels. After a period of several weeks, these flaps have attained sufficient independent vascularity from ingrowth of recipient tissue bed vessels to have their main axial vessels and pedicle transected.

Flaps impart greater mechanical durability and vascular supply than grafts. However, the choice of local flaps is predicated on the availability and quality of tissue and the complexity of the donor defect. Because there are often multiple options for a given defect, a certain creative flexibility in choice of reconstruction is present. For skin cancer defects, simple full-thickness defects without exposed vital structures can be reconstructed with local flaps. Being from adjacent territory, local flaps will have, in general, similar tissue color, thickness, and consistency and therefore match the donor site more precisely. However, the magnitude of the defect may prevent a simple transfer of local tissue. Tension imparted to the local flap may prevent a sufficient volume of tissue transfer; excessive tension can lead to ischemic flaps. The defect left by transfer of local flaps may be closed primarily, but on occasion this defect may itself necessitate graft or flap coverage. It may be advisable, if the defect is simple, to employ grafts to reconstruct larger defects (despite the disadvantages of a relative mismatch of tissue and prolonged healing).

If the imperative goal (functionally or cosmetically) is to match like with like tissue; then tissue expansion is a viable option. Silicone-lined expanders are placed subcutaneously near the defect and are subject to serial expansion with saline of overlying skin *(52)*. The excess skin is supported by a vascular capsule, which forms around the expander. This expanded skin can then be transferred to cover the defect in delayed fashion (coincident with removal of the expander).

The consequence of transferring local flaps is not limited to whether the ensuing defect can be closed primarily; careful consideration of the distortion of neighboring structures must be considered. A full-thickness defect of the upper cheek may be closed with a rhomboid flap, but depending on the orientation of the flap, distortion of the lower eyelid or nasofacial boundary may occur. A larger cheek advancement flap that distributes the tension more evenly along less distorting vectors could be an option in this case, with a judicious trade off between the larger flap and less distortion.

Frank failure of a local flap can be attributed to excessive tension and concomitant ischemia of the more distal portions of the flap. In addition to poor flap design, microcirculatory disorders from systemic illness, radiation, or tobacco use are potential contributory factors. Irradiated tissue is subject to a chronic vasculitis, which can predispose to flap (or skin graft) compromise *(53)*. Tobacco use is a well-established cause of ischemic insult to both flaps and skin grafts *(54,55)*. In select cases when local flaps will be used in the setting of antecedent radiation or significant tobacco use, a staged delay procedure may be an option *(56,57)*. Delay procedures re-define vascular territories by cutting off specified pre-existing vascular channels (by incisions or ligation of vessels) and opening up alternate pathways. The resultant flap has enhanced circulation and survival.

Aggressive or neglected skin cancer may result in defects with exposed bone, tendon, nerve, or vessels. A graft is normally not as durable a reconstruction, and a fasciocutaneous or musculocutaneous flap may be necessary to cover these vital structures and provide reasonable soft-tissue volume fill. Alternatively, when larger and complex defects are created by oncologic ablation, microvascular or distant pedicled staged transfer of tissue may be necessary. Preservation of function may also impact skin cancer defects that involve mobile areas. A simple skin graft will contract and may adhere to the underlying defect to inhibit motion. The use of more supple fasciocutaneous tissue from local or even distant recipient sites may ameliorate post-operative motion.

Conclusion

Skin cancers can yield reconstructive challenges both simple and complex. Preservation of form and function are the guiding principles. Conversely, the ability to reconstruct skin cancer defects allows the ablative surgeon to extirpate tumor with the security of knowing that techniques exist to reasonably restore form and function. This may allow a more aggressive surgical approach, which may impact disease-free survival (Figure 6.6) *(58)*. Moreover, novel technologies such as skin substitutes are being integrated into the armamentarium of reconstruction, which may yield alternatives for skin cancer reconstruction *(59,60)* (Figure 6.7). Although oncology determines the defect, the reconstruction is predicated on a calculus of defect dimension, exposed structures, and the magnitude and quality of donor tissue.

Acknowledgments: The author would like to acknowledge the work of Dennis E. Johnson for his artistic expertise.

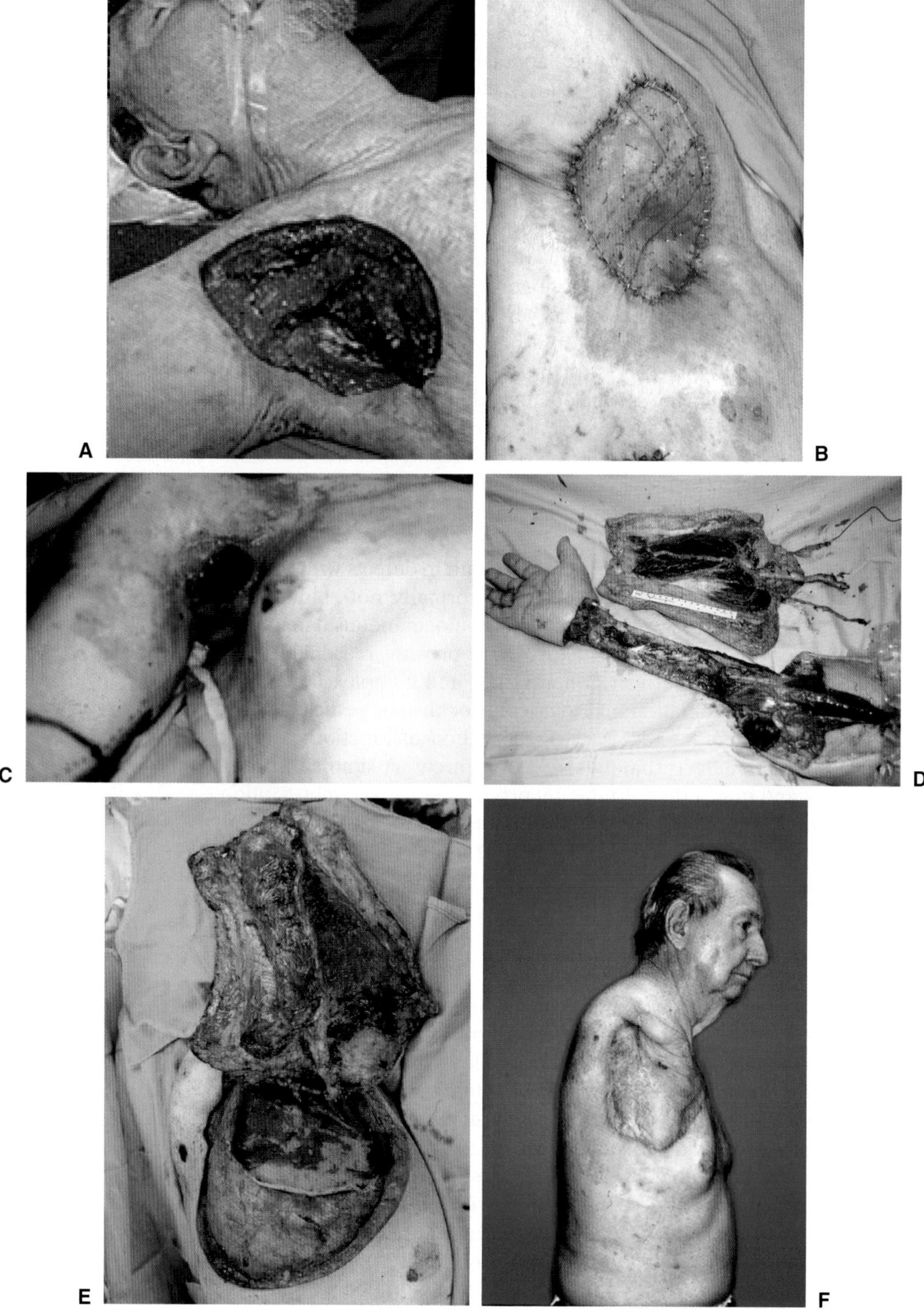

Figure 6.6. An example of complex, multi-stage reconstruction of skin cancer with long-term disease-free survival. **(A)** Recurrent axillary melanoma defect. **(B)** Defect reconstructed with pectoralis muscle flap with skin graft. **(C)** Another recurrence shown ulcerating through the prior reconstruction. **(D)** Radical resection resulting in forequarter amputation—a free fillet flap was taken from the amputated arm. **(E)** Inset of the free fillet flap to the subclavian vessels. **(F)** The patient at long-term follow-up with a healed wound; he is disease-free at 2 years (From Ref. 58, with permission).

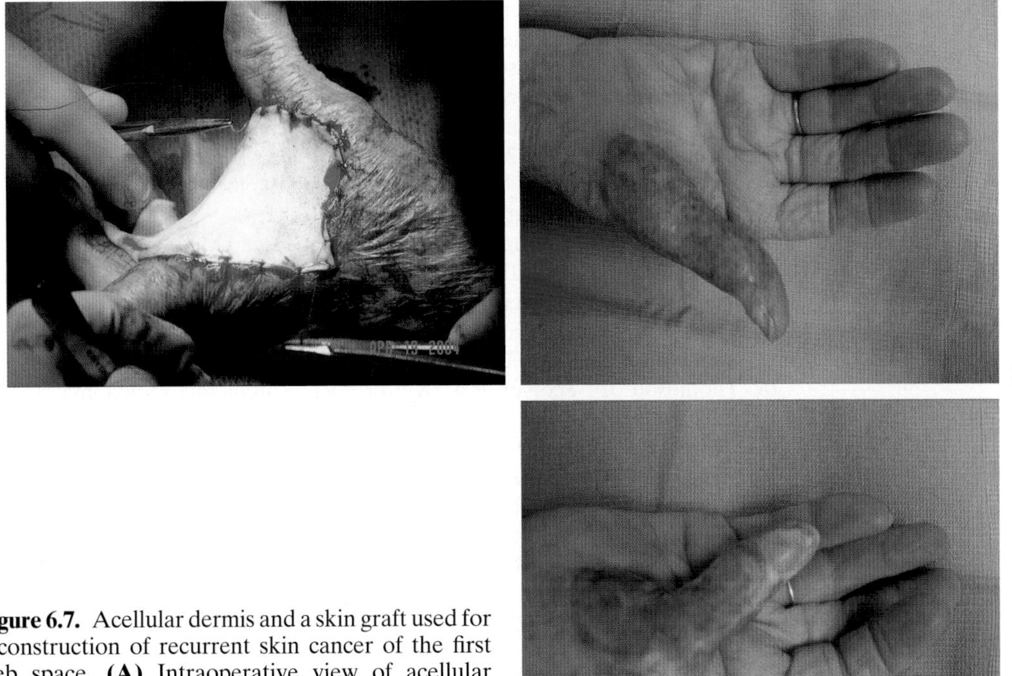

Figure 6.7. Acellular dermis and a skin graft used for reconstruction of recurrent skin cancer of the first web space. **(A)** Intraoperative view of acellular dermis applied to the web space defect of a patient; **(B and C)** Post-operative view of another patient who went on to have acellular dermis and STSG coverage showing functional restoration.

Reference

1. American Cancer Society. American Cancer Society Statistics 2005. www.cancer.org; accessed August 2005.
2. Chen JG, Fleischer AB Jr, Smith ED, et al. Cost of nonmelanoma skin cancer treatment in the United States. Dermatol Surg 2001;27(12):1035–1038.
3. Tsao H, Rogers GS, Sober AJ. An estimate of the annual direct cost of treating cutaneous melanoma. J Am Acad Dermatol 1998;38(5 Pt 1):669–680.
4. Acarturk TO, Edington H. Nonmelanoma skin cancer. Clin Plastic Surg 2005;32:237–248.
5. Ramsey ML. Basal cell carcinoma. Emedicine.com 2005. Accessed August 2005.
6. Alam M, Ratner D. Cutaneous squamous-cell carcinoma. N Engl J Med 2001;344:975–983.
7. Christenson LJ, Borrowman TA, Vachon CM, et al. Incidence of basal cell and squamous cell carcinomas in a population younger than 40 years. JAMA 2005;294(6):681–90.
8. Demers AA, Nugent Z, Mihalcioiu C, et al. Trends of nonmelanoma skin cancer from 1960 through 2000 in a Canadian population. J Am Acad Dermatol 2005;53:320–328.
9. Owens DM, Watt FM. Contribution of stem cells and differentiated cells to epidermal tumours. Nat Rev Cancer 2003;3:444–451.
10. Lovatt TJ, Lear JT, Bastrilles J, et al. Associations between ultraviolet radiation, basal cell carcinoma site and histology, host characteristics, and rate of development of further tumors. J Am Acad Dermatol 2005;52:468–473.

11. Black HS. Reassessment of a free radical theory of cancer with emphasis on ultraviolet carcinogenesis. Integrative Cancer Therapies 2004;3(4):279–293.
12. Tilli CMLJ, Van Steensel MAM, Krekels GAM, et al Molecular aetiology and pathogenesis of basal cell carcinoma. Br J Dermatol 2005;152:1108–1124.
13. Hussein MR. Ultraviolet radiation and skin cancer: molecular mechanisms. J Cutan Pathol 2005;32:191–205.
14. Sra KK, Babb-Tarbox M, Aboutalebi S, et al. Molecular diagnosis of cutaneous diseases. Arch Dermatol 2005;141:225–241.
15. Gawkrodger DJ. Occupational skin cancers. Occup Med 2004;54(7):458–463.
16. Lee E, Koo J, Berger T. UVB phototherapy and skin cancer risk: a review of the literature. Int J Dermatol 2005;44:355–360.
17. Gandini S, Sera F, Cattaruzza MS, et al. Meta-analysis of risk factors for cutaneous melanoma: II. Sun exposure. Eur J Cancer 2005;41(1):45–60.
18. Thompson JF, Scolyer RA, Kefford RF. Cutaneous melanoma. Lancet 2005;365:687–701.
19. Corona R, Dogliotti E, D'Errico M, et al. Risk factors for basal cell carcinoma in a Mediterranean population: role of recreational sun exposure early in life. Arch Dermatol 2001;137:1162–1168.
20. Netscher DN, Spira M. Basal cell carcinoma: an overview of tumor biology and treatment. Plast Reconstr Surg 2004;113(5):74E-94E.
21. Padgett JK. Cutaneous lesions: benign and malignant. Facial Plast Surg Clin N Am 2005;13:195–202.
22. Goldberg LH. Basal cell carcinoma. Lancet 1996;347:663–667.
23. Rudolph R, Zelac DE. Squamous cell carcinoma of the skin. Plast Reconstr Surg 2004;114(6):82–94(e).
24. Phillips TJ, Salman SM, Bhawan J. Burn scar carcinoma. Diagnosis and management. Dermatol Surg 1998;24(5):561–565.
25. Preston DS. Nonmelanoma cancers of the skin. N Engl J Med 1992;327:1649.
26. Cribier B, Asch P, Grosshans E. Differentiating squamous cell carcinoma from keratoacanthoma using histopathological criteria: is it possible? A study of 296 cases. Dermatology 1999;199:208–212.
27. Mendenhall WM, Zlotecki RA, Scarborough MT. Dermatofibrosarcoma protuberans. Cancer 2004;101:2503–2508.
28. Poulsen M. Merkel's cell cancer of the skin. Lancet Oncol 2004;5(10):593–599.
29. Brady MS. Current management of patients with merkel cell carcinoma. Dermatol Surg 2004;30(2 pt 2):321–325.
30. Pitman MJ. Merkel cell carcinoma of the skin. Emedicine.com 2005; accessed August 2005.
31. Swetter SM. Malignant melanoma. Emedicine.com 2005. Accessed August 2005.
32. Perniciaro C. Dermatopathologic variants of melanoma. Mayo Clinic Proc 1997;72(3):273–279.
33. Heasley DD, Toda S, Mihm MC Jr. Pathology of malignant melanoma. Surg Clinic North Am 1996;76(6):1223–1255.
34. Mohs FE. Moh's micrographic surgery. A historical perspective. Dermatol Clin 1989;7(4):609–611
35. Morton DL. Lymphatic mapping and sentinel lymphadenectomy for melanoma: past, present, and future. Ann Surg Oncol 2001;8(9 Suppl):S22-S28.
36. Epstein E. How accurate is the visual assessment of basal carcinoma margins? Br J Dermatol 1973;89:37–43.
37. Hallock GG, Lutz DA. A prospective study of the accuracy of the surgeon's diagnosis and significance of positive margins in nonmelanoma skin cancers. Plast Reconstr Surg 2001;107(4):942–947.
38. Damon T, King AR, Peat BG. Excision margins for non-melanotic skin cancer. Plast Reconstr Surg 2003;112(1):57–63.

39. Lang PG. The role of Mohs' micrographic surgery in the management of skin cancer and a perspective on the management of the surgical defect. Clin Plastic Surg 2004;31:5–31.
40. Campbell RM, Barrall D, Wilkel C, et al. Post-Moh's micrographic surgical margin tissue evaluation with permanent histopathologic sections. Dermatol Surg 2005;31(6):655–658.
41. Ghauri RR, Gunter AA, Weber RA. Frozen section analysis in the management of skin cancers. Ann Plast Surg 1999;43(2);156–160.
42. Manstein ME, Manstein CH, Smith R. How accurate is frozen section for skin cancers? Ann Plast Surg 2003;50(6):607–609.
43. National Comprehensive Cancer Network . National Comprehensive Cancer Network Melanoma Practice Guidelines 2005. www.nccn.org/professionals/physician_gls/PDF/melanoma. Accessed August 2005.
44. Veronesi U, Cascinelli N. Narrow excision (1-cm margin): a safe procedure for thin cutaneous melanoma. Arch Surg 1991;126:438–441.
45. Johnson TM, Sondak VK. Melanoma margins: the importance and need for more evidence-based trials. Arch Dermatol 2004;140:1148–1150.
46. Balch CM, Soong SF, Smith T, et al. Long-term results of a prospective surgical trial comparing 2 cm vs. 4 cm excision margins for 740 patients with 1–4 mm melanomas. Ann Surg Oncol 2001;8:101–108.
47. Ringborg U, Andersson R, Eldh J, et al. Resection margins of 2 versus 5 cm for cutaneous malignant melanoma with a tumor thickness of .8 to 2.0 mm: randomized study by the Swedish Melanoma Study Group. Cancer 1996;77: 1809–1814.
48. Bricca GM, Brodland DG, Ren D, et al. Cutaneous head and neck melanoma treated with Mohs micrographic surgery. J Am Acad Dermatol 2005; 52(1):92–100.
49. Cook J. Surgical margins for resection of primary cutaneous melanoma. Clin Dermatol. 2004;22(3):228–33.
50. Mathes SJ, Nahai F. Reconstructive Surgery Principles, anatomy & technique. Philadelphia: Elsevier. 1997:37–51.
51. Daniel RK, Kerrigan CL. Principles and physiology of skin flap surgery. In: Plastic Surgery ed. McCarthy J. Philadelphia: WB Saunders Company, 1990:275–328.
52. Margulis A, Bauer BS, Fine NA. Large and giant congenital pigmented nevi of the upper extremity: an algorithm to surgical management. Ann Plast Surg. 2004;52(2):158–67.
53. Kurul S, Dincer M, Kizir A, et al. Plastic surgery in irradiated areas: analysis of 200 consecutive cases. Eur J Surg Oncol 1997;23(1):48–53.
54. Kinsella JB, Rassekh CH, Wassmuth ZD et al. Smoking increases facial skin flap complications. Ann Otol Rhinol Laryngol. 1999 Feb;108(2): 139–42.
55. Goldminz D, Bennett RG. Cigarette smoking and flap and full-thickness graft necrosis. Arch Dermatol. 1991;127(7):1012–5.
56. Dhar SC, Taylor GI. The delay phenomenon: the story unfolds. Plast Reconstr Surg 1999;104(7):2079–91.
57. Fisher JC, Hurn I, Rudolph R et al. The effect of delay on flap survival in an irradiated field. Plast Reconstr Surg 1984;73(1):99–104.
58. Kim JYS, Ross MI, Butler CE. Reconstruction following radical resection of recurrent metastatic axillary melanoma. Plast Reconstr Surg 2006;117(5): 1576–1583.
59. Kim JY, Kloeters O, Oh SE, et al. Acellular dermis for reconstruction of recurrent squamous cell carcinoma of the 1st web space. Manuscript in preparation.
60. Sardesai MG, Tan AK. Artificial skin for the reconstruction of cutaneous tumour resection. J Otolaryngol 2002;31(4):248–252.

7

Lip, Cheek, and Scalp Reconstruction

Jeremy Waldman and Howard N. Langstein

Lip Reconstruction

History

Ancient Hindu descriptions of lip reconstruction date as far back as 3000 BC, but the first written account was by Susruta in 1000 BC *(1)*. Most of the surgical concepts still used today were developed during the mid-1800s and have been adapted and improved over the years. The idea of using like or similar tissues was introduced by Gillies in the 1920s and later modified by Karapandzic in 1974 *(2,3)*. Refinements by Burget and Menick, based on the subunit principle, placed further emphasis on lip aesthetics *(4)*. Even though new techniques continue to be introduced, the basic tenets of lip reconstruction remain largely unchanged.

Goals of Reconstruction

The lips are the dominating feature of the lower one-third of the face. They play an important functional as well as aesthetic role. Restoration of oral competence and aperture while maintaining sensation, mobility, and cosmesis should be the goal of the reconstructive surgeon.

Lip Neoplasms

Approximately 25% of all oral cavity carcinomas involve the lips *(5)*. Pathologic diagnosis will determine the planned resection and need for adjuvant therapy. Basal cell carcinoma is the most common upper lip malignancy, whereas squamous cell cancers predominate on the lower lip *(6)*. As such, lower lip tumors will most often require larger resection margins compared to the upper lip, and also consideration for evaluation of the draining lymph nodal basins.

Anatomy

Lips are three-layered structures that span horizontally between the oral commissures and vertically from the base of the columella to the chin.

Each is comprised of an outer layer of skin, a middle muscular layer, and an inner mucosal surface. The mucocutaneous junction, between the outer skin and inner mucosa, is referred to as the vermilion. The border of the vermilion, which separates the "red" lip from the "white" lip, is of great cosmetic importance because even minor errors in approximation are noticeable.

Burget and Menick emphasized a subunit approach to lip reconstruction *(4)*. Essentially, this entails reconstruction based on replacing the entire subunit to avoid a patch-like appearance to the viewer. With that in mind, the upper lip is divided into medial and lateral subunits. The two philthral columns extend from the base of the columella and define the border of these subunits as well as the central depression of the lip. As such, the upper lip is anatomically more complex than the lower lip, which is one large aesthetic unit.

The orbicularis oris is the principle muscle of the lip. Orbicularis fibers are oriented horizontally and provide sphincteric function for the oral cavity *(5)*. There are many other associated muscles that aid in the complex motions and functions. The modiolus is a paired fibrous structure located at the commissures that serves as an insertion site for the perioral musculature.

Blood supply to the lips is derived from the paired superior and inferior labial arteries. Both branch from the ipsilateral facial artery, which originates from the external carotid system.

Motor and sensory innervation is derived from branches of cranial nerves V and VII. The buccal and marginal mandibular branches of the facial nerve provide motor function to the upper and lower lips, respectively. The lower-lip sensation is provided by the mental nerve, which is the terminal branch of the inferior alveolar nerve from the mandibular division of the trigeminal nerve. Upper-lip sensation is via the infraorbital nerve from the maxillary division of the trigeminal nerve.

Lymphatic drainage of the lips is through the submandibular and submental basins. The upper lip, along with the lateral portions of the lower lip, drains primarily to the submandibular chain. The central portions of the lower lip preferentially drain to the submental nodes *(7)*.

Reconstruction

Reconstructive strategies in lip surgery are based on a thorough examination of the defect and consideration of patient factors. In particular, the reconstructive surgeon should note the size, location, and etiology of the defect as well as the age, gender, and comorbidities of the patient. In general, algorithms for lip reconstruction are based on the percentage of missing tissue, but it can be further simplified by dividing the defects into less than one-third, one-third to two-thirds, and greater than two-thirds. Special consideration is also given to defects isolated to the vermilion and involving the commissure.

Vermilion defects

Scars that remain within the borders of the vermillion without extending into the skin can be well hidden and difficult to notice. Therefore, when addressing defects within the vermilion, it can be advantageous to limit the placement of incisions to the red lip and mucosa. The labial mucosa can be advanced, for example with a V-Y flap, to cover vermillion defects with excellent functional and cosmetic results *(5,7,8)*. Smaller lesions can be treated with fusiform excision and primary closure even with horizontal orientation to avoid extending passed the vermilion border *(5,7)*. Larger lesions require a vertical orientation because horizontal shortening of the vermillion can cause a notched appearance. Incisions that cross the vermillion should do so perpendicularly.

Defects involving less than one-third

Defects that involve less than one-third of the total length of the upper or lower lip are generally amenable to primary closure with wedge, V-shaped, or W-shaped excisions. All incisions should be oriented along relaxed skin tension lines and closed in layers to approximate mucosa, muscle, and skin. Careful closure of the vermillion border is essential to the cosmetic outcome and is facilitated by marking of the vermillion with methylene blue dye *(5)*. This maneuver is also critical when repairing larger defects described in the following section.

As an adjunct to this technique, advancement flaps of both the upper and lower lip can be used to achieve closure. In the upper lip, this is aided by perialar crescent-shaped excisions to allow for advancement. On the other hand, in the lower lip, an incision placed along the mental crease provides the necessary release *(5,9)*.

Defects greater than one-third

Defects that measure more than one-third of the horizontal lip length are generally not able to be closed primarily. However, even with larger defects, techniques previously mentioned can be used in combination to enhance outcomes *(10,11)*.

For defects ranging from one-third to two-thirds, the cross-lip technique provides an excellent repair. Also known as a lip-switch or Abbe flap, this technique employs the transfer of tissue based on the labial artery of the unaffected lip to the defect of the opposite lip *(7)*. The pedicle is later divided in a second stage after it has developed independent vascularity, typically at 2–3 weeks *(11)*.

For defects that involve the commissure, the Estlander flap (a laterally based Abbe flap) is the best choice (Figure 7.1). The Estlander flap is similar to an Abbe flap, but it incorporates the commissure into its design. Both of these flaps allow for the simultaneous transfer of adjacent chin or cheek tissue to replace missing white lip, columella, and nasal sill *(11)*.

As defects grow larger, combinations of circumoral rotation-advancement flap techniques become useful. When the area of missing tissue is in the 60–80% of horizontal lip-length range, one can use the Bernard modification of the Webster procedure or Karapandzic flaps *(3,12–14)*. The Webster procedure and Bernard modification involves triangular nasolabial excisions combined with labiomental crease incisions to allow medial advancement of laterally based tissue (Figure 7.2). The Karapandzic flap advances and rotates segments of skin, orbicularis, and mucosa on neurovascular pedicle and can be used for defects of the upper or lower lip *(3)* (Figure 7.3). This procedure allows for the preservation of motor and sensory function, but is a technically difficult and can result

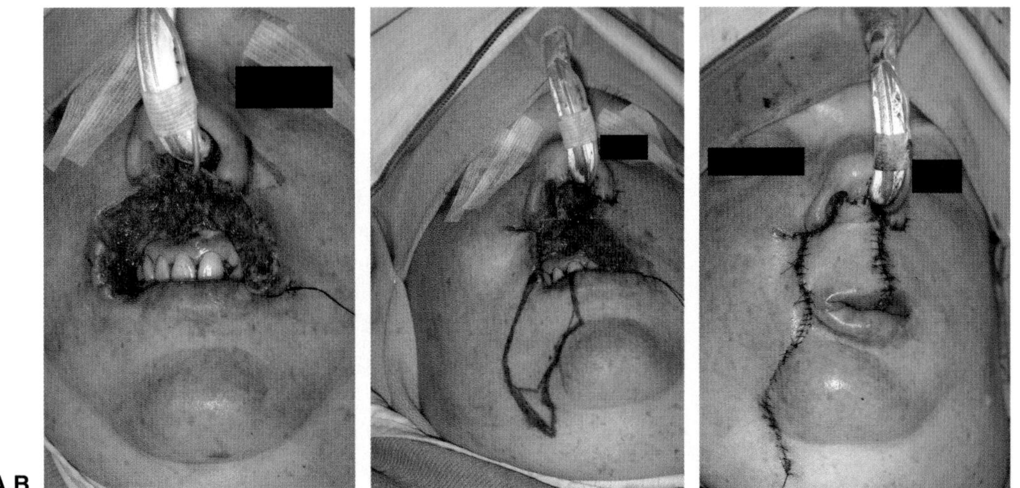

Figure 7.1. **(A)** Large defect of the upper lip following resection of invasive melanoma. **(B)** Intraoperative design of laterally based Abbe flap or Estlander flap with extension into the chin to replace nasal columellar tissue. **(C)** Inset of Estlander flap with defect closure, expected narrowing of oral sphincter.

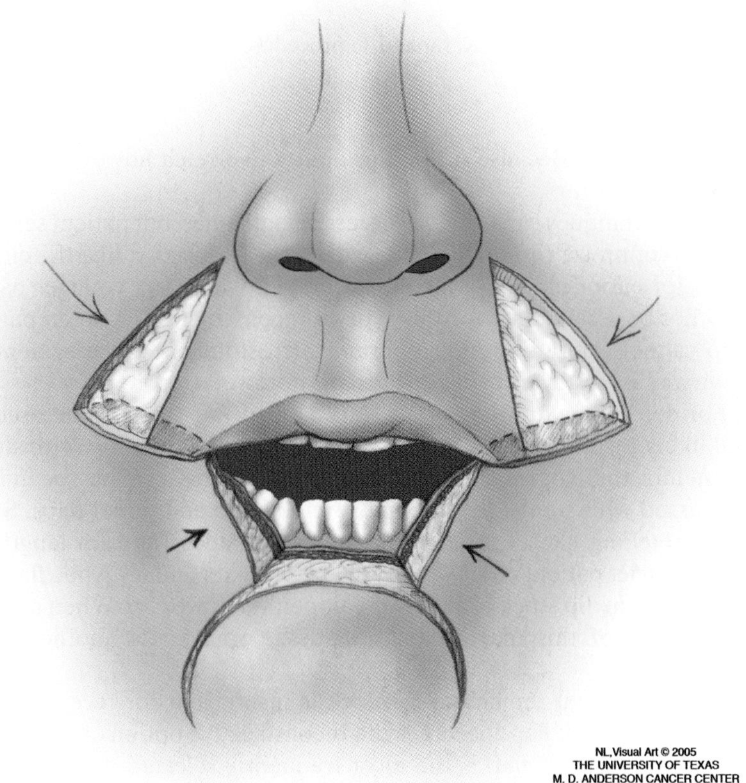

Figure 7.2. Diagram of Webster-Bernard procedure for large lower-lip defect.

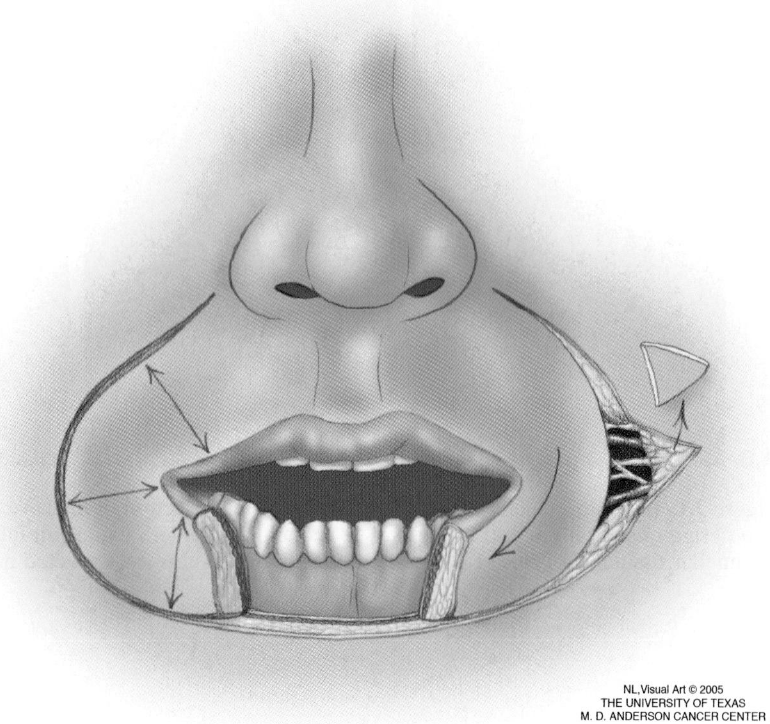

Figure 7.3. Diagram of Karapandzic procedure for large lower-lip defect.

in microstomia. Because of the lips ability to stretch however, this may only be temporary.

Both techniques can provide successful outcomes, but patient selection helps to optimize results. Patients with more skin laxity, like the elderly, allow for easier medial tissue advancement, whereas a younger patient may not be a candidate for this type of reconstruction. Also, in patients who cannot tolerate even temporary microstomia because of dentures or airway issues, Karapandzic flaps are not preferred.

For defects greater than 80%, Karapandzic flaps can still be used but will likely result in excessively flat and tight reconstructions with stomal diameters that may be less than 3 cm *(11)*. This can be secondarily addressed with stents, stretching exercises, and additional flaps. Stents and stretching can be used to augment the sulcus and lip length but require strict patient compliance (Figure 7.4). Secondary Abbe flaps can "balance" the lip stock between the upper and lower lip. When addressing defects of this magnitude, free tissue transfer is another viable tool.

When the total remaining lip stock is insufficient for reconstruction, transfer of distant flaps becomes the reconstructive option of choice. The free radial forearm flap is the most frequently selected donor site *(15)* (Figure 7.5). This provides thin pliable tissue flap that can be transferred as a composite with the palmaris longus tendon to aid in suspension.

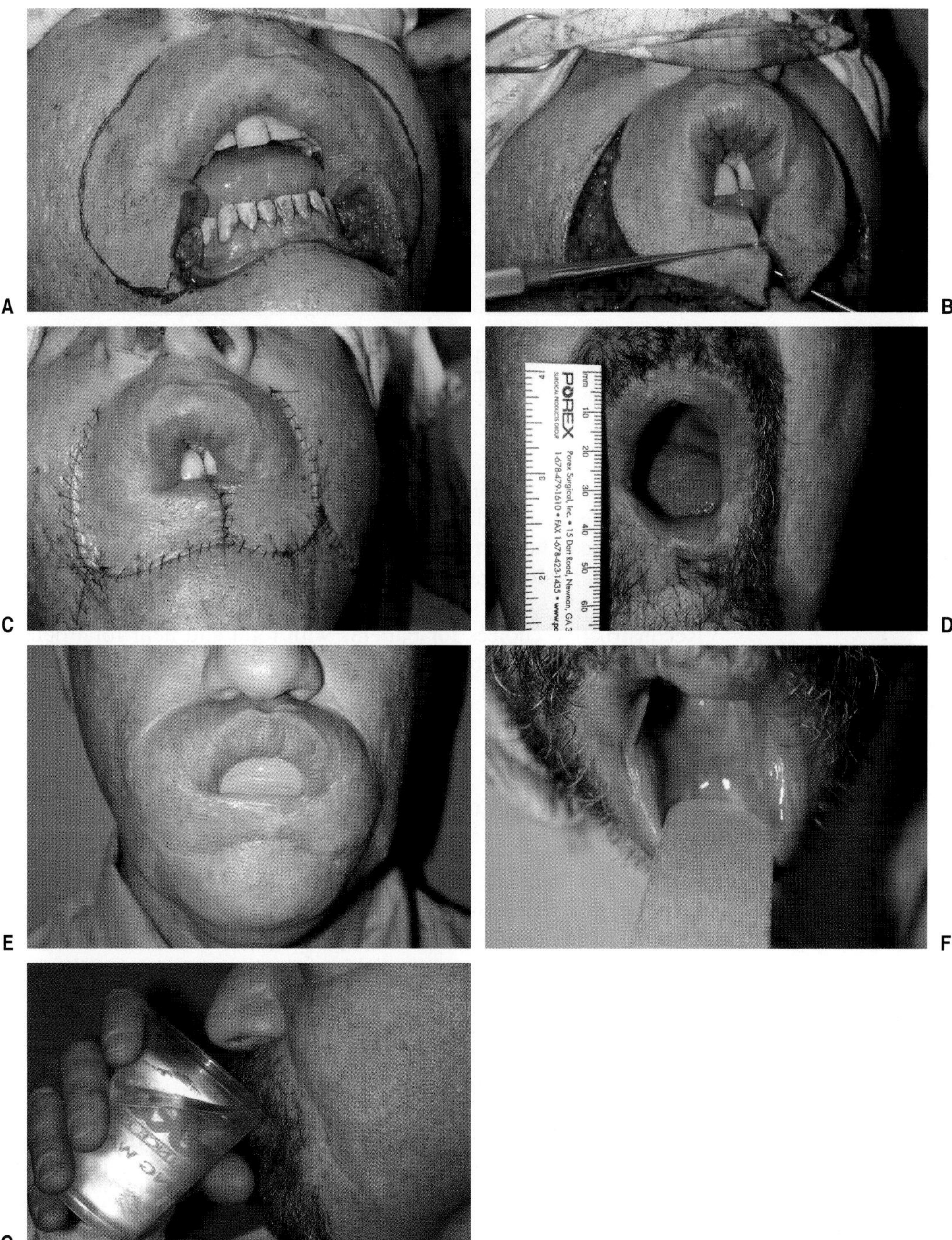

Figure 7.4. **(A)** Patient with near-complete lower-lip resection following removal of squamous cell cancer with markings for Karapandzic flaps. **(B)** Medial advancements of neurotized lip elements. **(C)** Immediate inset of flaps. **(D)** Post-operative view at 1 year, demonstrating sizable sphincteric opening. **(D)** Intra-oral soft splint in place, which was worn in order to deepen labiogingival sulcus. **(D)** Final result of sulcus. **(E)** Functional result at 1 year.

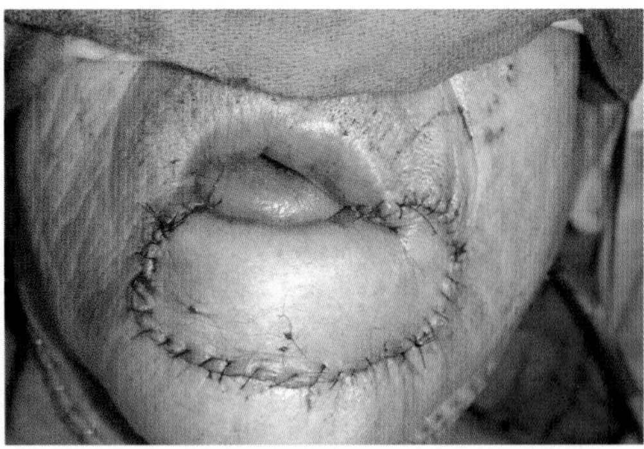

Figure 7.5. Entire lower lip reconstructed with radial artery forearm free flap and palmaris longus tendon suspension.

Successful reconstructions of both the upper and lower lip have been reported using the radial forearm *(15,16)*. Incorporating a sensory nerve with the flap can be performed, but may not be necessary as such flaps may spontaneously regain some sensation without nerve coaptation *(17)*.

Reconstructive choices for patients with total and near-total defects of the lip will ultimately be determined by both patient factors and surgeon experience and preference. Often several options can provide functional and cosmetic results.

Cheek Reconstruction

Introduction

Cheeks help to define the face by providing its lateral borders and are delineated by the contour of their underlying structures. The cheeks are intimately associated with the neighboring aesthetic units of the eyes, nose, and mouth. As a highly sun-exposed area, they are affected by many melanotic and non-melanotic skin cancers, resulting in the frequent need for reconstruction.

Defects range from simple excisions that can be primarily closed, to full-thickness areas that can include oral lining and require complex closures. The dimensions and appearance of the cheek varies with age and sex as well as hair position and style. Careful consideration should be given to these characteristics when planning reconstructions.

Goals of Reconstruction

Cheek reconstruction is unique because the surgeon must focus more on surface texture and color, rather than contour, to achieve the best aesthetic outcome *(18,19)*. Defects can be quite complex and may involve or abut other facial features. When performing a repair, one must consider the effect on adjacent structures including; eyelid, nose, lips, ear, and scalp. Even when these structures are not involved, excessive tension on wound closures can affect their aesthetics and function.

When analyzing defects, observation of the etiology, location, size, shape, and depth of the wound will allow for proper planning. Also, options will be affected be the amount of skin laxity and patterns of facial hair.

Anatomy

The cheeks form an aesthetic unit that is bordered laterally by the preauricular crease, medially by the nose and nasolabial fold, superiorly by the inferior orbital rim and zygomatic arch, and inferiorly by the by the border of the mandible *(20)*. Zide further divided this unit into three overlapping zones to help categorize reconstructive options *(21,22)*.

Zone 1: suborbital

This area extends from the sideburn laterally to the nasolabial fold medially, and from the lower eyelid skin superiorly to the gingival sulcus inferiorly. Furthermore, the zone is subdivided into three subunits (A, B, and C).

Zone 2: preauricular

The preauricular zone extends from the across the malar eminence and side burn to the superolateral junction of the helix and cheek. Inferiorly, its border is defined by the mandible.

Zone 3: buccomandibular

Zone 3 lies occupies the area inferior to Zone 1 and anterior to Zone 2. This extends from the gingival sulcus to the border of the mandible and lies adjacent to the chin and oral commisure. Tissue of this zone directly overlies the parotid masseteric fascia and parotid gland.

The parotid gland will often be encountered during reconstructive surgery of the cheek. It extends anterior and inferior from the external acoustic meatus between the ramus of the mandible and the mastoid process *(23)*. Care must be taken not to injure both its duct, which courses horizontally from the anterior border before entering the oral cavity, and facial nerve branches, which run within its substance.

Innervation and blood supply

Motor and sensory innervation to the cheek is intricate and has several areas of overlapping coverage. Sensation is provided mainly by the second and third divisions of the fifth cranial nerve via the infraorbital, mental, auriculotemporal and zygomaticofacial branches. Branches of the facial nerve (cranial nerve VII) provide motor innervation and must be remembered when performing deep plane dissections in the cheek area.

Blood supply to the cheek is via the facial artery and its branches, which originate from the external carotid artery.

Reconstruction

Skin grafts

Skin grafts are an important tool to the reconstructive surgeon. As previously stated, when performing cheek reconstruction, maintaining a texture and color match to the surrounding tissue is crucial to providing an aesthetic result. Skin grafting may provide a reasonable match but can often leave a patch-like appearance. Graft contracture can result in a significant deformity to adjacent structures and can be limited by selecting a full-thickness graft over a split-thickness graft. Even a full-thickness graft may not adequately fill defects that extend into the subcutaneous space. They should be avoided in wounds with a depth greater than 5 mm *(22)*. In general, full-thickness grafts are selected when local tissue is not available in small, nonirradiated wounds *(24)*. In selected cases, the entire cheek aesthetic unit can be replaced with a full-thickness skin graft with acceptable results (Figure 7.6).

Local and regional flaps

Because of the inherent skin laxity and availability of donor cheek, tissue local tissue reconstruction can adequately address many of the cheek defects.

Small lesions are often amenable to elliptical excision and primary closure without mobilizing large amounts of tissue. Incisions should be oriented along relaxed skin tension lines and can be designed to lie within the natural creases of the nasojugal groove, nasolabial fold, marionette lines, or preauricular fold *(25)*. This approach is applicable to defects in all zones.

Defects that cannot be closed primarily are often managed with local tissue rearrangement. Local flaps provide the best color and texture match to the surrounding tissue and can be designed to leave incisions in concealed locations. A useful solution is the Rhomboid flap, which employs the transfer of an adjacent rectangular flap while primarily closing the donor site. This approach allows the surgeon to orient the flap in a way that avoids conspicuous scars and unnecessary tension *(22)*. A slight modification of this technique described by Quaba increases this flaps flexibility when working with circular defects *(26)*. Bilobed flaps, V-Y advancement and swing side-plasty are also commonly used. If properly planned, these flaps can be used simultaneously for certain defects, and are definitely first-line choices for small and even some moderately sized cheek defects in zone 2.

Larger defects of the cheek require greater amounts of tissue mobilization and regional flap reconstruction. Rotation-advancement flaps can be designed to transfer cheek, neck, and anterior chest. These are essentially large random-pattern flaps designed either as anteriorly or posteriorly based advancements. They work well for defects in zones 1 and 3 since the incisions can be hidden along borders of the aesthetic units.

In designing this flap based anteriorly, an incision that originates at the superior portion of the defect passes horizontally to the preauricular crease, which is then followed inferiorly and then posteriorly into the occipital hairline *(18)* (Figure 7.7). Juri and Juri described elevating this

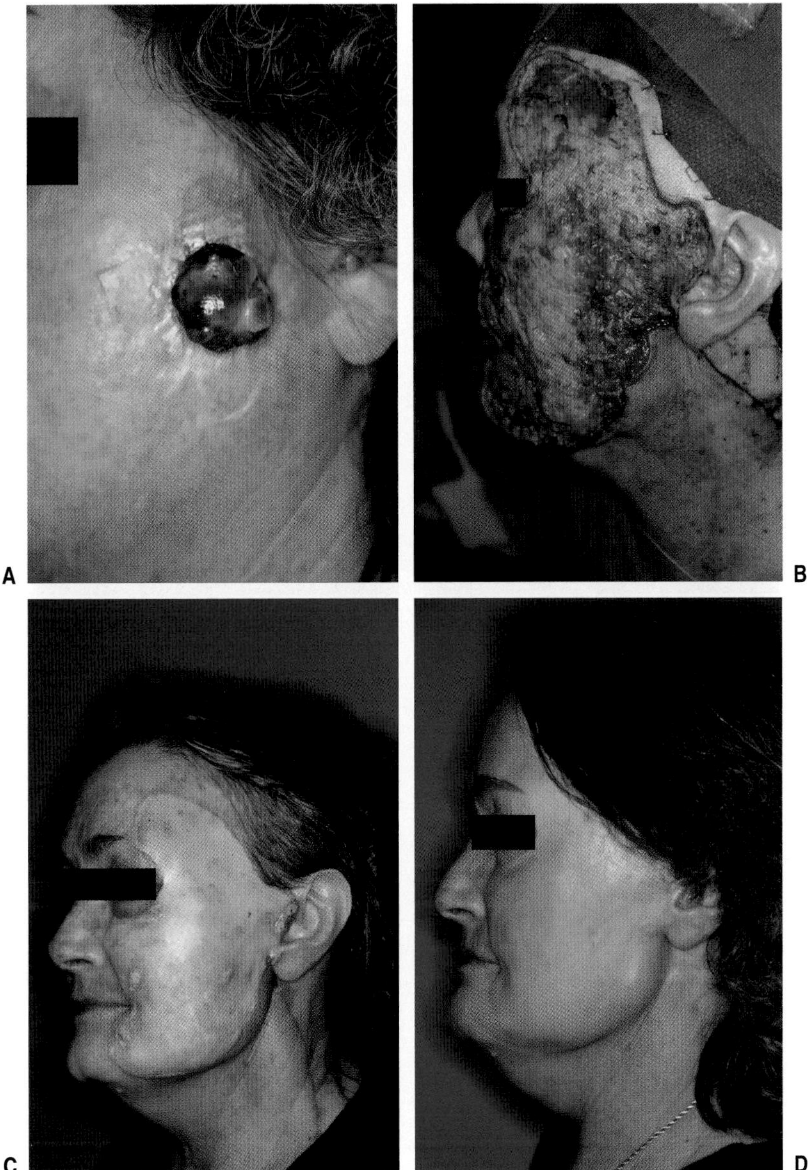

Figure 7.6. **(A)** Large invasive melanoma of left cheek, arising in scar tissue from distant scald burn scar. **(B)** Defect following melanoma resection involving lymph nodal dissection and removal of remainder of facial burn scar. Incision for lymph node dissection closed. **(C)** Large sheet of full-thickness skin successfully transferred to cheek, result at 6 months. **(D)** Improved texture of graft following camouflage cosmetic application.

flap in a subcutaneous plane based on the facial and submental arteries *(27,28)*. An extended version, called a cervicopectoral flap, can be designed by continuing the incision into the neck and onto the chest *(29–31)*. Elevation of this flap includes the platysma and deltopectoral fascia, which maintains the blood supply via the pectoral perforators. The blood supply to either flap can be further improved by elevating in a

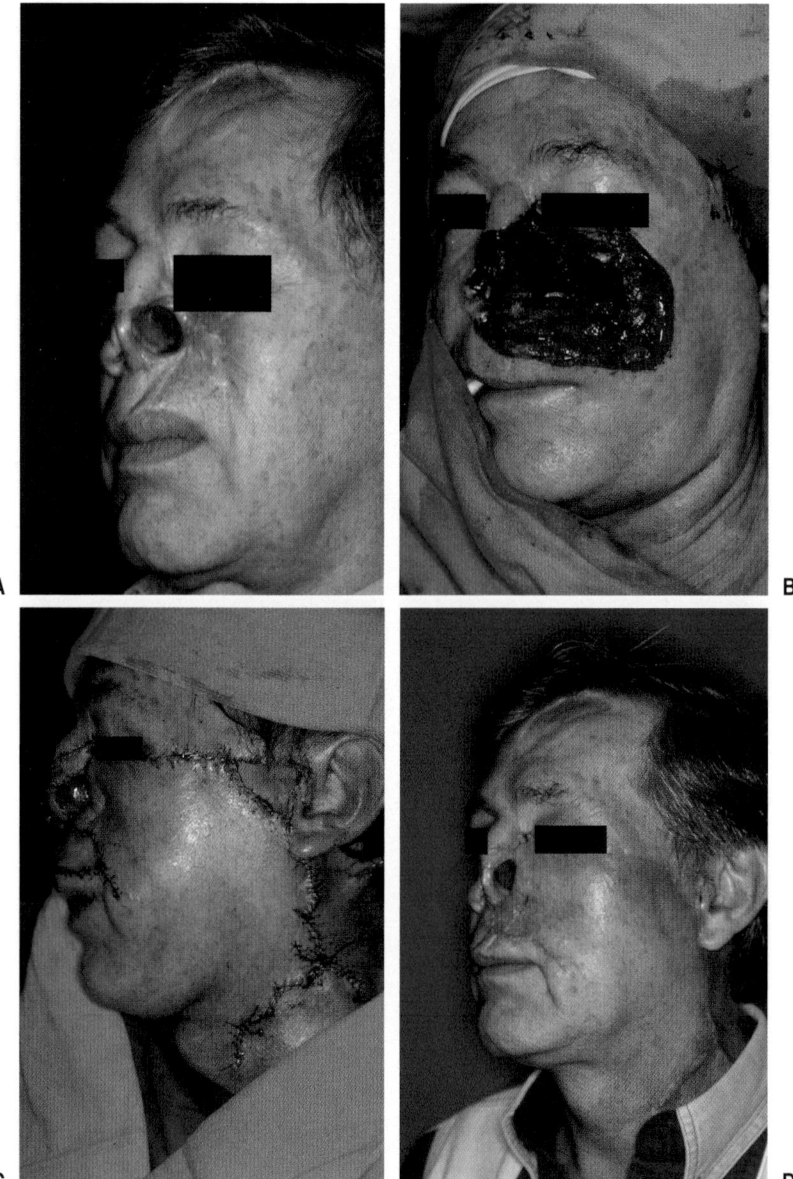

Figure 7.7. **(A)** Recurrent basal cell cancer medial cheek and nose following multiple resections. **(B)** Large defect of nose and medial cheek following tumor clearance. **(C)** Anteriorly based cervicofacial flap raised in deep plane used to reconstruct cheek. Nasal defect grafted and restored at a later date. Note small skin graft placed at preauricular region to reduce tension on suture line. **(D)** Early post-operative view showing full viability of cervical advancement flap.

deep plane, below the superficial musculoaponeurotic system (SMAS) as described by Kroll *(32)*. This improves flap viability, but the deep plane dissection is more technically challenging because of the risk of facial nerve injury.

A posterior-based flap is designed along the nasolabial fold and can continue across the jawline onto the neck and chest or turn superiorly toward the earlobe or mastoid *(33–35)*. This allows the flap to be vascularized by the superficial temporal, vertebral, and occipital vessels as well as perforators from the trapezius and thoracoacromial vessels when extending onto the chest *(18)*. Even though this design allows a better blood supply than the anteriorly based flap, it does have the disadvantage of placing the incision.

Distant flaps

Defects that extend into the oral cavity require oral lining reconstruction in addition to the cutaneous defect. Often, distant flaps are used in combination with local flap reconstruction. For example, the oral lining can be reconstructed by free tissue transfer and the cutaneous defect then covered with a large advancement flap. This circumstance would allow the surgeon to select well-vascularized tissue that can be easily contoured to be placed intra-orally and still provide excellent color match for the external defect. However, even in small defects, external skin affected by previous radiotherapy may not be available for local flap reconstruction, and a reconstruction that replaces both intra-oral and external layers is advised.

Distant tissue is available from regional flaps or by free tissue transfer. Regional options include the deltopectoral flap, pectoralis major myocutaneous flap, and trapezius musculocutaneous flap *(36–38)*. Free flap reconstruction may be more desirable in many circumstances because it offers composite flaps from outside of a potentially radiated field that can be more easily tailored and manipulated in three dimensions *(22)*. Some have argued that this method of reconstruction provides superior aesthetics and fewer complications *(39,40)*. Commonly selected flaps include the radial forearm, rectus abdominus, anterolateral thigh, and parascapular. All provide adequate soft tissue and have acceptable donor morbidity.

Scalp Reconstruction

History

Many techniques have been utilized throughout the years to reconstruct the different varieties of scalp defects. As far back as 1871, Netolitzky reported using a skin graft to repair the scalp *(41)*. Further advances in local flap reconstruction were later popularized and refined by Juri and Ortichochea *(42,43)*. With the advent of microsurgical techniques, Mclean and Buncke introduced free flap scalp reconstruction with omentum in 1972 *(44)*. Modern scalp reconstruction incorporates variations of these procedures, often in combination.

Goals of Reconstuction

The ideal scalp reconstruction consists of durable, thick, hair-bearing tissue that is properly oriented with respect to hair growth patterns. Furthermore, the reconstructed surface should safely cover potentially exposed skull and/or dura. When considering defects resulting from tumor extirpation, an additional concern is the ability to provide prompt and durable coverage that would allow patients to proceed with adjuvant therapy, such as radiation, if indicated.

Anatomy

Layers

The scalp is a single anatomic unit comprised of five distinct layers. Scalp skin is the thickest in the body and ranges from 3–8 mm as it moves from the forehead to the occiput *(45)*. Just deep to skin is the subcutaneous tissue that contains the nutrient vessels, which supply the scalp, as well as sensory nerves, lymphatics, and fibrous septae, which bind it to the galea (Figure 7.8).

The galea aponeurotica is a strong fibrous layer with extensive attachments. It is a continuation of the SMAS of the face and also joins the frontalis muscle anteriorly, occipitalis posteriorly, and the bilateral temperoparietal fascia. Beneath the galea and superficial to the pericranium is a layer of loose areolar tissue. This thin layer of connective tissue provides scalp mobility. Emissary veins cross through this space and provide a potential route of infection spread to the meninges *(46)*.

Pericranium, or periosteum of the skull, is the innermost layer. This tissue is densely adherent to the skull and contains a very rich blood supply.

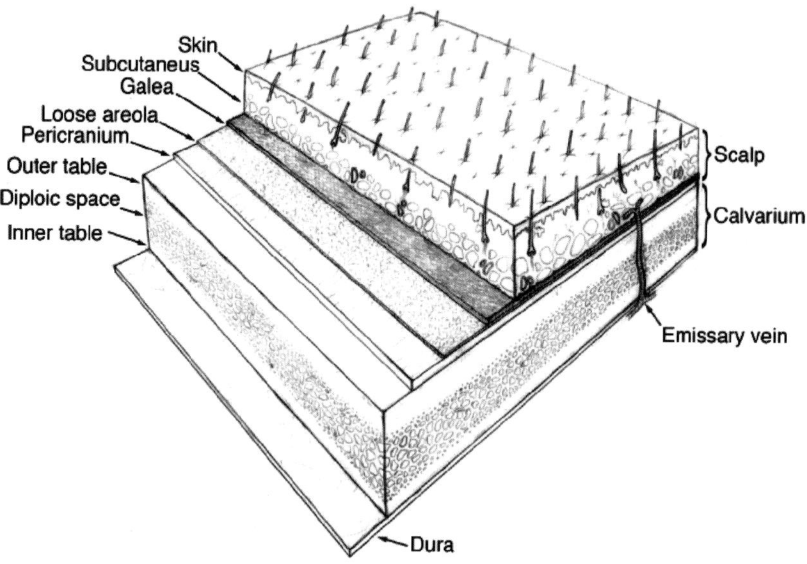

Figure 7.8. Layers of the scalp.

Blood supply

The scalp receives its blood supply from both the internal and external carotid systems. The principle supply originates from the external carotid artery and nourishes the scalp via the bilateral superficial temporal and occipital arteries. Lesser contributions are made form the posterior auricular as well as the supraorbital and supratrochlear branches of the internal carotid. As previously stated, these vessels course throughout the subcutaneous layer and form several anastomotic connections. As such, in cases of scalp avulsion injuries, the entire scalp can often survive on one major vessel.

Innervation

Sensory innervation to scalp has many sources. Anteriorly, the ophthalmic division of the fifth cranial nerve supplies sensation via the supraorbital and supratrochlear branches. Posteriorly, the greater and lesser occipital nerves, which originate from the second and third cervical nerves, provide coverage. The auriculotemporal branch of the maxillary division of the fifth cranial nerve accompanies the superficial temporal artery and innervates the temporal region.

Scalp Neoplasms

Scalp neoplasms occur with similar frequencies and cell origins as other cutaneous head and neck malignancies. Basal cell carcinoma occurs with greatest regularity, followed by squamous cell, melanoma, and other more unusual cutaneous tumors *(47)*.

Evaluation of the Defect

When planning scalp reconstruction, it is important to note not only the size and location but also depth of the defect. Presence or absence of the previously described layers can modify the algorithm and methods of repair. The excision of scalp neoplasms will often require inclusion of periosteum as well as calvarium and or dura mater in the specimen, thus creating complex composite wounds *(48)*. Also, patients who have previously been treated with local radiation therapy may demonstrate compromise of surrounding tissues, which can alter the availability of reconstructive options.

Reconstruction

Primary closure and skin grafting

In general, wounds less than 2–3 cm can be closed primarily, often requiring lateral undermining. Partial scalp defect on almost any size can be covered with skin grafts as long there is a healthy bed of tissue for the graft to lay upon. Robinson demonstrated in 1908 that pericranium alone is a suitable bed for grafting *(49)*. However, skin grafts do not provide very durable or hair-bearing coverage and may have difficulty withstanding post-operative radiation.

In defects where the periosteum has been resected, skin grafting can still be an option after removing the outer table of skull and allowing time for granulation *(50)*. This procedure may risk dural exposure, especially in children.

Even though there may be potential disadvantages, skin grafting is often a desirable option for covering scalp wounds. Frequently, the skin grafted wound can be secondarily reconstructed after contraction, with serial excision or flap coverage.

Local scalp flaps

Local flap coverage by tissue advancement or rearrangement remains the mainstay of treatment for small- to medium-sized defects (3–6 cm) *(51)*. Adjacent tissues can be elevated in a subgaleal plane and rotated, advanced, or transposed into the defect with primary closure or skin grafting of the donor site (Figure 7.9). Careful scoring of the

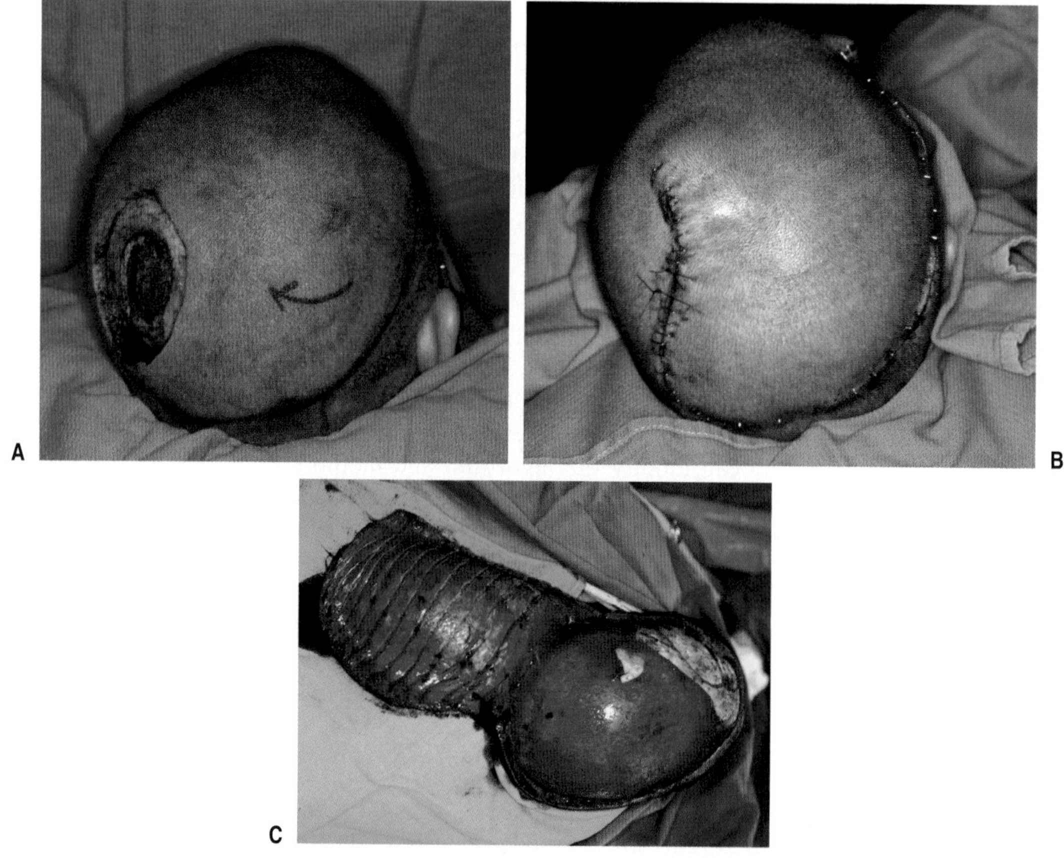

Figure 7.9. **(A)** Defect of scalp vertex following resection of melanoma. **(B)** Scalp flap used to close defect with primary closure of secondary defect. **(C)** Multiple scorings of galea in a different patient allowing for increased flap reach.

galea in a perpendicular plane allows further advancement and expansion of the flap, increasing the coverage area and the ability to close the donor area without a skin graft. If planned accordingly, this will often allow for the mobilization or hair-bearing tissue into the defect.

Some defects require elevation of multiple flaps to provide adequate coverage. This technique was first described and later modified by Ortichochea *(43,52)*. The Ortichochea three-flap technique uses two axial pattern flaps adjacent to the defect for wound closure and a third larger flap to close the donor site.

An axial pattern flap can also be designed based on the temperoparietal, occipital, or postauricular vessels and rotated to cover defects in many locations. Juri and Juri originally described the temperoparieto-occipital flap for anterior hairline reconstruction *(42)*. This flap is based on posterior branch of the superficial temporal vessels and may require delay procedures to ensure viability.

Tissue expansion can be a useful adjunct to local flap coverage *(53,54)*. Expansion increases the amount of local tissue available for flap coverage with hair-bearing skin. One or multiple tissue expanders are placed along the perimeter of the defect, inflated sufficiently, and then flaps are advanced. This strategy might not be appropriate for cancer defect reconstruction, as durable coverage is needed immediately and prior radiation renders the skin difficult to expand.

Scalp flaps are quite useful for reconstructing a variety of scalp defects, but they do have some potential drawbacks. To begin with, caution must be exercised in raising large flaps of tissue in areas of radiation or in smokers. Donor site defects can be difficult to close with large flaps and may require skin grafting. Furthermore, it remains to be seen if scalp flaps tolerate post-operative radiation without troubling wound problems. Hussussian et al. have presented a series of successful free flap scalp reconstructions and many of them were secondary reconstructions of failed local flaps after radiation *(48)*.

Free flaps

McLean and Bunke first described the free omental flap for scalp reconstruction in 1972 *(44)*. The omentum has largely been abandoned for the latissimus dorsi muscle free flap covered with a split-thickness skin graft (Figure 7.10). There are several other reports of successfully free flap reconstruction of scalp defects *(55–60)*. Other donor sites have been described including: rectus abdominus, serratus anterior, scapular, and radial forearm. This technique allows durable, well-vascularized tissue that has been shown to tolerate therapeutic doses of radiation to be transferred into the recipient site *(61–63)*. Variable donor sites allow the surgeon to plan a reconstruction with combinations of skin, muscle, fascia, and bone as determined by the defect. This does not provide hair-bearing skin and may be an aesthetically inferior reconstruction. Proponents would argue that this is far outweighed by the reliability and durability of these flaps *(48)*.

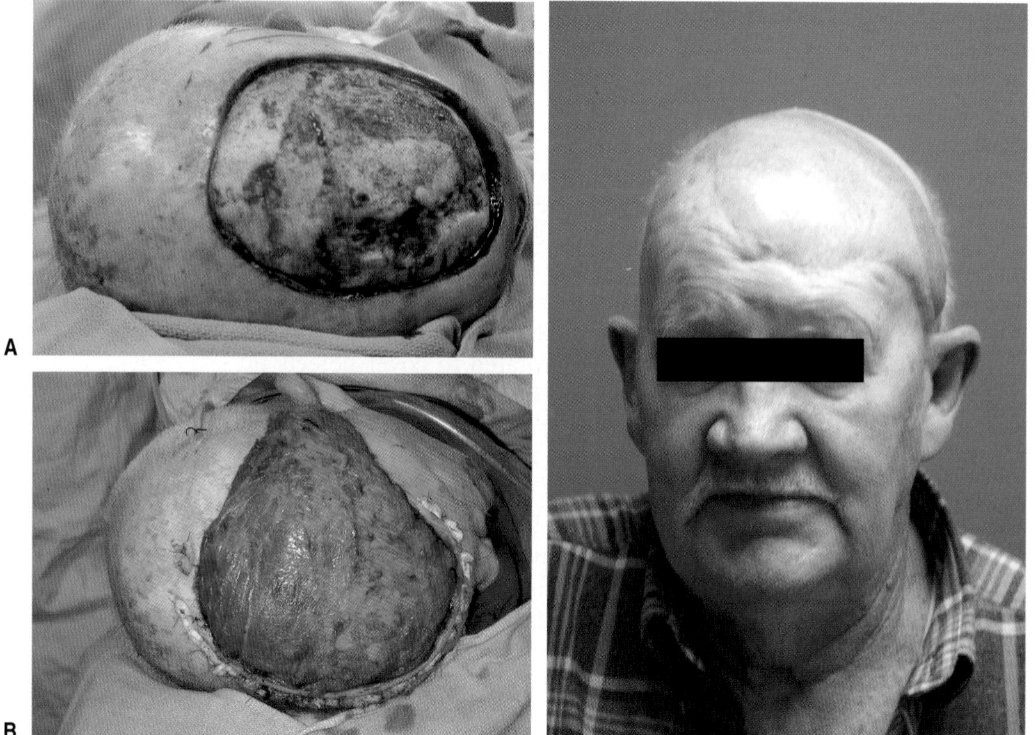

Figure 7.10. **(A)** Large defect of scalp with exposed cranium following unstable skin grafting and irradiation. **(B)** Intraoperative view of latissimus dorsi free flap transfer with microsurgical anastomoses to superficial temporal vessels, prior to application of split-thickness grafting. **(C)** Post-operative view at 1 year, demonstrating substantial flap atrophy and durable scalp coverage.

Calvarial defects

Tumor resection can often leave patients with calvarial defects in addition to the overlying soft tissue. This frequently warrants reconstruction to restore contour and protect the underlying intracranial contents. Autogenous bone grafting is the gold standard and material of choice for most plastic surgeons *(64)*. Donor site morbidity and post-operative resorption are the main drawbacks to selecting an autogenous reconstruction. The advantages include: resistance to infection, strength of the repair, and the ability of the graft to grow with the patient, especially in children. In cases of free tissue reconstruction, a composite flap with a bony segment can be selected to repair the entire defect. Conversely, bone grafting using split rib or calvarial bone grafts with soft-tissue coverage can be attempted.

Another alternative would be to use an alloplastic material to repair the bony defect. The two most commonly selected material are polymethylmethacrylate and hydroxyapatite cement *(65)*. Although these both spare the additional donor site, they increase the potential for problems with post-operative infection and material exposure. Perhaps with new innovations in tissue engineering, materials will soon be available that combine the advantages of both autologous and prosthetic repairs.

References

1. Hessler F. Commentarii et Annotationes in Susrutae Ayurvedam Enlager. Enke 1855;12.
2. Gillies HD. *Plastic surgery of the face.* London: Hodder & Stoughton; 1920.
3. Karapandzic M. Reconstruction of lip defects by local arterial flap. Br J Plast Surg 1974;27:93.
4. Burget GC, Menick FJ. The subunit principle in nasal reconstruction. Plast Reconstr Surg 1985;76:239.
5. Coppit GL, Lin DT, Burkey BB. Current concepts in lip reconstruction. Curr Opin Otolaryngol Head Neck Surg 2004;12(4):282–287.
6. Zide BM. Deformities of the lips and cheeks. In: McCarthy JG (ed.), *Plastic surgery, volume three.* Philadelphia: W.B. Saunders; 1990:2009–2056.
7. Zide BM, Stile FL. Reconstructive surgery of the lips. In: Aston SJ, Beasley RW, Thorne CHM, Grabb WC, Smith JW (eds.), *Grabb and Smith's plastic surgery, fifth edition.* Philadelphia: Lippincott-Raven; 1997:483–500.
8. Spira M, Stal S. V-Y advancement of a subcutaneous pedicle in vermillion lip reconstruction. Plast Reconstr Surg 1983;72:562.
9. Webster RC, Coffey RJ, Kelleher RE. Total and partial reconstruction of the lower lip with innervated muscle-bearing flaps. Plast Reconstr Surg 1960;25:360–371.
10. Calhoun KH. Reconstruction of small- and medium-sized defects of the lower lip. Am J Otolaryngol 1992;13:16–22.
11. Langstein HN, Robb GL. Reconstruction for extensive defects of the lip. Oper Tech Otolaryngol 2005;16(1):2–9.
12. Williams EF III, Setzen G, Mulvaney MJ. Modified Bernard-Burrow cheek advancement and cross-lip flap for total lip reconstruction. Arch Otolaryngol Head Neck Surg 1996;122:1253–1258.
13. Wechselberger G, Gurunluoglu R, Bauer T, et al. Functional lower lip reconstruction with bilateral cheek advancement flaps: revisitation of Webster method with a minor modification in the technique. Aesthetic Plast Surg 2002;26:423–428.
14. Yih WY, Howerton DW. A regional approach to reconstruction of the upper-lip. J Oral Maxillofac Surg 1997;55:383–389.
15. Sadove RC, Luce EA, McGrath PC. Reconstruction of the lower lip and chin with the composite radial forearm-palmaris longus free flap. Plast Reconstr Surg 1991;88:209–214.
16. Takada K, Sugata T, Yoshiga K, et al. Total upper lip reconstruction using a free radial forearm flap incorporating the brachioradialis muscle: report of a case. J Oral Maxillofac Surg 1987;45:959–962.
17. Ozdemir R, Ortak T, Kocer U, et al. Total lower lip reconstruction using sensate composite radial forearm flap. J Craniofac Surg 2003;14:393–405.
18. Menick F. Reconstruction of the cheek. Plast Reconstr Surg 2001;108(2):496–505.
19. Feldman J. Reconstruction of the burned face in children. In: Serafin D, Georgiade NG (eds.), *Pediatric plastic surgery.* St. Louis: Mosby; 1984.

20. Koch J, Hanasono M. Aesthetic facial analysis. In: Papel I (ed.), *Facial plastic and reconstructive surgery, second edition*. New York: Thieme; 2002: 135–144.
21. Zide BM. Deformities of the lips and cheeks. In: McCarthy JG (ed.), *Plastic surgery*. Philadelphia: Saunders; 1990:2009–2056.
22. Cabrera R, Zide BM. Cheek reconstruction. In: Aston SJ, Beasley RW, Thorne CH (eds.), *Grabb and Smith's plastic surgery*. Philadelphia: Lippincott-Raven; 1997:501–512.
23. Moore KL, Agur AM. Head. *Essential clinical anatomy*. Baltimore: Williams and Wilkins; 1995:342–408.
24. Kroll S. Reconstruction for large cheek defects. Oper Tech Plast Reconstr Surg 1998;5(1):37–49.
25. Roth DA, Longaker MT, Zide BM. Cheek surface reconstruction: best choices according to zones. Oper Tech Plast Reconstr Surg 1998;5(1):26–36.
26. Quaba AA, Sommerland BC. "A square peg into a round hole": a modified rhomboid flap and its clinical applications. Br J Plast Surg 1897;40:163.
27. Juri J, Juri C. Advancement and rotation of a large cervicofacial flap for cheek repairs. Plast Reconstr Surg 1979;64:692.
28. Juri J, Juri C. Cheek reconstruction with advancement-rotation flaps. Clin Plast Surg 1981;8:223.
29. Crow ML, Crow FJ. Resurfacing large cheek defects with rotation flaps from the neck. Plast Reconstr Surg 1976;58:196.
30. Becker DW. A cervicopectoral rotation flap for cheek coverage. Plast Reconstr Surg 1978;61:868.
31. Shestak KC, Roth AG, Jones NF, et al. The cervicopectoral rotation flap: a valuable technique for facial reconstruction. Br J Plast Surg 1993;46:375.
32. Kroll SS, Reece GP, Robb G, et al. Deep-plane cervicofacial rotation advancement flap for reconstruction of large cheek defects. Plast Reconstr Surg 1994;94:88.
33. Kaplan I, Goldwyn RM. The versatility of the laterally based cervicofacial flap for cheek repairs. Plast Reconstr Surg 1978;61:390.
34. Stark RB, Kaplan JM. Rotation flaps, neck to cheek. Plast Reconstr Surg 1972;50:230.
35. Garrett WS, Giblin TR, Hoffman GW. Closure of skin defects of the face and neck by rotation and advancement of cervicopectoral flaps. Plast Reconstr Surg 1966;38:342.
36. Bakamjian VY, Long M, Rigg B. Experience with the medially based deltopectoral flap in reconstructive surgery of the head and neck. Br J Plast Surg 1971;24:174.
37. Ariyan S. The pectoralis major myocutaneous flap, a versatile flap for reconstruction in the head and neck. Plast Reconstr Surg 1979;63: 73.
38. Panje W, Cutting C. Trapezius osteomyocutaneous island flap for reconstruction of the anterior floor of mouth and mandible. Head Neck Surg 1980; 3:66.
39. Kroll SS, Reece GP, Schusterman MA, et al. Comaprison of the rectus abdominus free flap to the pectoralis major myocutaneous flap for reconstruction in the head and neck. Am J Surg 1992;164:615.
40. Schusterman MA, Kroll SS, Weber RS, et al. Intraoral soft tissue reconstruction after cancer ablation: a comparison of the pectoralis major flap amd the free radial forearm flap. Am J Surg 1991;162:397–399.

41. Netolizky J. Zur Kasuistik der Hauttransplantation. Wien Med Wochenschr 1871;21:820.
42. Juri J, Juri C. Aesthetic aspects of reconstructive scalp surgery. Clin Plast Surg 1981;8:243.
43. Ortichochea M. Four-flap scalp reconstruction technique. Br J Plast Surg 1967;20:159.
44. McLean DH, Buncke HJ Jr. Autotransplatation of omentum to a large scalp defect with microsurgical revascularization. Plast Reconstr Surg 1972;49: 268.
45. Reed O, Argenta LC. The surgical repair of traumatic defects of the scalp. Clin Plast Surg 1982;9:131.
46. Cutting CB, Mcarthy JG, Bernstein A. Blood supply of the upper craniofacial skeleton: the search for composite calvarial bone flaps. Plast Reconstr Surg 1984;74:603.
47. Minor LB, Panje WR. Malignant neoplasms of the scalp. Etiology, resection, and reconstruction. Otolaryngol Clin North Am 1993;26(2): 279–293.
48. Hussussian CJ, Reece GP. Microsurgical reconstruction in patients with cancer. Plast Reconstr Surg 2002;109(6):1828.
49. Robinson EF. Total avulsion of the scalp. Surg Gynecol Obstet 1908;7: 663.
50. Stuzin JM, Zide BM. *Grabb and Smith's plastic surgery, fourth edition.* Boston: Little, Brown; 1991:401.
51. Wackym PA, Feurman T, Stasnick B, et al. Reconstruction of massive defects of the scalp, cranium, and dura, after resection of scalp neoplasms. Head Neck 1990;12:247.
52. Ortichochea M. New three-flap scalp reconstruction technique. Br J Plast Surg 1971;24:184.
53. Nordstrom RE, Devine JW. Scalp stretching with a tissue expander for closure of scalp defects. Plast Reconstr Surg 1985;75:578.
54. Wieslander JB. Repeated tissue expansion in reconstruction of a huge combined scalp-forehead avulsion injury. Ann Plast Surg 1988;20: 381.
55. Pennington DG, Stern HS, Lee KK. Free-flap reconstruction of large defects of the scalp and calvarium. Plast Reconstr Surg 1989;83:655.
56. Earley MJ, Green MF, Milling MA. A critical appraisal of the use of free flaps in primary reconstruction of combined scalp and calvarial cancer defects. Br J Plast Surg 1990;43:283.
57. Furnas H, Lineaweaver WC, Alpert BS, et al. Scalp reconstruction by microvascular free tissue transfer. Ann Plast Surg 1990;24:431.
58. Borah GL, Hidalgo DA, Wey PD. Reconstruction of extensive scalp defects with rectus free flaps. Ann Plast Surg 1995;34:281.
59. Lutz BS, Wei FC, Chen HC, et al. Reconstruction of scalp defects with free flaps in 30 cases. Br J Plast Surg 1998;51:186.
60. Lee B, Bickel K, Levin S. Microsurgical reconstruction of extensive scalp defects. J Reconstr Microsurg 1999;15:255.
61. Foote RL, Olsen KD, Meland NB, et al. Tumor-ablative surgery, microvascular free tissue transfer reconstruction, and postoperative radiation therapy for advanced head and neck cancer. Mayo Clin Proc 1994; 69:122.
62. Evans GR, Black JJ, Robb GL, et al. Adjuvant therapy: the effects on microvascular lower extremity reconstruction. Ann Plast Surg 1997; 39:141.

63. Zimmerman RP, Mark RJ, Kim AI, et al. Radiation tolerance of transverse rectus abdominis myocutaneous-free flaps used in immediate breast reconstruction. Am J Clin Oncol 1998;21:381.
64. McCarthy JG, Zide BM. The spectrum of calvarial bone grafting: introduction of the vascularized calvarial bone flap. Plast Reconstr Surg 1984;71:10.
65. Moreira-Gonzalez A, Jackson IT, Miyawaki T, et al. Clinical outcome in cranioplasty: critical review in long-term follow-up. J Craniofac Surg 2003;14(2):144–153.

8

Reconstruction of Mandible, Maxilla, and Skull Base

Peter C. Neligan and Joan E. Lipa

Head and neck reconstruction in patients with cancer presents unique challenges to the reconstructive surgeon. Because of its visibility, defects of any kind in the head and neck area are difficult to hide and the demands on our reconstructive skills are greater than they are elsewhere in the body, where cosmesis may be less vital and function less specialized. If life expectancy is limited, return to optimal quality of life as quickly as possible is of paramount importance.

The head and neck area includes both static and dynamic structures, as well as organs of special function. Whereas bony structures elsewhere in the body are related to structure and load, the bony skeleton of the head and neck area includes these functions but, in addition, includes the jaws, which have a very specialized function and unique reconstructive requirements. Reconstruction attempts to replicate tissue that has been resected in both form and function. The craniofacial skeleton fulfills several functions. It is responsible for the contour of the head and face. As well, it provides protection to vital structures, most notably the brain. Finally, the skeletal structures of the upper and lower jaws provide a very specialized functional role, that of mastication, which is unique in the body. The soft tissues of the face are also unique. They comprise external cover and translate emotions, and mucosal elements provide speech and assistance with mastication. Not infrequently, all of these elements have to be replaced. There are basic principles that guide us: (1) wherever possible, replace excised tissue with like tissue. This generally means local tissue and although this is not always available, we should, whenever possible, use it. Local tissue provides the best match both cosmetically and functionally. (2) Reconstruction should not interfere with treatment of the patient's main condition. If, for example the patient requires some sort of adjuvant therapy, we should ensure that our reconstructive choice would have healed satisfactorily in order not to delay that process. (3) Although the simplest treatment is not necessarily the best, an option that has a reasonable chance to succeed should be chosen. Technical feasibility alone is not an indication for any procedure.

Mandible

Introduction

Mandibular reconstruction has evolved since the 1980s to become a very reliable, though complex, procedure with the inception of microsurgical techniques, advanced plating systems, and the incorporation of reliable flaps for reconstruction. Furthermore, the concept of maintaining quality of life is paramount in the management of patients with cancer. Thus, even patients with a very limited life expectancy and extensive disease, so long as they are medically fit to tolerate a long operation, are routinely reconstructed if it is expected that their quality of remaining life would be significantly enhanced *(1)*.

The most common pathology in head and neck cancer that requires mandibular resection and reconstruction is squamous cell carcinoma (SCC) of oral mucosal origin. As such, the mandible is usually not reconstructed in isolation, but rather it is the major component of an ablation that includes the floor of mouth, parts of the tongue, and possibly external skin. The principles of oropharyngeal reconstruction are covered separately elsewhere, but it is important to note that this is a rather hostile environment for wound healing. It also follows that oropharyngeal SCCs involving the mandible are stage T4 tumors and will generally require adjuvant radiation therapy, making reconstruction with vascularized tissue essential. Therefore, non-vascularized bone grafts and osteoinductive compounds containing bone morphogenic protein-7 *(2)*, although encouraging in their use for smaller and often benign defects, are usually not appropriate in this setting. There may be a role in the future for tissue-engineered vascularized constructs *(3)*, but with our present level of expertise this is not our mainstay of treatment. At present, osseocutaneous free flaps contoured and secured with reconstructive titanium plates continue to be our foundation for mandibular reconstruction.

Classification of Mandibular Defects

The most elegant and clinically useful means of classifying mandibular defects as they relate to cancer resection and principles of reconstruction has been described by Boyd et al. *(4)*, as depicted in Figure 8.1. It is an evolution of the HCL method *(5)* and combines not only the location of the bony defect (H, C, L) but also the tissues that are missing and in need of reconstruction (o, m, s). H defects include lateral defects including the condyle but not significantly crossing the midline; L defects are the same only without the condyle; and C defects consist of the entire central segment containing the four incisors and the two canines. The letter o refers to a bony or osseous defect only (i.e., with neither a skin nor mucosal component); s refers to an accompanying skin defect and m denotes mucosal resection. Any defect for reconstruction can be described in terms of this combination of upper and lower case letters. For example, an angle-to-angle defect with floor of mouth resection would be denoted as LCLm. However, it is important to realize that

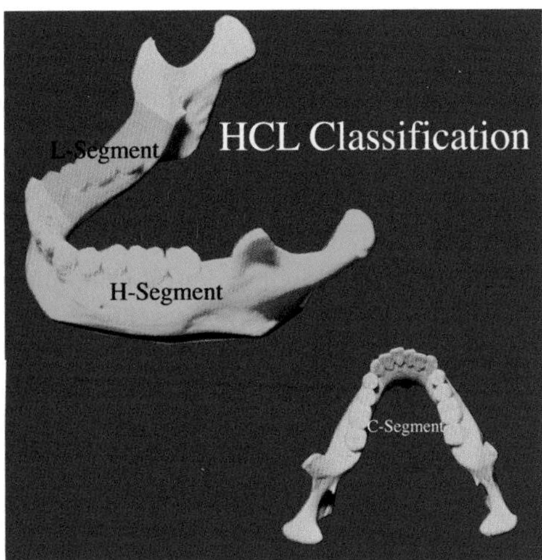

Figure 8.1. HCL classification of mandibular defects. H-segment defects include the condyle and can comprise the hemimandible, without crossing the midline; C-segment defects include the central mandible (four incisiors and two canines); and L-segment defects involve the lateral mandible without the condyle.

there is no one reconstruction that perfectly suits a described defect for all patients, and the reconstruction must be tailored taking into account all patient factors.

The cornerstone of the Boyd classification is the recognition of the significance of the C defect with respect to reconstruction. Whereas many modalities such as soft tissue alone or reconstruction plate alone can be used to reconstruct lateral or posterior defects, it is obligatory to use bone to reconstruct the C defect. This is as a result of detachment of the insertions of the mandibular retractors, the geniohyoids and digastrics that act unopposed on the soft tissues inferiorly and allow the mandibular reconstruction to ride upwards. The detached soft tissues also become ptotic and lower facial nerve damage may lead to poor oral sphincter tone. Any floor of mouth dead space that is not reconstructed may also contribute to contracture. It is, therefore, of utmost importance to attempt to normalize the positions of the soft tissues and re-suspend them to the mandibular reconstruction to avoid soft-tissue ptosis. A plate-only reconstruction placed in a C defect will be prone to exposure within the oral cavity *(6)*, also as a result of altered soft tissue mechanics.

Principles of Reconstruction

The goals of mandibular reconstruction are centered on restoring function (speech, deglutition, mastication, oral hygiene, airway maintenance) and cosmesis (soft-tissue support, contour) in single-stage surgery that will allow primary healing, rapid rehabilitation, and progression to adjuvant therapies, when indicated, without delay. A multi-disciplinary approach is necessary and pre-operative assessment should include adequate imaging, staging, and medical evaluation of fitness for surgery.

Because the most common defects in mandibular reconstruction involve an "m," or floor of mouth/tongue component *(7,8)*, it is also important to recognize that principles of reconstruction specific to this component must also be followed: avoidance of tongue tethering, avoidance of flap redundancy with subsequent "pocketing" of food, and thin soft-tissue coverage over the alveolus to allow for dental rehabilitation *(9)*.

Most patients undergoing mandibular resection for cancer ablation will require a temporary tracheostomy and nasogastric enteral feeding. These factors, in addition to the need for flap monitoring by trained personnel make these patients labor-intensive for post-operative nursing care.

For optimal post-operative dental rehabilitation, the occlusal relations of the maxillary and mandibular dentition must be maintained. Maxillo-mandibular fixation (MMF) with archbars is inadequate, not only because these patients are often edentulous, but more importantly because MMF does not control for rotation of a residual posterior non-tooth-bearing segment. Instead, the resected mandible is replaced with a replica of what has been removed in the form of template made prior to disruption of the mandible. There are several ways in which this can be done. The simplest method is to apply the reconstruction plate that will ultimately be used for fixation to the mandible before resection, with pre-drilling of at least three screws into remaining native mandible to ensure proper subsequent spatial orientation of the reconstruction plate. This ensures that when the plate is replaced with the reconstruction for which it serves as a template, the remaining elements of the mandible will be in exactly the same relative position as they were pre-operatively. Thus, optimal occlusion as well as undisturbed temporomandibular joint (TMJ) dynamics can be assured. The plate is therefore applied to the mandible, the holes are drilled and screws applied. The plate is then removed and used as a template for shaping the bony reconstruction, whichever flap is chosen for that purpose.

When the outer cortex of the mandible is involved, this pre-plating technique cannot be used as the reconstruction plate cannot be applied to the mandible prior to resection. Instead, the mandibular elements can be stabilized prior to resection of the bone by applying a bridging bar to the mandible, as shown in Figure 8.2. Once the mandible has been resected, the reconstruction plate can be bent to the shape of the mandible knowing that the remaining elements are once again held in the same relative position as pre-operatively, again maintaining occlusion and TMJ dynamics. Another elegant approach is to fashion a three-dimensional model of the mandible from pre-operative computed tomography (CT) scans. In particular, when the lesion does not cross the midline, the CT image can be reversed to provide a mirror-image of the uninvolved portion of mandible, the reconstruction plate can be shaped according to the model, sterilized, and then used as a template in the operating room to fashion a mandibular reconstruction with excellent symmetry to the uninvolved side with normal occlusion (*see* Figure 8.3).

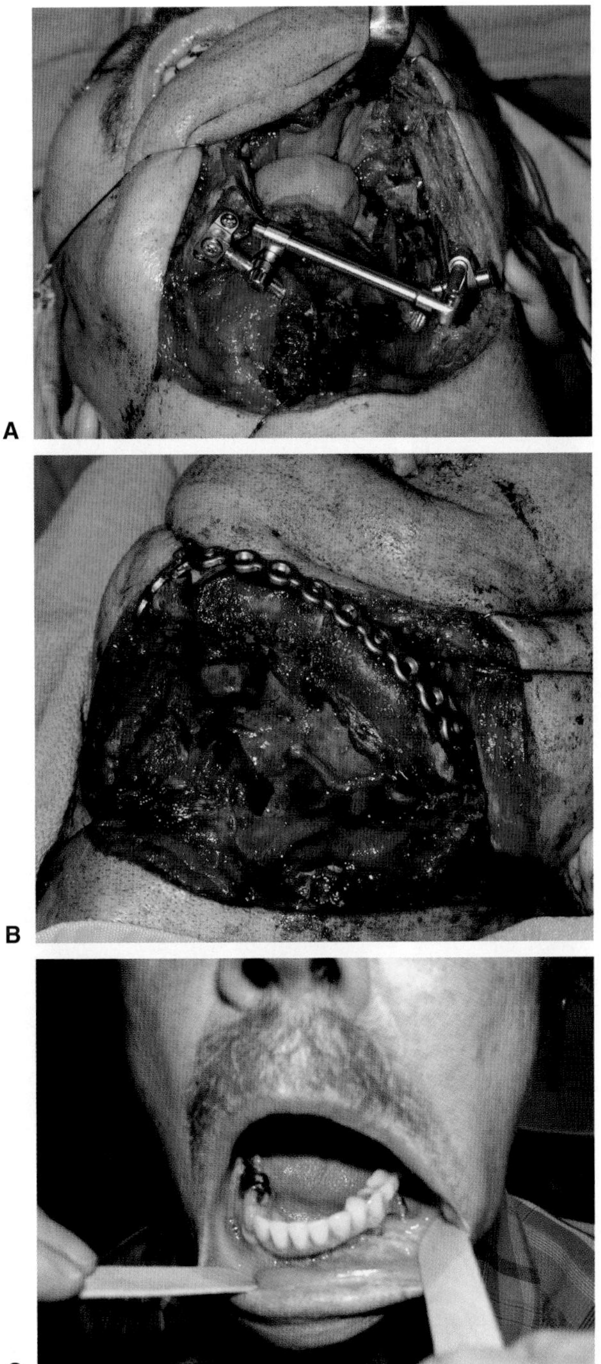

Figure 8.2. Reconstruction of a CL*o* mandibular defect. **(A)** Bridging bar applied prior to mandibular resection to stabilize remaining mandibular elements and preserve occlusal relationships. **(B)** Reconstruction plate for fixation of free fibular flap reconstruction. **(C)** Dental rehabilitation with osseointegrated dentures following free fibular flap mandibular reconstruction.

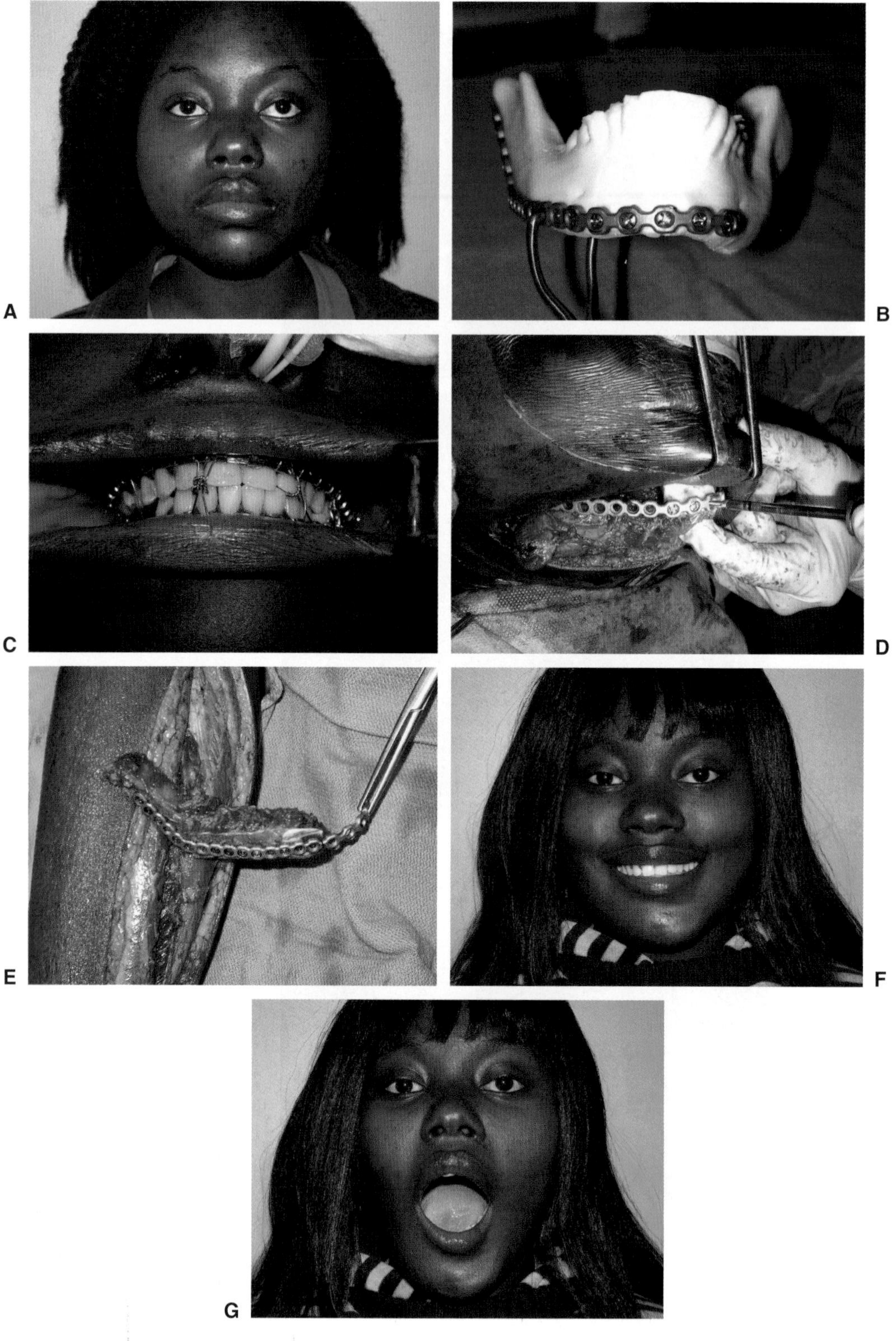
A
B
C
D
E
F
G

Shaping of the bone to the reconstruction plate can be time consuming with multiple osteotomies, so that ischemia time can be reduced by osteotomizing the flap *in situ* at the donor site and before the native blood supply is divided. Closing wedge osteotomies are preferable to opening wedge osteotomies in order to maintain maximal vascularized bone contact and avoid the need for bone grafts to fill in opening wedge osteotomy sites. Minimal periosteal stripping is carried out to avoid disruption of the periosteal blood supply to the flap. Unicortical fixation may also preserve maximal vascularity, and newer locking reconstruction plates avoid compression of the plate against the periosteum and theoretically are advantageous *(10)*.

Choice of Reconstruction

Although the high success rate of head and neck reconstructive procedures has allowed for significant improvement in both functional and aesthetic results, the ideal tissue for mandibular reconstruction does not exist. What we seek is a combination of the best bone stock with the best skin paddle combined in a package that produces least morbidity at both donor and recipient sites. The price paid for reconstruction is measured in terms of donor site morbidity, functional loss, and days of life lost. This latter concept was introduced by Boyd et al. in 1995 and is a valid one *(6)*. Given that the overall prognosis for many of these patients is limited, we must be sure that whatever intervention is performed is likely to succeed without complication. It follows that these technically demanding reconstructions should be performed only by those surgeons with a critical volume in microsurgical head and neck reconstruction to maintain excellence.

The choice of reconstruction depends on the post-ablative defect, prognosis, patient comorbidities, donor site availability and morbidity, and availability of recipient vessels. Although microsurgery has revolutionized mandibular reconstruction, there is still also a place for more traditional techniques, as alluded to earlier. Smaller bone defects (<4 cm in length) in well-vascularized, non-irradiated beds with good soft-tissue coverage can sometimes be reconstructed with non-vascularized bone grafts. Tissue engineering constructs may also play a role in this setting.

Figure 8.3. Reconstruction of an H mandibular defect. **(A)** Pre-operative appearance demonstrating expansile tumor of right mandible. **(B)** A mirror-image three-dimensional model has been constructed from CT images for pre-operative resection planning and bending of reconstruction plate. The pre-bent reconstruction plate can then be sterilized for intraoperative placement. **(C)** Placement of patient in MMF prior to resection. Elastic traction will be used post-operatively to facilitate maintenance of position of the condylar reconstruction, and it will facilitate early motion to prevent ankylosis. **(D)** Pre-bent plate is seated on the remaining central mandible and drill holes for this portion are placed. **(E)** Application of reconstruction plate to osteotomized fibular flap *in situ* to decrease ischemia time. Note that the periosteal sleeve condylar reconstruction has been created at the proximal end of the fibula flap, and a silk suture marks the location on the plate that corresponds to where it will be placed on the remaining cut surface of the central mandible. **(F)** Post-operative occlusion and mandibular contour. **(G)** Postoperative mandibular excursion is free of deviation with good interincisal opening.

Reconstruction plates, with or without additional soft tissue pedicled or free flaps, have been relegated to L defects in patients with poor prognosis (6). Complications of plate fracture and exposure still exist even in these patients *(11–13)*. It may even be acceptable not to reconstruct the bony defect in a small subset of patients, but instead to carry out a soft-tissue-only reconstruction. This has been advocated using either a rectus abdominis free flap *(14)* or pedicled pectoralis major myocutaneous flap *(15)*, usually in posterior defects. It can be particularly useful in cases of osteoradionecrosis with TMJ dysfunction with poor mouth opening, but in dentate patients occlusal shift is unpredictable and may be fraught with long-term functional and aesthetic impairment. Osteocutaneous free tissue transfer usually leads to improved outcome with decreased overall cost of care when compared with soft-tissue-only or plate and flap reconstructions *(15)*. As previously noted, the absolute indication for vascularized bony mandibular reconstruction in an otherwise relatively healthy patient is that of the central anterior mandibular defect.

Although rib *(16–18)*, metatarsal bone *(19,20)*, humerus *(21)*, and clavicle *(22,23)* have all been used in mandibular repair, the most widely used current donor sites include the fibula *(24–26)*, iliac crest *(27,28)*, scapula *(29–31)*, and radius *(32)*. Of these the fibula is by far the most popular and versatile.

Fibular osseocutaneous free flap

The fibula can provide up to 25 cm of uniform shaped bicortical bone. It can tolerate multiple osteotomies because of its profuse periosteal blood supply, and it does not need to have its nutrient artery preserved to maintain viability. The bone stock is adequate to support osseointegrated implants; however, the height of the neomandible is limited relative to that of the native dentate mandible. The skin island, based on the septocutaneous blood supply, is adequate in size and reliable in more than 90% of patients *(33)*. The skin has the potential for innervation, but its quality is intermediate in thickness and pliability and therefore ranks behind that of the radial forearm flap. The vascular pedicle is adequate in length and can be effectively lengthened by dissecting it off the proximal fibula. The flap can include portions of the flexor hallucis longus and/or soleus muscle to provide soft-tissue bulk where needed. Donor leg morbidity with or without skin grafting following fibula free flap harvest is minimal *(34,35)*. Routine angiography is not necessary, provided that clinical vascular examination of the extremity is normal *(36)*. However, patients with severe peripheral vascular disease or varicose veins are not ideal candidate for free fibula flap transfer and consideration for an alternate donor site should be made.

Iliac crest osseocutaneous flap

The ilium, based on the deep circumflex iliac artery (DCIA) and vein has a natural curvature not unlike that of the mandible. A total of 14–16 cm of bone can be harvested by extending the resection posteriorly to the sacro-iliac joint. This bone can be contoured to reconstruct the anterior mandibular arch with osteotomies through the outer cortex and it is well suited for placement of osseointegrated implants. The blood supply of the skin paddle of the osseocutaneous flap comes from an array of perforators that are located in a zone along the medial aspect of the iliac crest. It is important when insetting the skin paddle to maintain the relationship of skin to bone so as not to torque these perforators. Furthermore, the skin can be bulky and is not particularly pliable so it is usually less than the optimal choice for intra-oral reconstruction. Donor site morbidity can also be substantial. Patients are frequently slow to mobilize because of pain on walking. Moreover, abdominal wall weakness, frank herniation, and occasional gait disturbances can occur *(37)*. The donor defect of the DCIA can be minimized by splitting the ilium and taking only the inner table of the bone with the flap. In this manner, the crest itself is left and the abdominal repair is much more secure. Holes are drilled in the remaining crest to which the three layers of abdominal musculature are attached. Moreover, the muscles on the lateral side of the crest are undisturbed, further minimizing donor morbidity. Finally, the cosmetic defect of this maneuver is significantly less than when the traditional flap is used *(38)*. The iliac crest harvested with the internal oblique muscle is an alternative to using a skin paddle. The internal oblique can be used for intra-oral lining and be allowed to mucosalize. It is far less bulky than the DCIA skin paddle, and the amount of muscle harvested with the bone can be generous. This technique has found further application in the reconstruction of the maxillectomy defect, as will be discussed later in this chapter.

Scapular osseocutaneous flap

Based on the circumflex scapular artery, this flap has the advantage of providing an extensive expanse of skin as well as bone. Furthermore, the skin can be taken as separate skin paddles, a scapular as well as a parascapular flap based on the transverse and descending branches of the circumflex scapular artery, respectively. The bony perforators, which are direct short branches from the circumflex scapular artery, supply the lateral border of the scapula and provide approximately 8 cm of good bone stock. Medial scapula can also be harvested with this flap *(39)*, but harvesting lateral bone is more usual. Because of the anatomical characteristics of the vascular pedicle, the various elements of this flap (two skin paddles and bone) can all be manipulated independently of one another, as there is sufficient vascular length to facilitate this. This makes it very versatile for reconstructing complex three-dimensional defects. However, it has the disadvantage that the patient has to be turned in order to harvest this flap. Furthermore, although the bone stock is excellent it cannot safely be osteotomized. This limits its utility for larger bony defects. A further modification of the scapular osseocutaneous flap is to harvest the tip of the scapula. This provides an expanse of thin bone that can ideally be used to reconstruct midface defects such as those of the maxilla and the orbital floor *(40,41)*. The bone is supplied by an angular branch from the circumflex scapular artery.

Radial forearm osseocutaneous flap

The radial forearm flap provides probably the best-quality skin for intra-oral reconstruction. It is soft, thin, pliable, and can be harvested with the lateral antebrachial cutaneous nerve, making it an innervated flap by microneural connection to a recipient sensory nerve. The quality of this re-innervation has been well documented *(42)*. The radius itself provides a thin strip of bone that nevertheless is very strong and despite its size can tolerate osseointegrated dental implants *(32)*. When harvesting the bone, it is important to limit this harvest to approximately 30% of the circumference of the radius and to shape this harvest in the shape of a keel to minimize the risk of fracture of the residual radius. Despite these precautions, the incidence of fracture is reported as 15% (8), which is very high considering that up to 10% of patients will require a secondary surgical procedure to repair the radius fracture.

Special Considerations

Reconstruction of the condyle

For H defects (those involving the condyle), there is no consensus on condylar reconstruction. Although costochondral grafts are used frequently in the pediatric population in order to incorporate a growth center in the reconstruction *(43)*, this is not a priority for adult patients. Attempts have also be made to line the glenoid fossa with temporalis fascia *(44)* or dermis-fat grafts (45) in order to minimize the significant long-term problems with graft resorption, ankylosis, and reconstructive failure *(46)*. Furthermore, an additional donor site in our cancer patient population is to be avoided, and most ablative defects are not isolated solely to the condyle. These factors have led to strategies to accomplish maintenance of a functional TMJ while avoiding further morbidity.

Initial enthusiasm with condylar prostheses attached to reconstruction plates *(47)* has fallen out of favor because of late problems with heterotopic ossification, resorption of the glenoid fossa, and even erosion through the skull base, necessitating an unacceptably high revision rate *(48)*. In the past, condylar prostheses had been advocated by some on a temporary basis, until a definitive reconstruction could be carried out *(12)*, but this goes against the principle of one-stage reconstruction for our patients and should not be considered in our era of access to microvascular expertise.

Autotransplantation of the condyle can be used in cases where the tumor does not involve the condyle, but where there is insufficient neck and ramus remaining to allow for stable fixation of the remaining condylar segment to a bone graft reconstruction. This was initially described in combination with an iliac crest bone graft *(49)*; however, one could anticipate that the transplanted condyle on a bone graft would not provide the ideal situations for stable union and prevention of resorption. Instead, the avascular condyle can be mounted on the free vascularized bony reconstruction *(50)*. Resorption can still be a problem radiographically, but good functional outcome could still be obtained. Resorption implies that the autotransplanted condyle is merely serving as a spacer.

The authors' preferred reconstruction is to create a vascularized soft-tissue spacer in the form of a rolled periosteal sleeve at the condylar end of the fibula free flap. This is a simple reconstruction using tissue already elevated for reconstruction and avoids non-vascularized tissue. Excellent long-term functional results can be obtained with good occlusion, lack of mandibular deviation on mouth opening, and pain-free interincisal opening through a normal functional range (*see* Figure 8.3).

Dental rehabilitation

For patients undergoing mandibular reconstruction, prosthetic rehabilitation confers a better quality of life compared to those patient who do not go on to have a prosthesis *(51)*. However, it can still be difficult to fit and maintain a prosthesis because of a poor sulcus surrounding the neo-alveolus and xerostomia following radiation therapy *(52)*.

Osseointegrated implants have become the state of the art dental reconstruction *(53)* (*see* Figure 8.2). Although implants can be placed in all vascularized bone transfers, the free fibula bone stock has been shown to reliably allow for successful take of dental implants *(54)*. However, the vertical height of the fibula flap may be insufficient for implant placement and prosthesis fitting (55), and may require augmentation with either vertical distraction, which has been shown to be possible even in irradiated reconstructions *(56)*, or onlay iliac crest bone graft placement *(54)*. Alternatively, a "double-barrel" fibula free flap may be designed at the time of reconstruction in order to augment the vertical height *(57)*. Although implant abutment placement at the time of the fibula flap reconstruction is possible *(58)* and has been advocated for benign conditions *(59)*, the cost of dental implants is substantial and the microvascular reconstruction is already a lengthy operative procedure. One advantage to primary placement of osseointegrated implants is the theoretic advantage of initial healing and integration of the abutment before radiation is started, if needed. Delayed osseointegrated implant reconstruction is a more common practice that allows the patient to have recovered from their surgery, completed adjuvant treatment, and demonstrated disease-free survival. There is controversy as to whether implant survival is higher when placed in native mandible or in a bony free flap, but there is consensus as to the fact that there is a higher chance of failure when placed into irradiated bone, and, although frequently used, hyperbaric oxygen therapy has not been shown to improve outcome in this situation *(52,60)*.

Summary

The choice of reconstruction is determined by the characteristics of the defect. The fibula is the workhorse flap in most situations, as it supplies the greatest length of bone for reconstruction, carries reasonably thin and pliable skin for mucosal or skin coverage, allows for osteotomies to customize shaping, permits future dental rehabilitation with osseointegrated implants, and contributes little donor site morbidity. Although the iliac crest and radius have their proponents, they have, for the most part, been relegated to the position of secondary choice in those patients for whom the fibula, for whatever reason, is not an option. If soft-tissue bulk is a requirement, then the iliac crest may be a better option, and if extensive skin cover is required as, for example, in through-and-through defects then scapula may be a good option. The radial forearm flap, though it has many desirable characteristics, is associated with a high rate of fracture in the residual radius *(8)*.

Maxilla

Introduction

If there is any region in the head and neck where our reconstructive techniques are lacking it is in the maxillary defect. The maxilla is a unique six-sided, tetrahedron-shaped bone that provides support for the orbital contents above, fashions the roof of the mouth below, and the lateral wall of the nasal cavity medially. As well, it contains the maxillary antrum, which plays a significant role in the normal physiologic function of the upper airway. It is covered by skin on the outside, the orbicularis oculi muscle and eyelids superiorly, and mucosa elsewhere. It serves as the origin for many of the facial mimetic muscles.

This diversity of structural components is reflected in the etiology of tumors that affect the maxilla. They may originate from the paranasal sinuses, palate, nasal mucosal, orbital contents, overlying skin, or intra-oral mucosal. Whereas most malignant tumors affecting the mandible are SCCs, histopathology of tumors affecting the maxilla is heterogeneous and also includes osteosarcoma, melanoma, basal cell carcinoma, mucoepidermoid carcinoma, leiomyosarcoma, inverted papilloma, papillary adenocarcinoma, chondrosarcoma, adenoid cystic carcinoma, eccrine carcinoma, and malignant fibrous histiocytoma *(61)*. Malignancies arising from the maxillary sinus may be at an advanced stage at the time of detection. The maxilla is less commonly involved with cancer than the mandible, and thus experience in reconstruction has taken longer to accrue and perfect.

Classification

The techniques used in reconstruction of the maxillary defect have not yet reached the sophistication of state of the art mandibular reconstruction and are still evolving. In many instances we are, in effect, filling a hole. Although the type of reconstruction will obviously depend on the defect, maxillectomy defects remain difficult to classify and several classifications have arisen, driven largely by the need for prosthodontists to fashion obturators for rehabilitation and define outcomes when the palate is involved *(62–66)*. The emphasis on prosthetic reconstruction in the development of a classification system is an indicator that autogenous reconstruction of these defects has been lagging, partially because of the original perception that the ablative site should not be covered in order to allow for disease recurrence surveillance *(67)*. More recently, a classification has been developed by Cordeiro et al. that identifies the requirements of the bony reconstruction *(61)*. This serves as a useful basis for reconstruction, but the oncologic reconstructive surgeon must then take into account adjacent tissues that are affected (external covering, lining, specialized structures such as eye or nose or facial musculature). Other classification systems that take into account the extent of the horizontal and vertical resection have been developed *(68)*, but these are more complex and less likely to be used on a routine basis.

In Cordeiro's classification, there are four types of maxillectomy defects. This system serves as a useful guideline for reconstruction, helping to classify not only the bony defect but also the specific reconstructive goals.

Type I defects are "partial" or "limited" maxillectomies, consisting of anterior and/or medial walls, and may involve the lips, nose, or eyelids. These defects, if they involve the anterior wall, may involve sacrifice of branches of the facial nerve and muscular attachments. Usually skin resurfacing is the main objective of reconstruction, with little need for volume replacement. Static slings or nerve reconstruction may also be considered as needed.

Type II defects are "subtotal" maxillectomies, involving the lower five walls of the maxilla, including the palate but excluding the orbital floor. Contour as well as speech and swallowing are disrupted. The goal is to provide not only contour and volume, but also to recreate palatal separation and prevent velopharyngeal incompetence.

Type III defects are "total" maxillectomy defects (with removal of the orbital floor) and are further subdivided into IIIA defects that spare the orbital contents and IIIB defects that include the orbital contents. Type IIIA defects are the most challenging for the reconstructive surgeon with the main goals being prevention of functional loss of the eye, orbital dystopia, diplopia, enophthalmos, and ectropion. In addition, palatal closure and aesthetic contour may also be necessary.

Type IV defects involve the upper five walls of the maxilla, and may include the orbital contents and have exposed dura or brain. The palate is still intact. This becomes an issue of volume replacement and cranial base reconstruction, which will be covered in the next section.

Reconstructive Options

Reconstructive options will depend on the type of maxillectomy defect described in the previous section, which in turn defines which tissue is missing and goals of reconstruction.

Type I maxillectomies may not need any reconstruction if there is intact native soft-tissue cover. Bone grafts may be placed to maintain anterior projection, but caution should be exercised in cases where radiotherapy will be administered, as bone graft resorption may ensue. Because the anterior maxilla serves as the bony attachment for facial musculature associated with smiling, extensive soft-tissue degloving with loss of bony anchoring points may lead to changes in facial mimetic muscle function, and if muscle is resected then static sling support such as that used in facial paralysis cases may be a consideration. If a soft-tissue defect accompanies the partial maxillectomy defect, then the reconstruction becomes that of cheek resurfacing (possibly with the addition of lip, nose, or eyelid elements). Flaps with minimal bulk are most useful, and color match is important. However, even the scapula free flap may have poor color match. A useful exercise is to choose a flap of appropriate thickness for the defect, and that is logistically able to be raised concurrent with the ablation, such as an anterolateral thigh or radial forearm free flap. At a later date, the pale skin of the free flap can be removed and resurfaced with a scalp split-thickness skin graft that will provide optimal color match to the rest of the face. Of course, the best color match for the midface is local tissue and one must not forget the cheek rotation flap, cervicofacial flap, and the submental flap for coverage of limited areas of the cheek.

Type II ("subtotal") maxillectomies require a reconstruction that will allow for restoration of functional speech and swallowing. A dental obturator (with or without a skin graft placed on the deep surface of the cheek soft tissues) has been the classical treatment for these defects and although it works quite well, its success depends on the fit of the obturator. Patients occasionally may have mucositis or xerostomia with previous radiotherapy and may complain of excessive crustiness in the maxillectomy cavity; hygiene may be problematic. As well, there is a hollowing of the cheek that creates a cosmetic deformity that may or may not be significant but is quite variable and more pronounced when radiotherapy has been administered, as demonstrated in the case shown in Figure 8.4. These defects may also be reconstructed with a flap such as the rectus abdominis. This fills the cavity and can reconstruct the palate nicely; however, it may create difficulties for the prosthetist. Palatal reconstruction using this technique usually involves holding the palatal portion of the flap in position with a dental plate for 6 weeks post-operatively, during which time the muscle mucosalizes. Long-term results are variable because of the unpredictable amount of atrophy, which the muscle undergoes. This is particularly relevant in patients who undergo post-operative radiation. In these patients, muscle atrophy is compounded by fibrosis and contracture of the rectus muscle. Alternatives to this technique include the use of flaps such as the scapula, radial forearm, anterolateral thigh, or rectus abdominis myocutaneous flap with separate skin paddles for palate and lateral nasal wall. Alternatively, the iliac crest with internal oblique can also be used *(69)*, as demonstrated in Figure 8.5. This flap provides both bone, which may later be used as a platform for osseointegrated implants for dental rehabilitation, as well as the bulk of the internal oblique muscle. In this situation the muscle is, again, allowed to mucosalize intra-orally. Because of the bone the effects of muscle atrophy on contour are minimal.

When the soft palate requires reconstruction, thin sensate flaps such as the radial forearm are best suited to this area. Because the flap is not dynamic, however, velopharyngeal competence cannot be achieved unless the flap touches the posterior pharyngeal wall. Urken achieves this by fashioning a pharyngoplasty incorporated within his flap *(66)*. For large defects, and particularly those that include a pharyngeal defect, we have used two flaps in combination to close the defect; a radial forearm flap to provide pharyngeal closure with oral palatal reconstruction and a lateral arm flap anastomosed in sequence to provide nasal pharyngeal closure.

For type IIIA defects, reconstruction of the orbital floor is important if dystopia is to be avoided. This can be achieved with bone grafts such as split calvarial grafts, iliac crest, rib, or with titanium mesh. Using soft-tissue flaps alone to support the globe has proved disappointing, probably because of the subsequent muscle atrophy that has already been

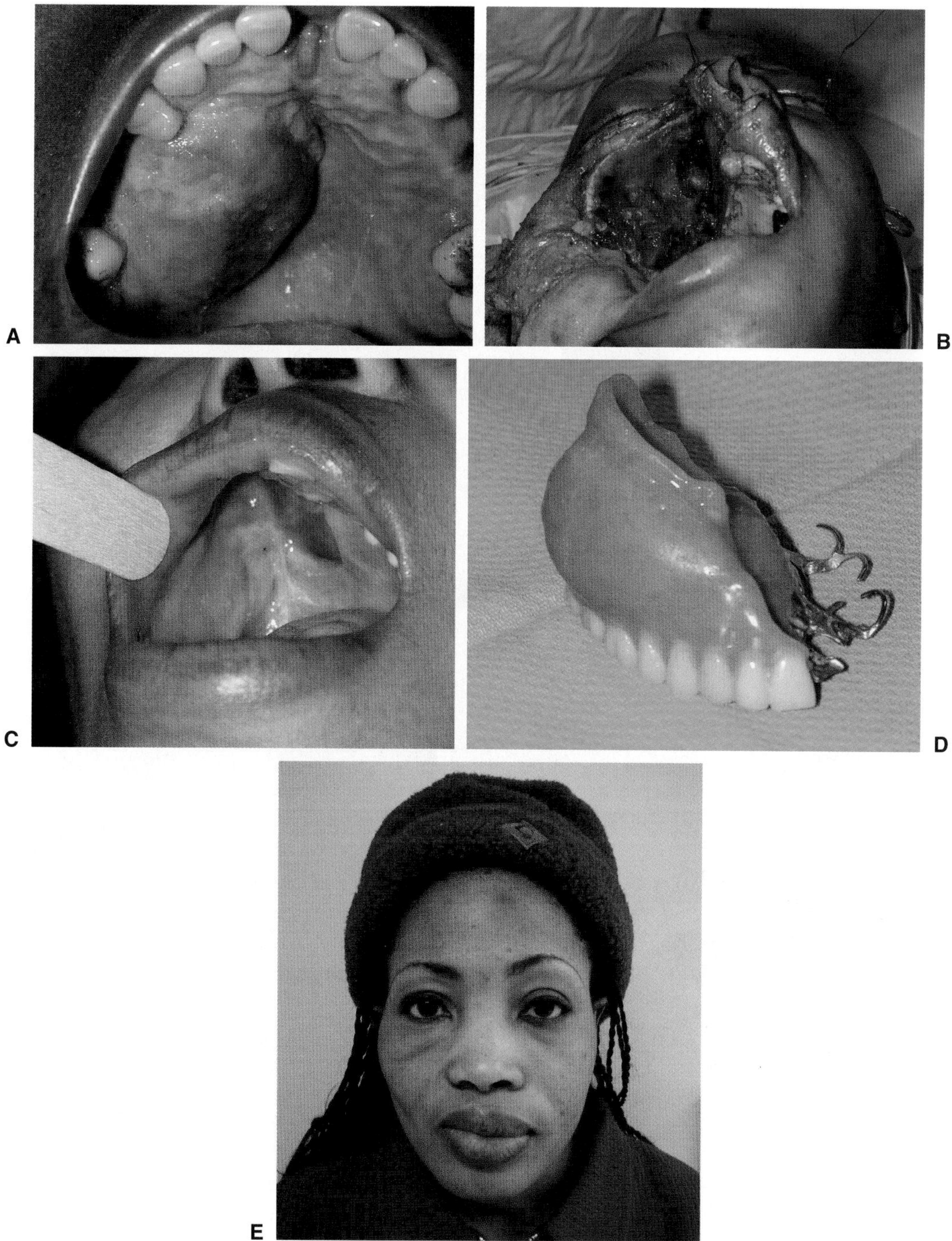

Figure 8.4. Type II maxillectomy defect with obturator reconstruction. **(A)** Tumor involves the right palate and maxillary sinus. **(B)** Resulting defect. **(C)** Mucosalized maxillectomy cavity. **(D)** Obturator reconstruction. **(E)** Post-operative appearance with poor support of cheek soft tissues.

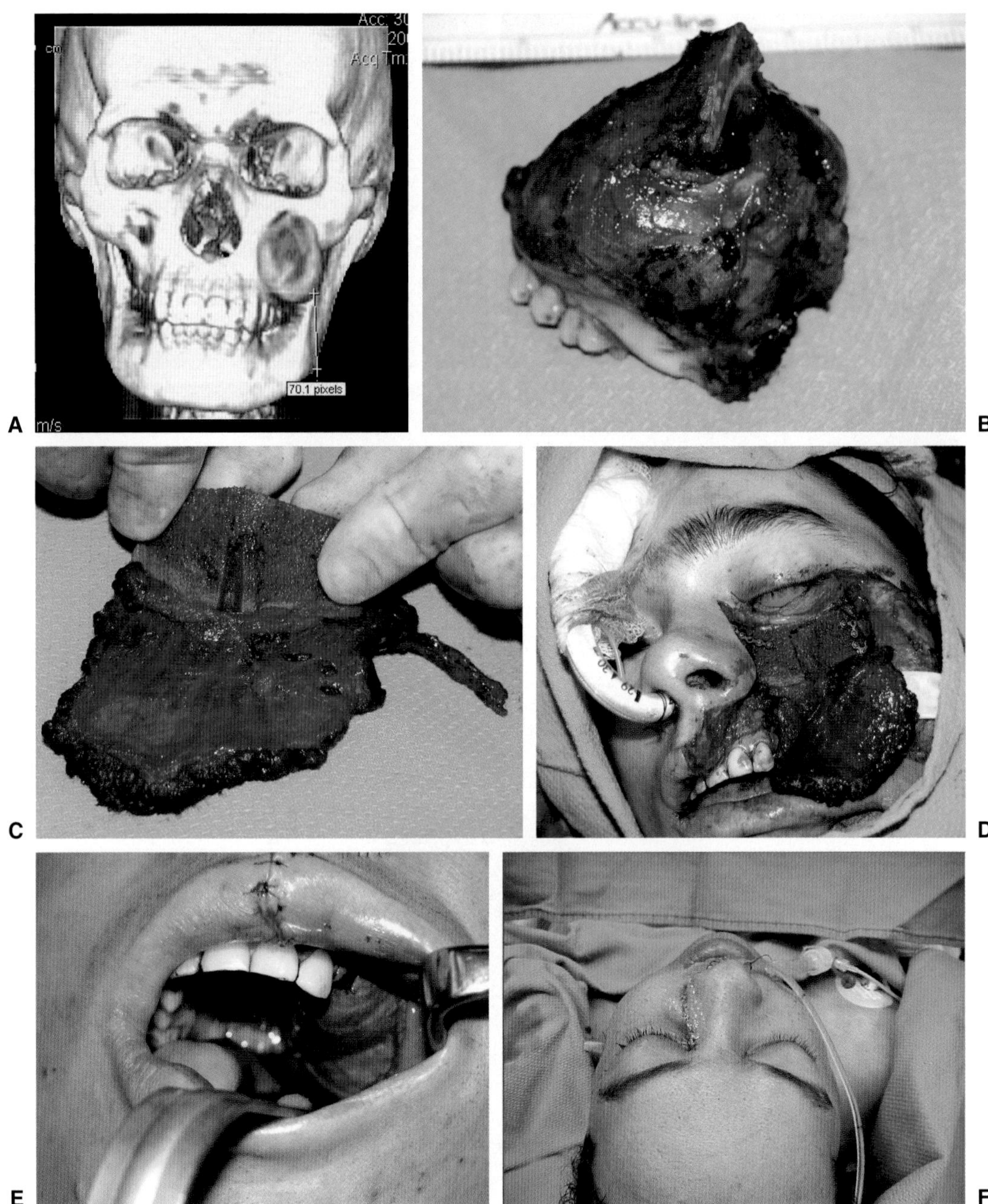

Figure 8.5. Type II maxillectomy defect reconstructed with iliac crest and internal oblique muscle flap. **(A)** Pre-operative three-dimensional-CT scan of left maxillary tumor. **(B)** Resection __. **(C)** Internal-table iliac crest free flap with internal oblique muscle, showing single osteotomy. **(D)** Inset of flap for preservation of anterior cheek contour, and muscle for palate reconstruction. **(E)** Intra-oral appearance of palate reconstruction. Internal oblique muscle has been left to mucosalize. **(F)** External contour.

discussed. However, when bone grafts or mesh are placed, surrounding well-vascularized tissue such a rectus abdominis flap is necessary, and may also be useful for closing a palatal defect. Once again, a useful alternative is to use vascularized iliac crest for contour, with additional bone graft where necessary, and to use the internal oblique to aid with bulk or palatal closure. In situations where a free flap is to be avoided but vascularized bone is desirable for orbital floor reconstruction because of the need for subsequent radiotherapy, a pedicled temporoparietal fascia flap with vascularized calvarium can be used, with or without temporalis muscle for additional bulk. Type IIIB and IV defects are often large defects, requiring bulk and possible dural repair and are usually reconstructed with rectus abdominis myocutaneous flaps to achieve coverage and separation of the cranial contents from the aerodigestive tract.

Special Considerations

To reach the ipsilateral neck vessels, a free flap pedicle length from the midface must be approximately 10cm. This is achievable with radial forearm and anterolateral thigh flaps. The pedicle length for a rectus abdominis flap can be increased by intramuscular dissection *(70)*.

Skull Base

Introduction

A cranial base lesion, for purposes of this discussion, is defined as one that requires both an intracranial and extracranial approach for its ablation. Tumors requiring this combined approach for ablation were previously considered unresectable prior to the advent of reliable reconstruction and advances in diagnostic and interventional radiology. The intracranial surface of the skull base is formed by the floor of the anterior, middle, and posterior cranial fossae. Extracranially, the skull base forms the roof of the orbits, sphenoid sinus, nasopharynx, and infratemporal fossa. Therefore, our reconstructive goals for cranial base lesions are very specific because, almost by definition, this type of resection leaves the dura exposed to the upper aerodigestive tract. These resections frequently also involve resection and repair of the dura and this repair is, in turn, exposed to the aerodigestive tract.

Principles of Reconstruction

When the dura is reconstructed, it is necessary to obtain a water-tight seal between the cranial contents and the aerodigestive tract in order to avoid contamination with resultant ascending meningitis or brain abscess. The dural repair must be covered by well-vascularized tissue, which will aid with maintaining the dural seal and must obliterate dead space. Therefore, local pedicled flaps have been supplanted by free flaps now that free flap reliability is upwards of 95%, and this avoids the downfall

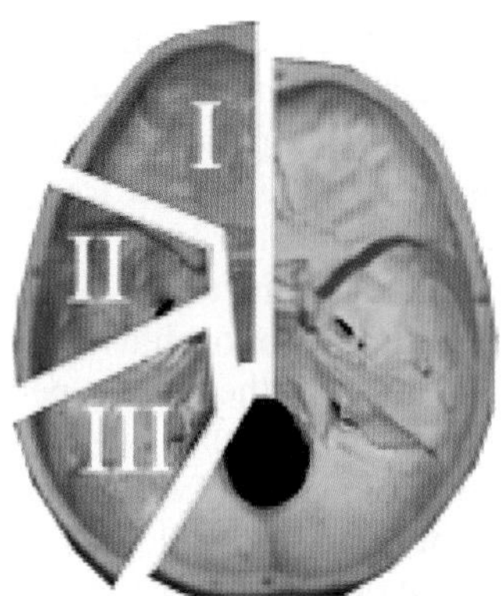

Figure 8.6. Classification of skull base defects. Region I tumors extend to involve the anterior cranial fossa and include the clivus; Region II tumors extend to the middle cranial fossa; and Region III tumors involve the posterior cranial fossa.

of pedicled flaps in which the portion of the flap that is critical for reconstructive success is the most vulnerable to partial flap failure. Finally, the type of flap reconstruction is guided by the region of the skull base to be reconstructed.

Classification

Multiples classifications have been devised for skull base reconstruction *(71–73)*, but the classification developed by Irish et al. *(73)*, based upon anatomic boundaries and tumor growth patterns of skull base neoplasms within the different zones, divides the skull base into three regions (Figure 8.6) relevant to surgical approach and reconstruction.

Region I tumors arise from the sinuses, orbit, and other local structures anteriorly and extend to involve the anterior cranial fossae. These are resected through an anterior craniofacial approach (frontal craniotomy through a coronal incision, usually combined with a lateral rhinotomy and possibly maxillectomy), as are tumors that arise from the clivus and extend posteriorly to the foramen magnum (craniotomy with mandibulotomy with possible palatal split).

Region II tumors primarily involve the infratemporal and pterygopalatine fossa with extension to the middle cranial fossa, and originate in the lateral skull base. Whereas Zone I tumors are the most common, Zone II tumors are the rarest and are associated with the worst prognosis *(73)*. Surgical access is through an infratemporal approach with a hemicoronal incision and preauricular extension, possibly combined with a mandibulectomy or mandibulotomy; through a transtemporal approach requiring a hemicoronal incision with a post-auricular extension with transection of the external auditory canal; or, alternatively, through a frontotemporal craniotomy.

Region III tumors arise around the ear, parotid, and temporal bone and extend intracranially to involve the posterior cranial fossae *(73)*.

Reconstructive Options

There are several options for repairing the dura. The commonly used options in our practice are: (1) the pericranial (vascularized scalp periostium) flap; (2) fascia harvested from the anterior rectus sheath; (3) tensor fascia lata grafts; and (4) fibrin sealants. The latter is used as an adjunct to the other techniques to ensure that the dura is truly sealed and the risk of cerebrospinal fluid (CSF) leak minimized. The pericranial flap when used is raised prior to the craniotomy and protected during the case so that it can be used to seal the dura at the end of the procedure. This is usually applicable to anterior dural defects. It is important to remember that when the bone flap is being replaced, the blood supply of the pericranial flap is not compromised. For this reason, space has to left between the bone ends to accommodate the pericranial flap (*see* Figure 8.7). One of the most important functions of the reconstructive flap is to obliterate dead space, and to this end it is important to suspend the flap from the cranial base to ensure that the flap is

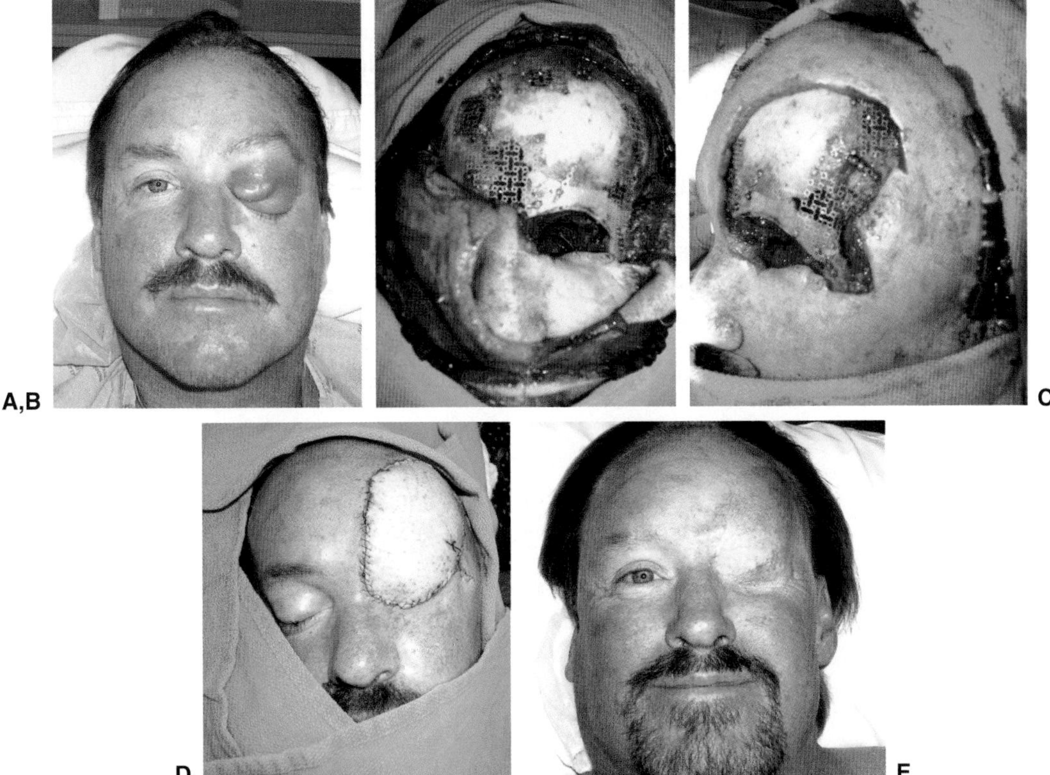

Figure 8.7. Region I cranial base reconstruction with pericranial flap and free anterolateral thigh flap. **(A)** Pre-operative appearance. **(B)** Obliteration of the communication of the intracranial contents and aerodigestive tract was accomplished with a pericranial flap passed through bony defects left prior to replacement of the frontal bone flap and replacement of the orbital bar. **(C)** Residual external defect. **(D)** Coverage with a free anterolateral thigh flap. **(E)** Post-operative appearance.

directly in apposition to the dural repair *(74)*. The use of free tissue transfer in the cranial base has minimized the risk of CSF leak, meningitis, and abscess formation and allows us to operate on and ablate tumors that were previously considered unresectable *(75)*. The workhorse flap in this area is the rectus abdominis, usually as a muscle flap but occasionally as a myocutaneous flap. The malleability of the muscle allows it to conform to irregularly shaped defects and aid in the obliteration of dead space and maintenance of a water-tight seal *(76)*. The tendinous intersections of this muscle can be used as a means of placing secure sutures in the flap by which it can be suspended from the skull base. Region III defects often require extensive external coverage without a major requirement to fill dead space, and in these situations the anterolateral thigh flap may be useful.

Special Considerations

Free flaps for cranial base reconstruction are usually revascularized from the superficial temporal vessels or, alternatively, from vessels in the neck. Vein grafts are rarely necessary. Because the flap reconstructions are often buried, they may not be amenable to clinical monitoring and an implantable Doppler probe may be considered. Bony reconstruction is often unnecessary, but titanium mesh can be a useful adjunct, as it is inert, does not interfere with post-operative imaging, and is relatively resistant to infection.

Conclusion

Defects resulting from oncologic ablation of the mandible, maxilla, and cranial base are varied in their etiology and prognosis. Similarly, reconstructive efforts must be customized to the defect. However, the common goals of optimizing functional and aesthetic outcome while minimizing complications and need for further surgery prevail.

References

1. Boyd JB, Morris S, Rosen IB, et al. The through-and-through oromandibular defect: rationale for aggressive reconstruction. Plast Reconstr Surg 1994; 93(1):44–53.
2. Toriumi DM, Kotler HS, Luxenberg DP, et al. Mandibular reconstruction with a recombinant bone-inducing factor. Functional, histologic, and biomechanical evaluation. Arch Otolaryngol Head Neck Surg 1991; 117(10):1101–1112.
3. Warnke PH, Springer IN, Wiltfang J, et al. Growth and transplantation of a custom vascularised bone graft in a man. Lancet 2004;364(9436):766–770.
4. Boyd JB, Gullane PJ, Rotstein LE, et al. Classification of mandibular defects. Plast Reconstr Surg 1993;92(7):1266–1275.
5. Jewer DD, Boyd JB, Manktelow RT, et al. Orofacial and mandibular reconstruction with the iliac crest free flap: a review of 60 cases and a new method of classification. Plast Reconstr Surg 1989;84(3):391–403; discussion 404–405.

6. Boyd JB, Mulholland RS, Davidson J, et al. The free flap and plate in oromandibular reconstruction: long-term review and indications. Plast Reconstr Surg 1995;95(6):1018–1028.
7. Urken ML, Weinberg H, Vickery C, et al. Oromandibular reconstruction using microvascular composite free flaps. Report of 71 cases and a new classification scheme for bony, soft-tissue and neurologic defects. Arch Otolaryngol Head Neck Surg 1991;117(7):733–744.
8. Thoma AR, Khadaroo O, Grigenas, et al. Oromandibular reconstruction with the radial-forearm osteocutaneous flap: experience with 60 consecutive cases. Plast Reconstr Surg 1999;104(2):368–378.
9. Thoma A, Levis C, Young JEM. Oromandibular reconstruction after cancer resection. Clin Plast Surg 2005;32(3):361–375.
10. Alpert B, Gutwald R, Schmelzeisen R. New innovations in craniomaxillofacial fixation: the 2.0 lock system. Keio J Med 2003;52(2):120–127.
11. Boyd JB. Use of reconstruction plates in conjunction with soft-tissue free flaps for oromandibular reconstruction. Clin Plast Surg 1994;21(1):69–77.
12. Schoning H, Emshoff R. Primary temporary AO plate reconstruction of the mandible. Oral Surg Oral Med Oral Pathol Oral Radiol Endod 1998; 86(6):667–672.
13. Arias-Gallo J, Maremonti P, Gonzalez-Otero T, et al. Long term results of reconstruction plates in lateral mandibular defects. Revision of nine cases. Auris Nasus Larynx 2004;31(1):57–63.
14. Kroll SS, Robb GL, Miller MJ, et al. Reconstruction of posterior mandibular defects with soft tissue using the rectus abdominis free flap. Br J Plast Surg 1998;51(7):503–507.
15. Talesnik A, Markowitz B, Calcaterra T, et al. Cost and outcome of osteocutaneous free-tissue transfer versus pedicled soft-tissue reconstruction for composite mandibular defects. Plast Reconstr Surg 1996;97(6): 1167–1178.
16. Netscher D, Alford EL, Wigoda P, et al. Free composite myo-osseous flap with serratus anterior and rib: indications in head and neck reconstruction. Head Neck 1998;20(2):106–112.
17. Guelinckx PJ, Sinsel NK. The "Eve" procedure: the transfer of vascularized seventh rib, fascia, cartilage, and serratus muscle to reconstruct difficult defects. Plast Reconstr Surg 1996;97(3):527–535.
18. Millard DR Jr, Maisels DO, Batstone JH. Immediate repair of radical resection of the anterior arch of the lower jaw. Plast Reconstr Surg 1967;39(2):153–161.
19. Duncan MJ, Manktelow RT, Zuker RM, et al. Mandibular reconstruction in the radiated patient: the role of osteocutaneous free tissue transfers. Plast Reconstr Surg 1985;76(6):829–840.
20. Rosen IB, Bell MS, Barron PT, et al. Use of microvascular flaps including free osteocutaneous flaps in reconstruction after composite resection for radiation-recurrent oral cancer. Am J Surg 1979;138(4):544–549.
21. Martin D, Breton P, Henri JF, et al. [Role of osteocutaneous external brachial flap in the treatment of composite loss of substance of the mandible]. Ann Chir Plast Esthet 1992;37(3):252–257.
22. Seikaly H, Calhoun K, Rassekh CH, et al. The clavipectoral osteomyocutaneous free flap. Otolaryngol Head Neck Surg 1997;117(5):547–554.
23. Siemssen SO, Kirkby B, O'Connor TP. Immediate reconstruction of a resected segment of the lower jaw, using a compound flap of clavicle and sternomastoid muscle. Plast Reconstr Surg 1978;61(5):724–735.
24. Hidalgo DA. Fibula free flap: a new method of mandible reconstruction. Plast Reconstr Surg 1989;84(1):71–79.

25. Hidalgo DA. Fibula free flap mandibular reconstruction. Clin Plast Surg 1994;21(1):25–35.
26. Hidalgo DA, Rekow A. A review of 60 consecutive fibula free flap mandible reconstructions. Plast Reconstr Surg 1995;96(3):585–596; discussion 597–602.
27. Taylor GI. Reconstruction of the mandible with free composite iliac bone grafts. Ann Plast Surg 1982;9(5):361–376.
28. Taylor GI. The current status of free vascularized bone grafts. Clin Plast Surg 1983;10(1):185–209.
29. Nakatsuka T, Harii K, Yamada A, et al. Surgical treatment of mandibular osteoradionecrosis: versatility of the scapular osteocutaneous flap. Scand J Plast Reconstr Surg Hand Surg 1996;30(4):291–298.
30. Swartz WM, Banis JC, Newton ED, et al. The osteocutaneous scapular flap for mandibular and maxillary reconstruction. Plast Reconstr Surg 1986;77(4):530–545.
31. Coleman JJ III, Wooden WA. Mandibular reconstruction with composite microvascular tissue transfer. Am J Surg 1990;160(4):390–395.
32. Mounsey RA, Boyd JB. Mandibular reconstruction with osseointegrated implants into the free vascularized radius. Plast Reconstr Surg 1994; 94(3):457–464.
33. Jones NF, Monstrey S, Gambier BA. Reliability of the fibular osteocutaneous flap for mandibular reconstruction: anatomical and surgical confirmation. Plast Reconstr Surg 1996;97(4):707–716; discussion 717–718.
34. Daniels TR, Thomas R, Bell TH, et al. Functional outcome of the foot and ankle after free fibular graft. Foot Ankle Int 2005;26(8):597–601.
35. Shpitzer T, Neligan P, Boyd B, et al. Leg morbidity and function following fibular free flap harvest. Ann Plast Surg 1997;38(5):460–464.
36. Disa JJ, Cordeiro PG. The current role of preoperative arteriography in free fibula flaps. Plast Reconstr Surg 1998;102(4):1083–1088.
37. Hartman EH, Spauwen PH, Jansen JA. Donor-site complications in vascularized bone flap surgery. J Invest Surg 2002;15(4):185–197.
38. Shenaq SM, Klebuc MJ. The iliac crest microsurgical free flap in mandibular reconstruction. Clin Plast Surg 1994;21(1):37–44.
39. Thoma A, Archibald S, Payk I, et al. The free medial scapular osteofasciocutaneous flap for head and neck reconstruction. Br J Plast Surg 1991;44(7): 477–482.
40. Batchelor AG, Sully L. A multiple territory free tissue transfer for reconstruction of a large scalp defect. Br J Plast Surg 1984;37(1):76–79.
41. Gucer T, Oge K, Ozgur F. Is it necessary to use the angular artery to feed the scapular tip when preparing a latissimus dorsi osteomyocutaneous flap? Case report. J Reconstr Microsurg 2000;16(3):197–200.
42. Boyd B, Mulholland S, Gullane P, et al. Reinnervated lateral antebrachial cutaneous neurosome flaps in oral reconstruction: are we making sense? Plast Reconstr Surg 1994;93:1350.
43. Munro IR, Phillips JH, Griffin G. Growth after construction of the temporomandibular joint in children with hemifacial microsomia. Cleft Palate J 1989;26(4):303–311.
44. Kaban LB, Perrott DH, Fisher K. A protocol for management of temporomandibular joint ankylosis. J Oral Maxillofac Surg 1990;48(11):1145–1151; discussion 1152.
45. Dimitroulis G. The interpositional dermis-fat graft in the management of temporomandibular joint ankylosis. Int J Oral Maxillofac Surg 2004; 33(8):755–760.

46. Medra AM. Follow up of mandibular costochondral grafts after release of ankylosis of the temporomandibular joints. Br J Oral Maxillofac Surg 2005;43(2):118–122.
47. Vuillemin T, Raveh J, Sutter F. Mandibular reconstruction with the THORP condylar prosthesis after hemimandibulectomy. J Craniomaxillofac Surg 1989;17(2):78–87.
48. Lindqvist C, Soderholm AL, Hallikainen D, et al. Erosion and heterotopic bone formation after alloplastic temporomandibular joint reconstruction. J Oral Maxillofac Surg 1992;50(9):942–949; discussion 950.
49. Rossi G, Arrigoni G. Reimplantation of the mandibular condyle in cases of intraoral resection and reconstruction of the mandible. J Maxillofac Surg 1979;7(1):1–5.
50. Hidalgo DA. Condyle transplantation in free flap mandible reconstruction. Plast Reconstr Surg 1994;93(4):770–781; discussion 782–783.
51. Teoh KH, Huryn JM, Patel S, et al. Prosthetic intervention in the era of microvascular reconstruction of the mandible—a retrospective analysis of functional outcome. Int J Prosthodont 2005;18(1):42–54.
52. Shaw RJ, Sutton AF, Cawood JI, et al. Oral rehabilitation after treatment for head and neck malignancy. Head Neck 2005;27(6):459–470.
53. Jacob RF, Reece GP, Taylor TD, et al. Mandibular restoration in the cancer patient: microvascular surgery and implant prostheses. Tex Dent J 1992; 109(6):23–26.
54. Kramer FJ, Dempf R, Bremer B. Efficacy of dental implants placed into fibula-free flaps for orofacial reconstruction. Clin Oral Implants Res 2005; 16(1):80–88.
55. Levin L, Carrasco L, Kazemi A, et al., Enhancement of the fibula free flap by alveolar distraction for dental implant restoration: report of a case. Facial Plast Surg 2003;19(1):87–94.
56. Klesper B, Lazar F, Siessegger M, et al. Vertical distraction osteogenesis of fibula transplants for mandibular reconstruction–a preliminary study. J Craniomaxillofac Surg 2002;30(5):280–285.
57. Bahr W, Stoll P, Wachter R. Use of the "double barrel" free vascularized fibula in mandibular reconstruction. J Oral Maxillofac Surg 1998;56(1):38–44.
58. Sclaroff A., Haughey B, Gay WD, et al. Immediate mandibular reconstruction and placement of dental implants. At the time of ablative surgery. Oral Surg Oral Med Oral Pathol 1994;78(6):711–717.
59. Chana JS, Chang YM, Wei FC, et al. Segmental mandibulectomy and immediate free fibula osteoseptocutaneous flap reconstruction with endosteal implants: an ideal treatment method for mandibular ameloblastoma. Plast Reconstr Surg 2004;113(1):80–87.
60. Teoh KH, Patel S, Hwang F, et al. Implant prosthodontic rehabilitation of fibula free-flap reconstructed mandibles: a Memorial Sloan-Kettering Cancer Center review of prognostic factors and implant outcomes. Int J Oral Maxillofac Implants 2005;20(5):738–746.
61. Cordeiro PG, Santamaria E. A classification system and algorithm for reconstruction of maxillectomy and midfacial defects. Plast Reconstr Surg 2000;105(7):2331–2346.
62. Aramany MA. Basic principles of obturator design for partially edentulous patients. Part I: classification. J Prosthet Dent 1978;40:554–557.
63. Spiro RH, Strong EW, Shah JP. Maxillectomy and its classification. Head Neck 1997;19:309–314.
64. Umino S, Masuda G, Ono S, et al. Speech intelligibility following maxillectomy with and without a prosthesis: an analysis of 54 cases. J Oral Rehab 1998;25:153–158.

65. Okay DJ, Genden E, Buchbinder D, et al. Prosthodontic guidelines for surgical reconstruction of the maxilla: a classification system of defects. J Prosthet Dent 2001;86(4):352–363.
66. Genden EM, Wallace DI, Okay D, et al. Reconstruction of the hard palate using the radial forearm free flap: indications and outcomes. Head Neck 2004;26(9):808–814.
67. Jones NF, Hardesty RA, Swartz WM, et al. Extensive and complex defects of the scalp, middle third of the face, and palate: the role of microsurgical reconstruction. Plast Reconstr Surg 1988;82(6):937–952.
68. Brown JS, Rogers SN, McNally DN, et al. A modified classification for the maxillectomy defect. Head Neck 2000;22(1):17–26.
69. Brown JS. Deep circumflex iliac artery free flap with internal oblique muscle as a new method of immediate reconstruction of maxillectomy defect. Head Neck 1996;18(5):412–421.
70. Cordeiro PG, Disa JJ. Challenges in midface reconstruction. Semin Surg Oncol 2000;19(3):218–225.
71. Jackson IT, Hide TAH. A systematic approach to tumors of the base of the skull. J Maxillofac Surg 1982;10(2):92–98.
72. Jones NF, Schramm VL, Sekhar LN. Reconstruction of the cranial base following tumour resection. Br J Plast Surg 1987;40(2):155–162.
73. Irish J, Gullane PJ, Gentili F, et al. Tumors of the skull base: outcome and survival analysis of 77 cases. Head Neck 1994;16(1):3–10.
74. Neligan PC, Boyd JB. Reconstruction of the cranial base defect. Clin Plast Surg 1995;22(1):71–77.
75. Neligan PC, Mulholland S, Irish J, et al. Flap selection in cranial base reconstruction. Plast Reconstr Surg 1996;98(7):1159–1166.
76. Gullane PJ, Lipa JE, Novak CB, et al. Reconstruction of skull base defects. Clin Plast Surg 2005;32(3):391–399.

9

Pharynx, Cervical Esophagus, and Oral Cavity Reconstruction

Michael J. Miller

Defects of the oral cavity, pharynx, and cervical esophagus pose a particular challenge in reconstructive surgery for patients with cancer because of their unique tissue elements, structure, integrated function, bacterial contamination, and proximity to other vital structures. The oropharynx and cervical esophagus are composed of specialized voluntary and involuntary muscles and fibrous connective tissue. The epithelial surfaces are thin, pliable mucosa coated with a film of saliva that supplies moisture, provides lubrication, initiates digestion, and controls bacterial flora. These tissues form elegant, compact, anatomically complex structures that have no exact autologous analogs to use for replacement. They are functionally integrated to coordinate speech, mastication, swallowing, and breathing. Impairment of one function necessarily affects each of the others to some degree. Complicating matters is the high level of bacterial colonization normally present in the oral cavity. Ordinarily, these bacteria are non-virulent but become so with surgery and/or radiotherapy-associated changes in the microenvironment. Finally, the carotid artery, internal jugular vein, and portions of cranial nerves V, VII, IX, X, XI, and XII are located immediately adjacent to the pharynx and cervical esophagus. These must be preserved and protected if they have not been removed with the tumor resection. Local donor tissue options available for transfer into the defect are usually limited. Typically, they do not afford a suitable amount of tissue or are impaired by scarring or radiation injury *(1)*.

All these technical challenges are combined with a variety of social issues. Many patients with head and neck cancer have a history of tobacco use and alcohol abuse that complicates post-operative management and renders some surgical techniques less reliable. All patients can expect alterations in appearance and function that can have adverse social and emotional consequences. The key to successful reconstruction of the oral cavity, pharynx, and cervical esophagus is to understand the anatomic relationships and functional requirements of the involved structures and consider a full range of reconstructive techniques in each case.

Reconstructive Requirements

The aerodigestive tract is anatomically divided into the oral cavity, pharynx, and cervical esophagus. The principal task of reconstruction is to restore a three-dimensional surface within the osseous confines of the mandible, palate, maxilla, and vertebral column while preserving adjacent neurovascular structures. The fundamental goals are primary wound healing and protection of vital structures. Furthermore, the reconstruction should not interfere with tumor surveillance or delivery of adjuvant radiotherapy and/or chemotherapy. Each region presents slightly different issues in the restoration of function and aesthetics. For example, the soft-tissue defect resulting from ablation of an advanced tumor often includes bone; thus, reconstruction must involve restoration of the maxilla, mandible, or even vertebral column. Rarely can all the issues be addressed without trade-offs, and patients must be made aware of these. Optimal functional results may require more than one operation. As with all cancer-related reconstructive surgeries, the methods used must have a high degree of reliability. Techniques prone to failure result in increased need for medical care and hospitalization. These patients often have a limited life expectancy, and consuming their remaining life with repeated hospitalizations, clinic visits, or treatments for surgical complications adversely affect quality of life (QOL). Besides these general requirements, each region of the aerodigestive tract has additional unique considerations.

Oral Cavity

The oral cavity extends from the junction of the lip vermillion and skin to an imaginary vertical plane defined by the junction of the hard and soft palates and the circumvallate papillae of the tongue. It includes the lip vermillion, maxillary and mandibular labial sulci, alveolar ridges and sulci, buccal mucosa, floor of the mouth, hard palate, retromolar trigone, and oral (mobile) tongue. Functional issues relate to mastication, speech, swallowing, and facial appearance.

Typical reconstructive problems include the appearance and competence of the lips; recreation of the alveolar ridge and retromolar trigone contours; maintenance of tongue mobility; restoration of a compliant buccal surface, possibly including the external skin; and separation of the oral and nasal cavities. Ideally, the lips should have symmetric vermillion, with sufficient sensation and tone to allow mastication and speech and prevent saliva drooling. The reconstruction should not tether the lips and should provide adequate tissue to allow for subsequent scar contracture, especially in patients who undergo post-operative radiotherapy. The alveolar sulci should be sufficiently deep and mechanically stable to facilitate dental restoration. Overly shallow sulci allow tongue, lip, or cheek motion to dislodge dental prostheses during speech and mastication. The tongue must retain maximum mobility. It should be able to protrude to contact the lips, deviate laterally to the buccal surfaces, and reach the hard palate to facilitate manipulation of the food bolus during mastication, initiate swallowing, and help produce intelligible speech. The retromolar trigone requires thin, pliable soft tissue that reliably protects the mandible but does not impair jaw motion. The restoration must be sufficiently thin to avoid impinging jaw closure yet pliable to prevent trismus. Defects of the buccal mucosa may require repair full-thickness reconstruction including mucosa, buccinator muscle, and external cheek skin. In these circumstances, consideration must be given to restoring the cheek aesthetic units and matching the surrounding skin color.

The palate serves two purposes. It separates the nasal and oral cavities and provides a rigid surface for the tongue to push against during speech and swallowing. Palatal reconstruction often cannot be accomplished with autologous tissue alone, and a prosthesis is usually necessary. Thus, palate reconstruction requires multi-disciplinary planning. It is best to plan the reconstruction in close collaboration with the prosthodontist. The tissue portion of the reconstruction must be designed to accommodate the shape of the prosthesis and provide a mechanically stable platform for it. A properly fashioned prosthesis satisfies the dual purpose of obturating the palate and positioning the roof of the mouth to facilitate contact by the tongue.

Pharynx

The pharynx lies posterior to the oral cavity and extends to the cricopharyngeus muscle at the level of the hyoid bone. It includes the tonsillar pillars, soft palate and uvula, base of the tongue, pharyngeal walls, vallecula, and piriform sinuses. Defects involving the vallecula and piriform sinuses are clinically related more closely to the laryngeal defects and will not be discussed here. The pharynx may be divided into three distinct regions: the oropharynx, nasopharynx, and hypopharynx. These designations are useful for referring to the primary tumor location and guiding resection, but ablative defects are rarely limited to one area. Tissue loss in any of these three regions results in similar functional and reconstructive problems, so the regions must be considered together.

The functional concerns in pharyngeal reconstruction relate to preserving the airway, speech, and swallowing. In addition, the major cervical vessels and cranial nerves immediately adjacent to the pharynx must be protected. In the oropharynx, the soft palate and posterior pharyngeal walls must be restored close enough together to permit air passage into the nasopharynx without nasal emission during speech or escape of liquids during swallowing. Accurate restoration of the base of the tongue and adjacent pharyngeal walls is essential to prevent aspiration, perhaps the most vexing problem that results from defects in this area. Loss of normal soft-tissue contours, pliability, and motor coordination often makes chronic aspiration unpreventable when the defect involves this area. When full functional restoration is not possible, a permanent tracheostomy is necessary, and the patient must be informed of this possibility.

Complete healing is especially important in pharyngeal reconstruction because of the proximity of the carotid artery. Fistulas at this level tend to drain into the neck, bathing the carotid artery with heavily contaminated saliva. This can lead to sudden carotid artery rupture, or "carotid blowout," a life-threatening complication with a mean reported mortality rate of 40% *(2)*. Patients who have undergone radiotherapy are especially at risk. The ideal soft-tissue restoration provides a thin, pliable epithelial lining that is able to tolerate a moist, contaminated environment. The importance of well-vascularized tissue cannot be overemphasized. Marginal necrosis of tissue at the inset of the flap may be trivial in other settings but can result in fistula formation and progress to carotid artery injury in pharyngeal reconstruction. Good surgical techniques are important when insetting the flap to prevent edge necrosis. The epithelial edges should be carefully everted, and the sutures should be tied under proper tension to approximate tissues without impairing the blood supply.

Cervical Esophagus

The cervical esophagus begins after the cricopharyngeus muscle, which inserts to the thyroid and cricoid cartilages and is the most inferior muscle of the pharynx. The cervical esophagus descends in the midline posterior to the larynx and trachea and then passes behind the sternal notch and into the thorax. The recurrent laryngeal nerves are located laterally and posteriorly to the walls of the cervical esophagus and are a concern only in cases in which the larynx is preserved. Primary tumors limited to the cervical esophagus are rare. Most tumors directly invade from the larynx, thyroid, or parathyroid glands or extend from more distal tumors of the thoracic esophagus. Thus, defects isolated to the cervical esophagus are unusual. Typically, esophageal reconstruction also requires repair of a laryngeal defect. Primary tumors of the cervical esophagus often extend for long distances beneath the mucosa and are treated with total esophageal resection and reconstruction. In these cases, the surgical team should include a thoracic surgeon.

The primary functional consideration in cervical esophageal reconstruction is preservation of swallowing. A second issue is voice restoration because resection nearly always includes a laryngectomy. Aspiration is not a concern after a laryngectomy or when the larynx and cricopharyngeus muscles have been preserved, keeping the upper esophageal sphincter intact. As in the pharynx, reliable healing without fistula formation is of paramount importance because of the adjacent carotid artery.

Esophageal defects may be limited, requiring only a portion of the circumference of the esophagus to be repaired. In other cases, there may be insufficient remaining esophageal tissue to salvage, and a circumferential reconstruction is needed. The repair of circumferential defects requires planning to accommodate a luminal diameter of 1.5–2.0 cm. In addition, careful attention to surgical technique during the procedure is essential to avoid stricture formation. Strictures result from excessive tissue turned in at the suture line or from flap edge necrosis that leads to secondary healing, scar formation, and contraction. Post-operative strictures can be treated with serial endoscopic dilation, but often they must be repaired surgically to prevent recurrence. A chronic, recurrent stricture impairs swallowing and severely reduces the patient's QOL because of dietary restrictions and repeated treatments. A full discussion of voice restoration is beyond the scope of this chapter, but if a tracheoesophageal puncture is anticipated, optimal voice quality will require stable cervical esophageal walls lined with minimal mucus. This allows for a vibrating column of air above the puncture to provide a steady voice tone and volume.

Finally, cervical esophageal reconstruction may require replacing the overlying skin, especially in patients with recurrent tumors and a history of surgery or radiotherapy. At times, the tumor may directly erode the skin, but more often, there simply is insufficient skin to cover the added tissue required to restore the esophagus. There is little space in the neck, especially in nutritionally depleted patients, and soft-tissue scarring and fibrosis further limit the ability of the skin to expand and accommodate added volume. In these cases, it is best not to close the skin completely with excessive tension, but instead to replace open areas with a split-thickness skin graft or a suitable flap.

Surgical Planning

Selecting the best surgical option in oral cavity and pharyngoesophageal reconstruction requires a systematic thought process tailored to each patient's circumstances (Figure 9.1). Planning begins in the pre-operative clinic, with a careful evaluation of the patient's overall health and the extent of the tumor. After a physical examination, imaging studies, and a discussion with the ablative surgeon, the reconstructive surgeon makes his or her best estimate of the extent of resection. A list of possible reconstructive options is formulated and discussed thoroughly with the patient. The reconstructive surgeon plans for the defect that is most likely to result from tumor resection as well as the most extensive defect that could occur. Once the various reconstructive options are explained to the patient, permission is obtained to select the final option during

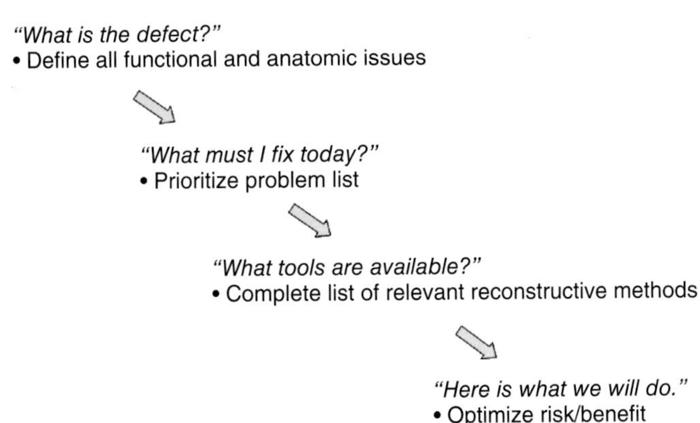

Figure 9.1. Systematic thought process for reconstructive surgery of the oral cavity, pharynx, and cervical esophagus.

surgery after negative margins have been confirmed and the actual reconstructive needs have been clearly determined. It is best to discuss the possibility of competing functional priorities (e.g., optimal speech versus swallowing) with the patient, the patient's family, and members of the multi-disciplinary team prior to surgery. It is important to understand, as clearly as possible, the patient's reconstructive preferences.

After the pre-operative preparations have been completed, surgery is performed. Major head and neck cancer surgery is best performed with separate ablative and reconstructive surgery teams operating together. The reconstructive plan for the reconstruction is finalized intraoperatively on completion of the ablative procedure. In choosing the final method for reconstruction, the surgeon should answer three questions.

Question 1: What is the defect?

When the ablative surgery has been completed, the defect is examined carefully. The reconstructive surgeon makes a list of the specific anatomic and tissue elements of the defect and the resulting functional problems. The dimensions of the soft-tissue defect and proximity of critical surrounding structures are assessed. The ideal reconstructive plan would resolve every problem in a single operation, but this is never possible—leading to the next question to ask in planning the reconstruction.

Question 2: What must I fix today?

Because it is never possible to simultaneously address every problem, the next step is to prioritize each problem on the list. Some must be immediately addressed, and others can safely be dealt with at another time or even left unrepaired. Top-priority issues are ones that will be life-threatening or cause unacceptable morbidity if not repaired. Reliable wound healing and protection of vital structures are necessary. Next in importance are functional issues such as speech and swallowing. The lowest priority issues are usually related strictly to aesthetic appearance. However, the specific ranking can vary on the basis of associated medical conditions and the patient's personal preferences, especially regarding aesthetics.

Question 3: What tools are available?

Each option is considered systematically, proceeding from the simple to the complex. Discipline in this thought process prevents the clinician from falling into the habit of using the same technique for every defect rather than choosing the best one on the basis of the associated advantages and disadvantages. The best solution is the simplest and most reliable method that addresses the maximum number of high-priority concerns with the least risk. Lower priority issues can be addressed during subsequent surgeries or, for practical reasons, not be repaired at all.

The key in making the final decision is optimization of the risks and benefits of the procedure. The best solution may not be the most technically simple one because of the overall total balance of concerns, especially if the simplest solution is also more prone to failure. If the consequences of failure are unacceptable (e.g., exposure of vital structures), a more complicated procedure (e.g., free tissue transfer) is indicated if it has a higher probability of success than a simpler one (e.g., pectoralis major muscle flap). Deciding on a final reconstructive plan requires a multi-disciplinary approach. It also requires flexibility. The clinician must have a back-up plan in case the final defect created by tumor ablation is different than anticipated.

Reconstructive Options

After answering the previous questions, the surgeon decides whether to use primary closure, secondary closure, skin grafting, local flaps, regional flaps, free tissue transfer, or a combination of these procedures in the reconstruction.

Primary and Secondary Closure

Closing a defect primarily or simply allowing it to heal without repair (secondary closure) is generally not suitable for large defects, but these options may be appropriate under specific circumstances and should always be considered in the decision-making process. Both methods depend on the use of local tissue. In primary closure, the surgeon directly advances the local tissues; in secondary closure, natural wound contraction and epithelial cell migration accomplish the same result. Because of this, these methods should be used only when local tissue is healthy, well vascularized, and able to be advanced without distorting or restricting adjacent mobile structures.

Primary closure is most often a realistic option for mucosal defects limited to the buccal surface or the tongue, two areas of relative tissue excess in the oral cavity. It is important to avoid excessive tension at the wound edges and not to leave empty space beneath the mucosa, particularly if the defect extends into the alveolar sulci or floor of the mouth. Fluid contaminated by oral flora collects in submucosal spaces and may ultimately lead to infection, wound breakdown, and fistula formation. When primary closure is possible, it is associated with higher scores in post-operative performance in terms of eating in public, intelligibility of speech, and normalcy of diet *(3)* compared to other forms of repair. This reflects the fact that defects amenable to primary closure are associated with a minimal derangement of intra-oral anatomy and function.

Secondary closure may be suitable for limited, non-irradiated mucosal defects involving the mandibular or maxillary alveolar ridges, hard palate, or posterior pharyngeal wall. In these locations, the underlying bone stabilizes the soft tissues, allowing granulation and mucosalization without limiting tongue motion, lip configuration, jaw opening, or swallowing. Secondary closure requires meticulous oral hygiene.

Skin Grafting

A split-thickness skin graft may be appropriate for repair when there is no history of irradiation and the defect involves primarily the mucosal surface with minimal sacrifice of the underlying tissue *(4)*. In oral cavity defects that include a maxillectomy, the skin graft may be placed on the remaining bone and soft tissues and the reconstruction completed using maxillary prosthetics. In all cases, a successful graft requires a well-vascularized tissue bed that contains no vital structures. A split-thickness graft is preferred because of its greater pliability and thus improved adherence to intra-oral contours, leading to a higher likelihood of successful revascularization or skin graft "take." As in other locations, success requires complete immobilization of the graft on the wound bed during the critical 5-day post-operative period of revascularization. In the oral cavity, it is also important to prevent saliva from dissecting beneath the graft and separating it from the wound bed. This can be accomplished using a variety of surgical stents and bolster dressings made from dental acrylic, soft dental liners, or gauze coated with antibiotic ointment and sutured over the graft *(5)*.

There is always a component of wound contraction associated with skin grafting, although less so than with secondary wound closure. The absolute amount of contracture is related to the completeness of successful skin graft revascularization and healing. For this reason, the same basic principles apply to skin grafting as to other methods that use local tissue, in terms of ideal locations in the oral cavity and pharynx. Large defects involving the undersurface of the tongue are not amenable to primary closure or secondary healing but can be successfully repaired by skin grafting. Although a well-healed skin graft can tolerate post-operative radiotherapy, it is best to consider alternatives to skin grafts when radiotherapy is planned because of the possibility of functionally limiting soft-tissue contractures. Circumferential grafting, used for pharyngeal reconstruction in the past *(6,7)*, is of historical interest only; this is because contemporary techniques using tissue flaps less prone to stricture and fistula formation.

Dermal grafting, using either autologous dermis *(8)* or an acellular processed dermal allograft *(9)*, has been used to reduce the amount of wound contraction while allowing mucosalization of the surface. These grafts are applied in a fashion similar to epidermal skin grafts. After healing, the wound is allowed to epithelialize by migration from the surrounding mucosa. The use of mucosal cells expanded in tissue culture to repair the intra-oral lining has been described previously *(10)*, but this technique is unproven for general clinical use at this time.

Local Flaps

Large defects in the oral cavity and pharyngoesophagus require tissue transfer for reconstruction. The first transfers to consider are local flaps from the tongue, local mucosa surfaces, or the external skin of the face and neck.

Tongue flaps were described for use in reconstructing the oral cavity in the 1950s and remain a useful alternative *(11)*. The abundant blood supply of the tongue makes possible many different flap designs from the dorsum, lateral borders, or ventral surface. Posteriorly based dorsal flaps easily reach the retromolar trigone or tonsillar fossa. Anteriorly based flaps reach defects on the buccal mucosa, lips, floor of the mouth, or palate. Bipedicled flaps oriented transversely can be used for the lips or the floor of the mouth. The principal disadvantage of tongue flaps is the limited amount of tissue available and possible adverse consequences related to speech and mastication.

Mucosal flaps are useful for a variety of small intra-oral defects. Multiple random designs are possible because of the rich blood supply of the submucosa (Figure 9.2). An axial pattern flap may be designed based on the facial artery (a facial artery musculomucosal flap) *(12)*. This flap is harvested from non-irradiated tissue on the buccal surface, the principal site of relative tissue excess in the oral cavity other than the tongue. Although the arterial supply is predictable, venous drainage is variable, and the flap must be harvested with care to preserve adequate venous outflow *(13)*. It may be transferred within the oral cavity to repair defects of the hard and soft palate, alveolus *(14)*, upper and lower lips *(15)*, or the floor of the mouth. Care must be taken during harvest to avoid injuring the parotid duct. The long pedicle length also permits transfer into the neck for limited repairs of the cervical esophagus or pharynx *(16)*. Mucosal flaps may be harvested from the larynx when the larynx is not involved with tumor but must be resected because intractable aspiration is anticipated. Laryngeal transposition flaps are based on the superior laryngeal arteriovenous pedicle and are created by skeletonizing the laryngeal mucosa and transferring the soft tissue into the defect *(17)*.

A variety of local skin flaps have been used for repair of the oral cavity, pharynx, and cervical esophagus. These flaps include flaps from the forehead, nasolabial area, submandibular area, and cervical skin. Some random pattern rotational and bipedicled flap designs have been replaced with newer techniques that are less deforming and permit single-stage

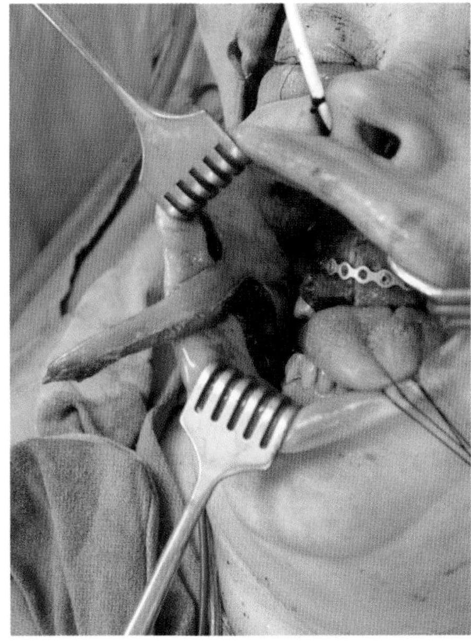

Figure 9.2. Buccal musculomucosal flap used in combination with a free tissue bone transfer for maxillary reconstruction.

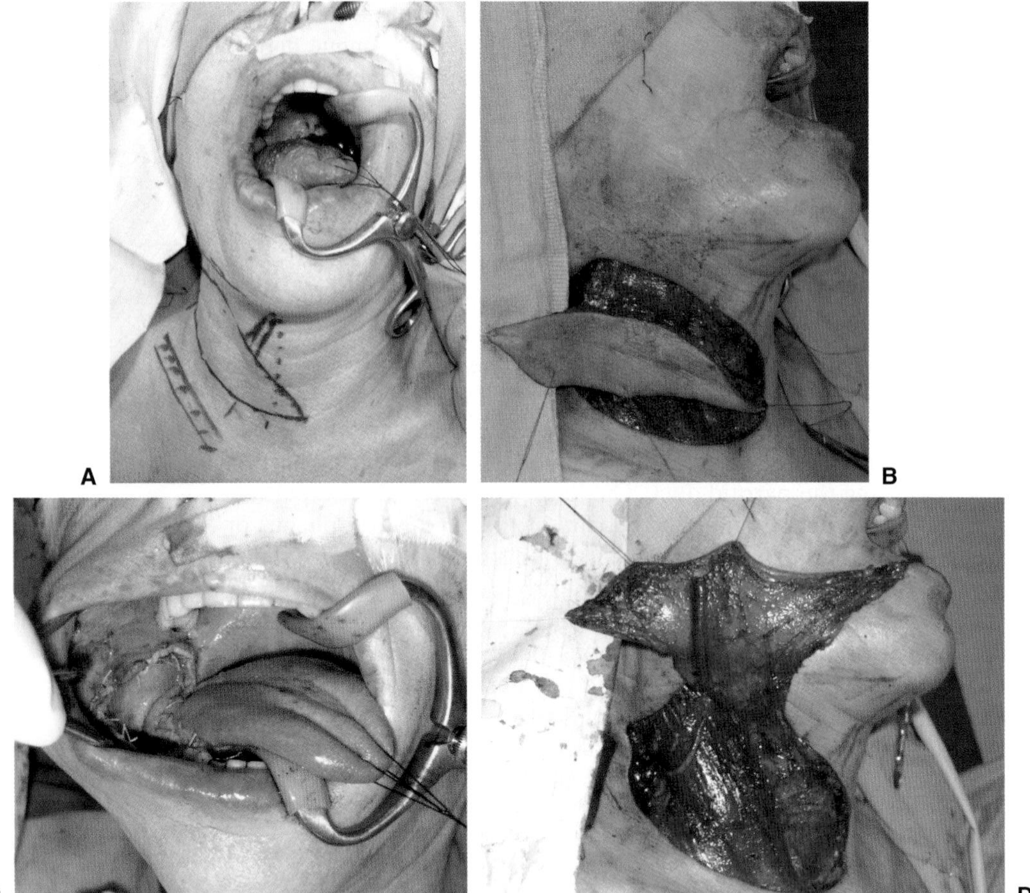

Figure 9.3. Platysma musculocutaneous rotation flap for repair of right cheek and gingivobuccal sulcus. **(A)** Flap design. **(B)** Appearance of flap after mobilization. **(C)** Appearance after cephalad rotation for passage into the oral cavity. **(D)** Flap after inset into defect.

reconstruction, but local skin flaps remain useful for limited defects and are particularly beneficial when combined with other techniques to restore individual anatomic units *(18)*. Nasolabial flaps have been used to repair a wide variety of oral defects, particularly those of the floor of the mouth and labial mucosa *(19,20)*. The submental island flap, an axial pattern flap based on the submental artery, is a useful flap for limited defects nearly anywhere in the oral cavity *(21,22)*. The anatomic basis for this flap has been well described *(23,24)*. It is a versatile flap with a long vascular pedicle and results in minimal deformation of the donor site.

Another useful local skin flap is a musculocutaneous unit based on the platysma muscle (Figure 9.3). The anatomic basis of this flap was described in detail by Hurwitz and coworkers *(25)*, who found that the platysma and overlying skin are supplied by several vascular sources, including the post-auricular and occipital arteries of the upper lateral neck, the facial and submental arteries of the upper medial neck, and the transverse cervical arteries of the midlateral neck. The cervical skin can be transferred on any one of these direct cutaneous vessels, and it is ideal for thin coverage in the oral cavity. Its primary disadvantage is limited availability in patients with a history of neck irradiation.

Regional Flaps

Many defects of the head and neck have tissue replacement needs in excess of what is available from the methods described previously. Regional flaps are the next alternative. The principal regional flaps used to reconstruct the oral cavity and pharyngoesophagus are the deltopectoral and the pectoralis major musculocutaneous flaps.

The deltopectoral flap was introduced by Bakamjian et al. in the 1960s *(26)*. It is an axial pattern flap based on perforating vessels from the internal mammary artery and vein at the lateral border of the sternum. These vessels run obliquely across the upper chest toward the shoulder, allowing the distal skin to be mobilized and reach into the oral cavity and pharyngoesophageal area. The deltopectoral flap provides thin tissue that can be used for oral lining or tubed to repair the cervical esophagus (Figure 9.4). The reliability of the distal skin can be

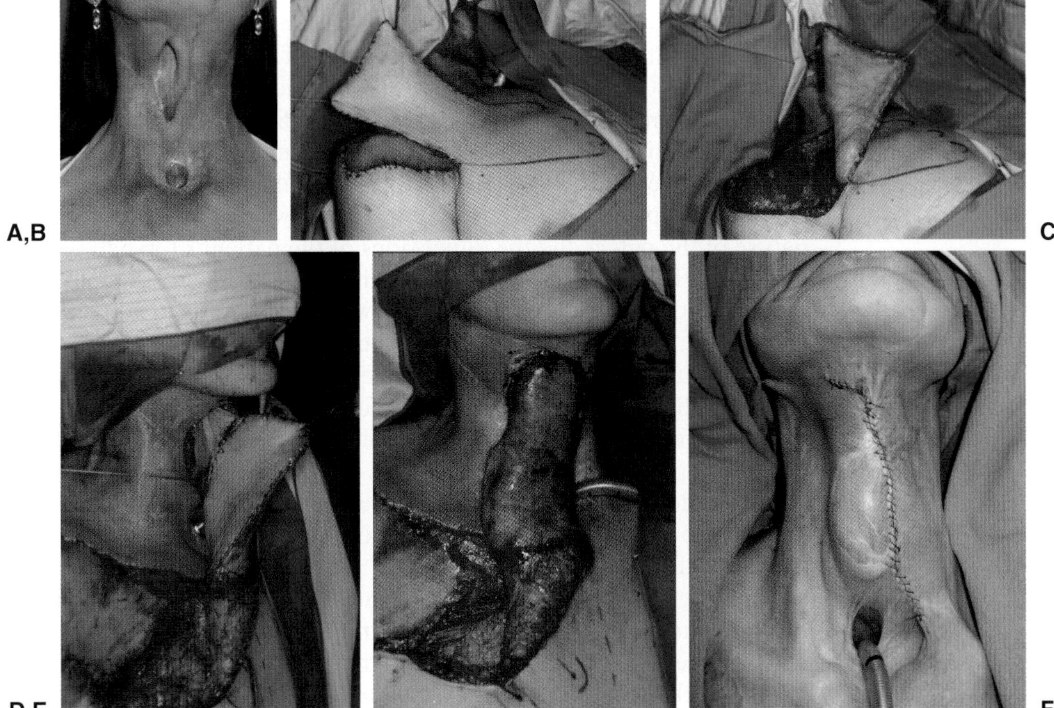

Figure 9.4. Deltopectoral flap for delayed repair of chronic cervical esophageal defect. **(A)** Pre-operative appearance of established cervical esophagus defect. **(B)** The flap is designed with a base over the internal mammary perforators at the sternal margin. The distal half of the flap is mobilized in Stage I (delay procedure) to increase the reliability. **(C)** The undersurface may be skin grafted to prefabricate a bilaminated flap to reconstruct both the esophageal lumen and cervical skin cover simultaneously. **(D, E)** At Stage II the flap is completely elevated and transferred into the defect. **(F)** Appearance after Stage III when the pedicle to the flap is divided and inset completed.

enhanced by performing a delay procedure. This technique also allows prefabrication of a flap with two opposing epithelial surfaces by placing a split-thickness skin graft on the deep surface of the flap that will heal during the period of delay. On the basis of xenon-133 clearance studies, the optimal time to complete elevation and transfer of the flap appears to be approximately 14 days after the delay procedure for most flap designs *(27)*. The primary disadvantage of this technique is that a staged reconstruction is required, in which the tip of the flap is inset into the head and neck defect and later the flap pedicle is divided at the sternum after healing and revascularization have occurred at the recipient site. For many indications, this flap has been replaced by the pectoralis major flap and various free tissue transfers, but it remains a valuable alternative in selected circumstances *(28,29)*.

The greatest single advance in head and neck reconstruction prior to the advent of microvascular surgery was the introduction of the pectoralis major musculocutaneous flap in 1979 *(30)*. Flaps designed using the latissimus dorsi or trapezius muscles will be restricted by pedicle length, excessive bulk, and cervical contour deformities, and trapezius muscle flaps cause shoulder drop when harvested in a transverse direction. For these reasons, the pectoralis major flap has been the primary workhorse for major head and neck reconstruction since its introduction. It provides adequate amounts of well-vascularized tissue for many defects (Figure 9.5). Other advantages are minimal donor site morbidity, consistent anatomy, and generally satisfactory pedicle length. This flap does not require microvascular expertise and equipment and usually requires less operative time compared to microvascular tissue transfers. The pectoralis flap has several disadvantages, however, depending on the nature of the defect and the dimensions of the patient's torso. It affords less design flexibility in terms of epithelial surface area, tissue bulk, and arc of rotation. For example, patients with short chests may have difficulty with the flap reaching beyond the floor of the mouth. Flaps with thick subcutaneous tissue or well-developed pectoralis major muscles may be difficult to fit into the tight confines of the mandible arch. Breast tissue in some women can restrict the amount of skin surface area available for flap harvesting. The procedure can also result in the creation of a contour deformity in the neck because of the muscle bulk passing over the clavicle and through the subcutaneous plane of the lower neck. The muscle will atrophy over time, but it can become shortened by scar contracture, creating a web-like deformity and causing some limitation of neck extension, tightness, and discomfort months later. These problems can be minimized by harvesting the flap as an island, dividing the muscle in the superior aspect of the flap and passing only the vascular pedicle over the clavicle, a maneuver that has the added benefit of increasing the arch of rotation. Despite its limitations, the pectoralis major musculocutaneous flap remains a good solution to many reconstructive situations, especially in patients who are not candidates for microsurgery because of previous surgery, radiotherapy, or comorbid conditions.

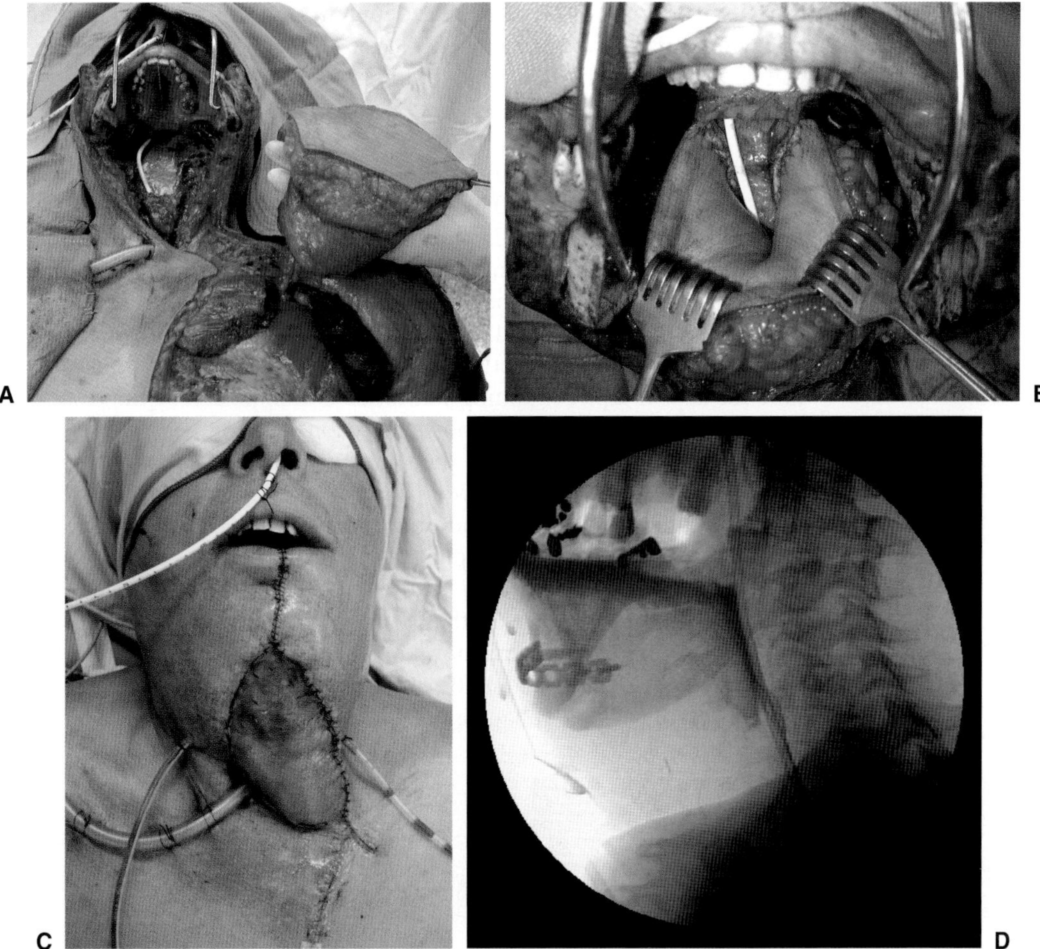

Figure 9.5. Total cervical esophageal reconstruction using a pectoralis major musculocutaneous rotation flap. **(A)** Appearance of the defect (exposed using a mandible splitting procedure) and the pectoralis major flap prepared for transfer. Note the pedicle vessels isolated at the base to reduce the amount of soft tissue passed over the clavicle. **(B)** Formation of the cervical esophagus by tubing the skin paddle. **(C)** Final appearance with a split-thickness skin graft on the muscle. This will contract and atrophy over ensuing weeks to improve neck contour. **(D)** Barium swallow demonstrating satisfactory function of restored cervical esophagus.

Free Tissue Transfer

For large, complex defects, microvascular flaps clearly provide the best means of reconstruction. Free tissue transfer for head and neck reconstruction is perhaps the greatest advance in head and neck surgery in the past two decades. These techniques permit the introduction of specialized tissue into the defect with a reliable blood supply, resulting in a reconstruction that most closely resembles the normal anatomy. Neck discomfort and contour deformities can be avoided by eliminating bulky muscle pedicles. Furthermore, immediate, single-stage restoration of complex defects is usually possible.

Several donor sites are available, depending on the nature of the defect and the patient's body habitus. Mucosal defects of practically any size can be restored using thin, pliable skin harvested from the volar forearm (Figure 9.6) or thigh (Figure 9.7). Full-thickness defects of the buccal mucosa and cheek skin can be repaired with a scapular perforator flap because of the superior color match between the skin of the upper back and the face (Figure 9.8). The anterolateral thigh flap in particular has become common in oral and pharyngoesophageal reconstruction because of the large amount of thin pliable tissue available, minimal donor site morbidity, opportunity to perform the flap elevation at the same time as the ablative procedure, and high reliability *(31)*. Defects requiring more bulk are well suited for rectus abdominis or latissimus dorsi musculocutaneous flaps. Flaps containing soft tissue and bone can be harvested for composite defects, allowing one-stage reconstruction.

Free visceral transfers have become the standard in cases in which vascularized mucosa is preferred (Figure 9.9). Jejunal segments can be used to repair the lining of the oral cavity and pharynx *(32)* and completely restore the cervical esophagus *(33)*. Although the use of vascularized colon and gastric mucosa have been described and are favored by some, most surgeons believe the jejunum is the ideal portion of bowel to use as a free visceral transfer to the head and neck: harvesting the jejunum is technically straightforward, the lumen closely matches the size of the cervical esophagus, the intraluminal flora is less hazardous,

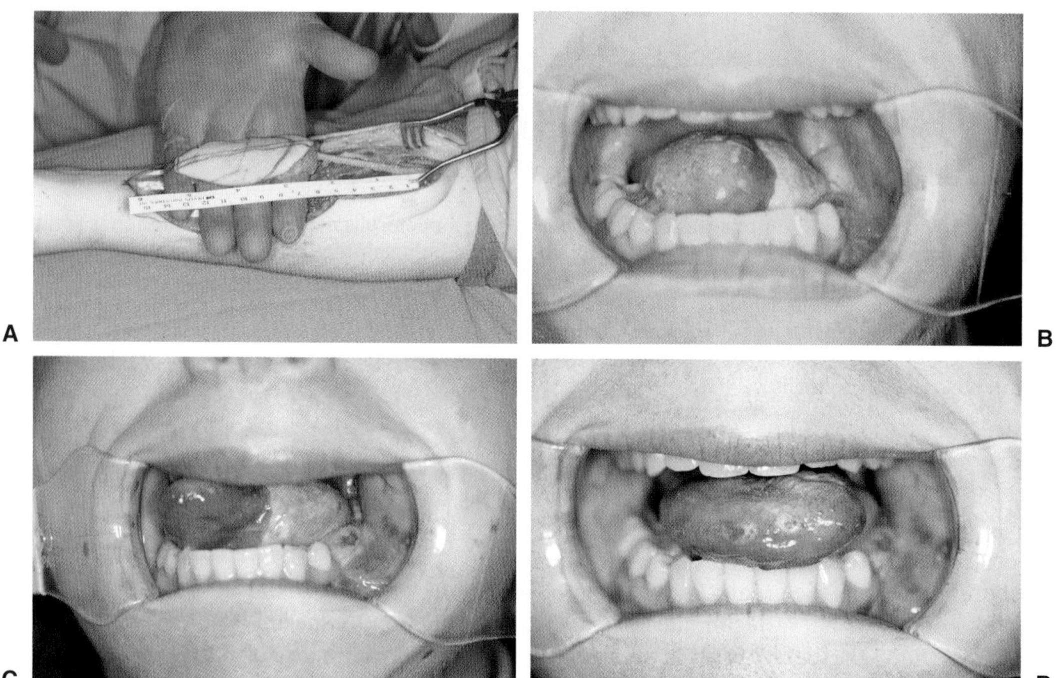

Figure 9.6. Reconstruction of the left lateral mobile tongue and floor of the mouth using a radial forearm free flap in a 33-year-old woman. **(A)** Flap prepared for transfer. Thin soft-tissue replacement permits maximum function as demonstrated by mobility with tongue in anterior **(B)**, right **(C)**, and left **(D)** protrusion.

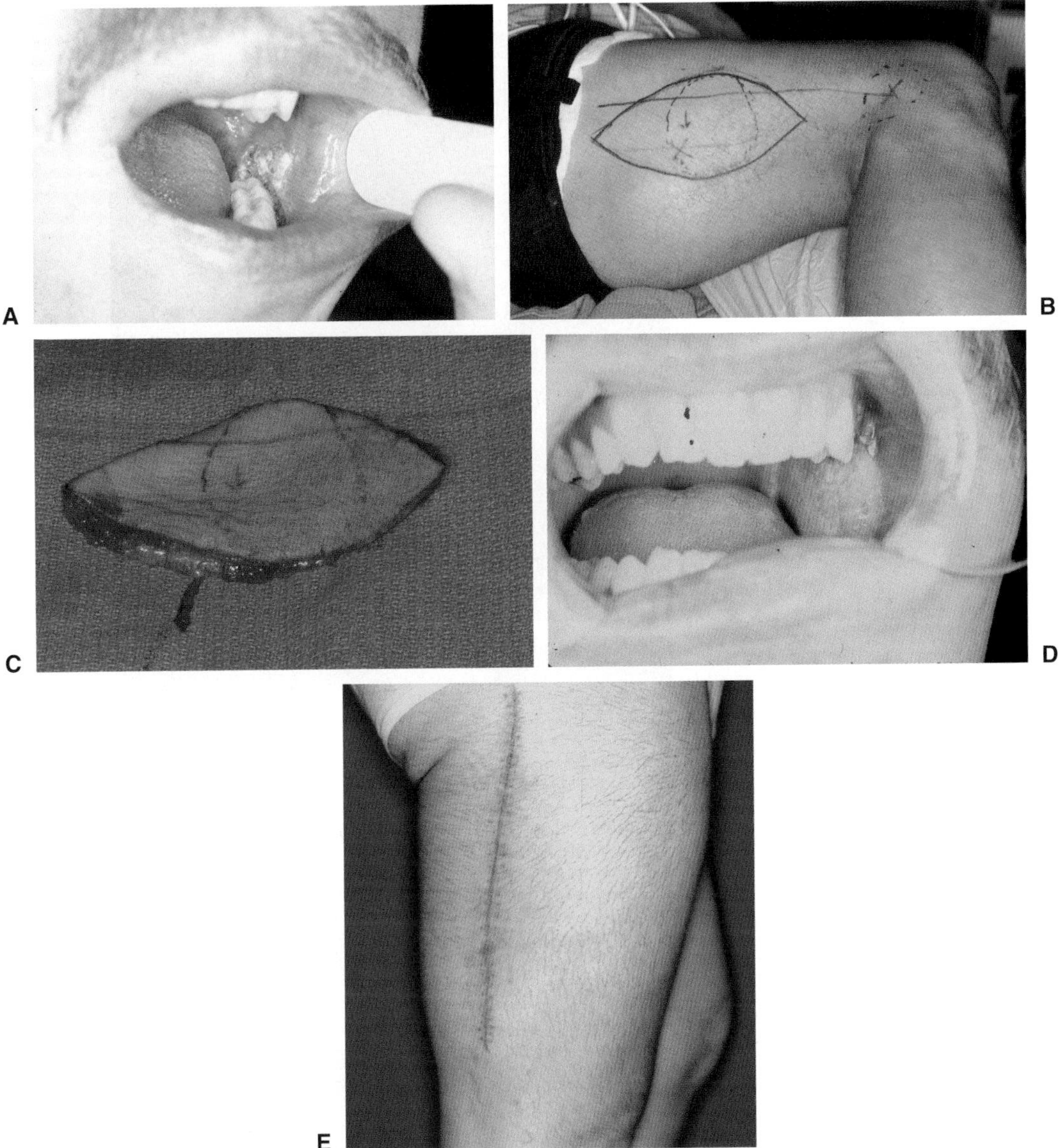

Figure 9.7. Reconstruction of the left buccal surface using a lateral thigh perforator flap. **(A)** Appearance of the tumor prior to resection. **(B)** The flap is designed on the posterolateral thigh based on the third profunda femoris artery perforator. Appearance of the flap ready for transfer **(C)** and 3 months postoperatively **(D)** healed into restored buccal surface. **(E)** Donor sites on the thigh can provide large amounts of thin skin without the need for skin grafting.

and the jejunum has a large and reliable vascular pedicle. Furthermore, the jejunal flap retains motor and secretory function after being transferred.

The many advantages of reconstructive microsurgery for oral and pharyngoesophageal defects, combined with advances in surgical technique that afford a technical success rate of more than 95%, make

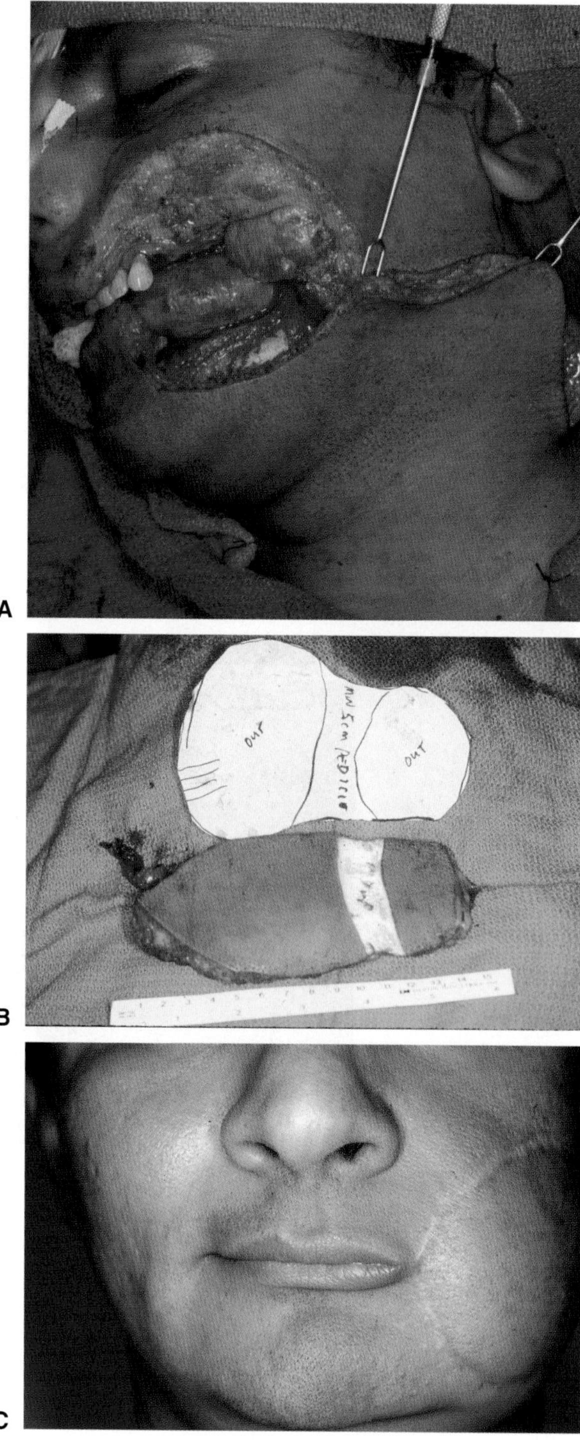

Figure 9.8. Full-thickness cheek reconstruction using a scapula flap based on a perforator from the circumflex scapular artery. **(A)** Appearance of full-thickness defect of the cheek with loss of buccal mucosa, buccinator muscle, and skin. The transverse incision was used for access to the neck for cervical lymph node dissection and flap revascularization. **(B)** Scapular flap designed for folding to restore both intra-oral and external cheek surfaces. **(C)** Final appearance 8 months after surgery and completion of radiotherapy, demonstrating good skin color match between skin from the upper back and face.

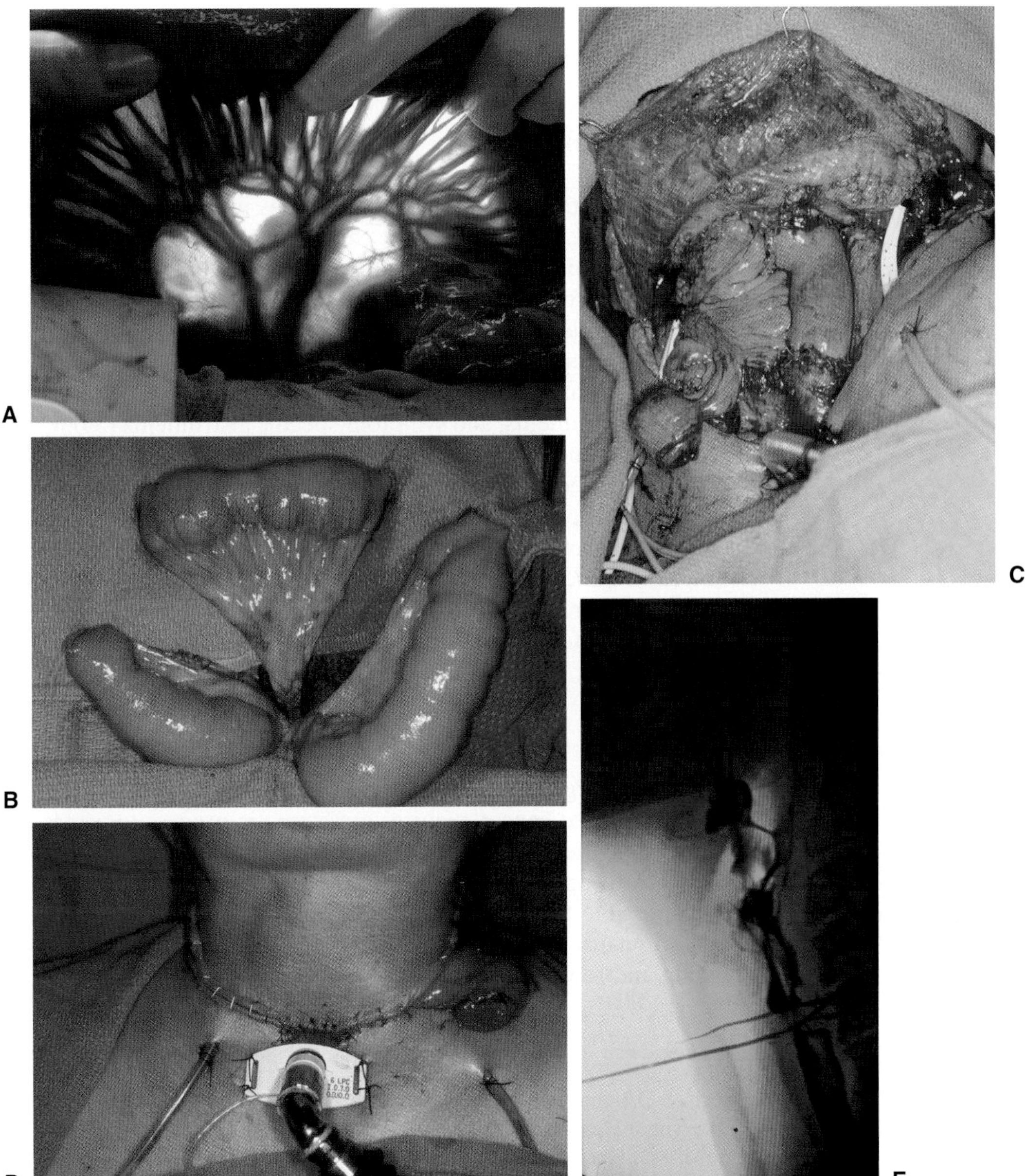

Figure 9.9. Cervical esophageal reconstruction using a free jejunal transfer following total laryngectomy. **(A)** Appearance of the mesenteric blood supply by transillumination during surgery. **(B)** Jejunal flap isolated and ready for transfer. **(C)** Flap inset (anastomosed to the pharynx superiorly and the distal cervical esophageal stump inferiorly) and revascularized. **(D)** Appearance of completed reconstruction demonstrating exposure of redundant segment of jejunum to facilitate flap perfusion monitoring during the post-operative period. This piece of tissue is removed by ligating and dividing the mesentery at skin level at the bedside after 7 days. **(E)** Post-operative barium swallow study demonstrating restoration of function with patient flow and no leaks.

microvascular reconstruction the most appropriate means of managing many major head and neck defects.

Assessing Outcomes

The clinical value of reconstructive surgery lies in improved functional outcome and QOL. Recent decades have been marked by increased awareness of the importance of functional outcomes and QOL in cancer patients after treatment. A variety of tools are available to objectively assess QOL in patients with head and neck cancer. These tools can be classified as instruments that measure general health-related QOL, general QOL for patients with cancer, disease-specific instruments, treatment-specific instruments, and symptom-specific instruments *(34)*. Compared to pre-treatment levels, patients treated for head and neck cancer have a persistent reduction in QOL and function long after the completion of treatment, particularly in terms of normalcy of eating in public, understandability of speech, and normalcy of diet. Low QOL has also been found in patients with head and neck cancer who are concerned about tumor recurrence *(35)*. In addition, the method of reconstruction has a significant effect on QOL *(36)*.

Conclusion

Reconstructive surgery for defects resulting from ablation of oral and pharyngoesophageal cancer requires a systematic process to assess the defect, prioritize the problems, and select the best reconstructive option. The goals are to optimize function and QOL, returning the patient as closely as possible to his or her pre-morbid condition, free of disease. Reconstruction after surgery for head and neck cancer is one of the most challenging and rewarding areas of reconstructive surgery in oncology.

References

1. Sabri A. Oropharyngeal reconstruction: current state of the art. Curr Opin Otolaryngol Head Neck Surg 2003;11(4):251–254.
2. Citardi MJ, Chaloupka JC, Son YH, Ariyan S, Sasaki CT. Management of carotid artery rupture by monitored endovascular therapeutic occlusion (1988–1994). Laryngoscope 1995;105(10):1086–1092.
3. Malone JP, Stephens JA, Grecula JC, Rhoades CA, Ghaheri BA, Schuller DE. Disease control, survival, and functional outcome after multimodal treatment for advanced-stage tongue base cancer. Head Neck 2004; 26(7):561–572.
4. Zieske LA, Johnson JT, Myers EN, Schramm VL Jr, Wagner R. Composite resection reconstruction: split-thickness skin graft—a preferred option. Otolaryngol Head Neck Surg 1988;98(2):170–173.
5. Qureshi SS, Chaukar D, Dcruz AK. Simple technique of securing intraoral skin grafts. J Surg Oncol 2005;89(2):102–103.
6. Rob CG, Bateman GH. Reconstruction of the trachea and cervical oesophagus; preliminary report. Br J Surg 1949;37(146):202–205.

7. Edgerton MT. Reconstruction of the hypopharynx and the cervical esophagus after removal of cancer. Proceedings of the National Cancer Conference 1960;4:685–687.
8. Smiler D, Radack K, Bilovsky P, Montemarano P. Dermal graft—a versatile technique for oral surgery. Oral Surg Oral Med Oral Pathol 1977;43(3): 342–349.
9. Rhee PH, Friedman CD, Ridge JA, Kusiak J. The use of processed allograft dermal matrix for intraoral resurfacing: an alternative to split-thickness skin grafts. Arch Otolaryngol Head Neck Surg 1998;124(11):1201–1204.
10. Tsai CY, Ueda M, Hata K, et al. Clinical results of cultured epithelial cell grafting in the oral and maxillofacial region. J Craniomaxillofac Surg 1997;25(1):4–8.
11. Bakamjian V. *Lingual flaps in reconstructive surgery for oral and perioral cancer.* Philadelphia: W.B. Saunders Company; 1990.
12. Pribaz J, Stephens W, Crespo L, Gifford G. A new intraoral flap: facial artery musculomucosal (FAMM) flap. Plast Reconstr Surg 1992;90(3): 421–429.
13. Dupoirieux L, Plane L, Gard C, Penneau M. Anatomical basis and results of the facial artery musculomucosal flap for oral reconstruction. Br J Oral Maxillofac Surg 1999;37(1):25–28.
14. Hatoko M, Kuwahara M, Tanaka A, Yurugi S. Use of facial artery musculomucosal flap for closure of soft tissue defects of the mandibular vestibule. Int J Oral Maxillofac Surg 2002;31(2):210–211.
15. Pribaz JJ, Meara JG, Wright S, Smith JD, Stephens W, Breuing KH. Lip and vermilion reconstruction with the facial artery musculomucosal flap. Plast Reconstr Surg 2000;105(3):864–872.
16. Sasaki TM, Taylor L, Martin L, Baker HW, McConnell DB, Vetto RM. Correction of cervical esophageal stricture using an axial island cheek flap. Head Neck Surg 1983;6(1):596–599.
17. Spiro RH, Sobol SM, Gerold F. Laryngeal transposition flap for reconstruction of large oral cavity defects. Laryngoscope 1983;93(1):32–35.
18. Ducic Y, Burye M. Nasolabial flap reconstruction of oral cavity defects: a report of 18 cases. J Oral Maxillofac Surg 2000;58(10):1104–1108.
19. Varghese BT, Sebastian P, Cherian T, et al. Nasolabial flaps in oral reconstruction: an analysis of 224 cases. Br J Plast Surg 2001;54(6):499–503.
20. Napolitano M, Mast BA. The nasolabial flap revisited as an adjunct to floor-of-mouth reconstruction. Ann Plast Surg 2001;46(3):265–268.
21. Martin D, Pascal JF, Baudet J, et al. The submental island flap: a new donor site. Anatomy and clinical applications as a free or pedicled flap. Plast Reconstr Surg 1993;92(5):867–873.
22. Vural E, Suen JY. The submental island flap in head and neck reconstruction. Head Neck 2000;22(6):572–578.
23. Magden O, Edizer M, Tayfur V, Atabey A. Anatomic study of the vasculature of the submental artery flap. Plast Reconstr Surg 2004;114(7):1719–1723.
24. Atamaz Pinar Y, Govsa F, Bilge O. The anatomical features and surgical usage of the submental artery. Surg Radiol Anat 2005;27(3):201–205.
25. Hurwitz DJ, Rabson JA, Futrell JW. The anatomic basis for the platysma skin flap. Plast Reconstr Surg 1983;72(3):302–314.
26. Bakamjian VY, Long M, Rigg B. Experience with the medially based deltopectoral flap in reconstructuve surgery of the head and neck. Br J Plast Surg 1971;24(2):174–183.
27. Tsuchida Y, Tsuya A, Uchida M, Kamata S. The delay phenomenon in types of deltopectoral flap studied by xenon-133. Plast Reconstr Surg 1981;67(1):34–41.

28. Sharma RK, Panda N. Old is still gold: use of deltopectoral flap for single-stage pharyngeal reconstruction. Plast Reconstr Surg 2006;117(2):691–692.
29. Andrews BT, McCulloch TM, Funk GF, Graham SM, Hoffman HT. Deltopectoral flap revisited in the microvascular era: a single-institution 10-year experience. Ann Otol Rhinol Laryngol 2006;115(1):35–40.
30. Ariyan S. Further experiences with the pectoralis major myocutaneous flap for the immediate repair of defects from excisions of head and neck cancers. Plast Reconstr Surg 1979;64(5):605–612.
31. Lin DT, Coppit GL, Burkey BB. Use of the anterolateral thigh flap for reconstruction of the head and neck. Curr Opin Otolaryngol Head Neck Surg 2004;12(4):300–304.
32. Ichioka S, Nakatsuka T, Yoshimura K, Kaji N, Harii K. Free jejunal patch to reconstruct oral scar contracture following caustic ingestion. Ann Plast Surg 1999;43(1):83–86.
33. Chang DW, Hussussian C, Lewin JS, Youssef AA, Robb GL, Reece GP. Analysis of pharyngocutaneous fistula following free jejunal transfer for total laryngopharyngectomy. Plast Reconstr Surg 2002;109(5):1522–1527.
34. Fung K, Terrell JE. Outcomes research in head and neck cancer. ORL J Otorhinolaryngol Relat Spec 2004;66(4):207–213.
35. Smith GI, Yeo D, Clark J, et al. Measures of health-related quality of life and functional status in survivors of oral cavity cancer who have had defects reconstructed with radial forearm free flaps. Br J Oral Maxillofac Surg 2006;44(3):187–192.
36. Chandu A, Smith ACH, Rogers SN. Health-related quality of life in oral cancer: a review. J Oral Maxillofac Surg 2006;64(3):495–502.

10

Concepts in Nasal Reconstruction

Elisabeth K. Beahm, Robert L. Walton, and Gary C. Burget

Introduction: The Challenge of Nasal Reconstruction

The nose dominates the central face, and when it is deformed it may cause a profound loss of the facial aesthetic and sense of self. Although a spectrum of procedures has been advocated for nasal reconstruction, several tenets are commonly accepted as being essential: (1) Autologous tissues represent the gold standard for a successful nasal reconstruction; (2) Optimal results are usually achieved through staged surgical interventions requiring several separate and temporally remote operative steps; and (3) aesthetic reconstruction of a nose is best accomplished through restoration of the missing components. Reconstruction of the nose is a complex and challenging endeavor that continues to evolve. The creation of a thin, refined nasal construct with a functional airway and an aesthetically pleasing three-dimensional shape that resists gravity and remains stable over time remains a daunting surgical challenge.

History of Nasal Reconstruction

Rhinoplasty and nasal reconstruction have been practiced for several thousand years, with origins in ancient India, when amputation of the nose was often used as punishment for a number of offenses. The highly visible nature of the amputated nose was a strong impetus for innovation in nasal reconstruction. It was quickly recognized that grafts alone were inadequate. For reconstruction of large, composite defects of the nose, well-vascularized flaps with their own blood supply were essential. The first detailed description of a nasal reconstruction appears to be the repair of an amputated nose with a forehead flap in the *Sushrutas Samhita* (circa 600–800 BC), commonly known as the Indian method *(1)*. Although there are subsequent reports of early Greeks and Romans using the forehead flap for nasal reconstruction, it was not until much later that the forehead flap came to prominence in Europe. The French used cheek tissues *(2,3)*. The Italians, such as the Branchas of Sicily in the mid 15th century, used arm flaps for nasal reconstruction, as documented and popularized by Gaspare Tagliacozzi in 1597 *(4,5)*. The first introduction of the Indian method of reconstruction to the Western world was likely a report in a London magazine in 1794 in which a central forehead flap was used to reconstruct the mutilated nose of a driver of the English army whose nose and one of his hands were amputated in India as a penalty of war *(5,6)*. Joseph Carpue's subsequent report of a midline forehead flap in 1816 appears to be a pivotal impetus for the application of this technique in Europe (Figure 10.1) *(7)*.

As experience with nasal reconstruction in Europe began, surgeons initially focused their attention on employing flaps to restore the most obvious defect, the missing nasal skin cover. As experience matured, however, it was noted that when the nasal lining was missing or not restored, the nasal reconstructions fared rather poorly. Surgeons came to realize that in additional to the external covering, functional, stable reconstructions required a multi-laminate approach including the restoration of the nasal lining and placement of a rigid substructure to support the soft tissues of the reconstruction and render the aesthetic details. Over the intervening century, a number of practitioners attempted to address these critical issues in nasal reconstruction, and their approaches were carefully reviewed and synthesized by Blair *(8)*. He is largely credited with the concept of promoting the restoration of all the components of the missing nose including the use of a forehead flap for skin cover in conjunction with well-vascularized lining and bone and cartilage structural support. Although numerous refinements including the use of free tissue transfer have been applied to nasal reconstruction, the tenets laid

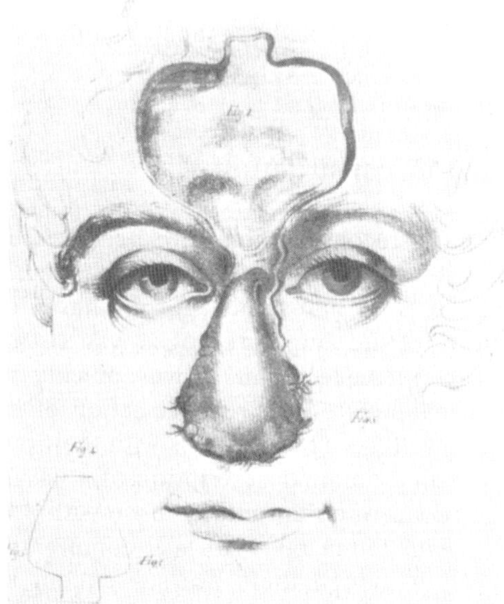

Figure 10.1. Successful transfer of a midline forehead flap for nasal reconstruction. (From ref. *4*, reprinted with permission)

down in Blair's early treatise remain the basis for modern nasal reconstruction.

Nasal Anatomy

The reconstructive requirements for correction of a nasal defect is assessed by careful study of the skin, nasal lining, and supporting skeletal structure that is specific to different anatomic regions of the of the nose. If the nose is divided by thirds, different characteristics are evident. In terms of underlying structural support, the proximal one-third of the nose rests over the nasal bones, the middle one-third over the upper lateral cartilages, and the distal one-third (the tip region) is supported by paired alar cartilages, which overlay the membranous septum. The columella is supported by the medial crura of the lower lateral cartilages. The soft triangle is the region of skin and lining that spans the apical junction of the medial and lateral crura of the lower lateral cartilage. The skin quality of the nose also varies by location. The superior one-third of the nose has thin, loosely fixed skin, whereas the tip area has sebaceous, thick, fixed skin, and the columella/soft triangle portion has thin, fixed skin.

The external appearance of the nose reflects the influence of the three-dimensional underlying cartilage/bone framework on the overlying soft-tissue cover, and this will vary in proportion to the specific characteristics of the structural and soft-tissue elements. Concavity or convexity of the nose results in reflections of light and shadow, specific to each nasal region. These visual/anatomic segments of the external nose have been defined as "subunits," a concept initiated and refined by Burget and Menick, and are used as a basis for nasal reconstruction (Figure 10.2) *(9–11)*. Regional subunits can provide anatomic borders that may guide the most aesthetic placement of scars. Scars appear most obvious when there are differences in color or in contour compared to the surrounding tissues. The transition areas between the aesthetic subunits are visually noted as areas of shadow, where placement of a scar will make it less visible to the eye. Reconstructions based on the subunit principle call for extending the defect within a particular subunit to include the entire subunit so as to obtain an optimal contour and visual appearance of the reconstructed part. Strict adherence to the subunit principle, therefore, may result in sacrifice of significant amounts of existing nasal tissue and this has emerged as a highly debatable issue in nasal reconstruction. A number of surgeons more favorably endorse the concept of "hemi-units" as an alternative *(12)*. In this approach, resection of partitions of the subunits, or "hemi-units," in areas such as the nasal sidewall or dorsum, which are linear, can favorably camouflage the juncture between flap and native nasal tissues while retaining portions of the existing native nasal subunit. Although maximal retention of the existing nasal tissues is appealing, the surgeon must be strongly cautioned against the temptation to preserve poor quality or unfavorably positioned native nasal tissues (such as those on a convex or

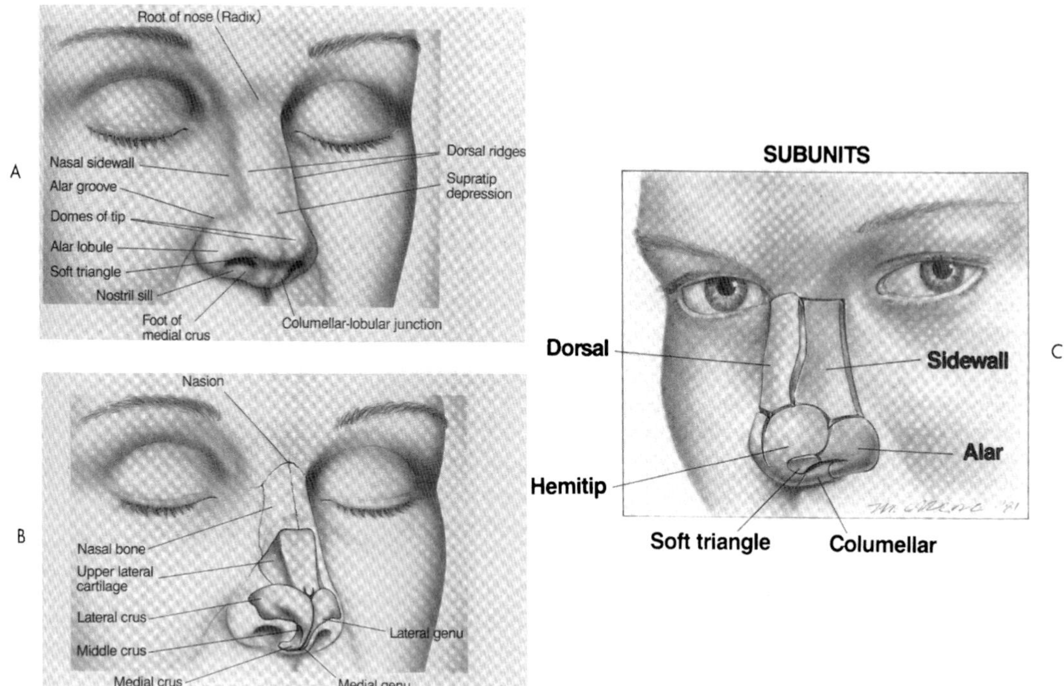

Figure 10.2. Nasal anatomy: subunits and underlying support. The nuanced appearance of the external nose results from a synthesis of the characteristics of the external skin cover and underlying skeletal support. The distinctive appearance of each anatomic region may be classified by topographic areas of light and shadow termed subunits. (From ref. *9*, reprinted with permission)

concave surface), as this may yield an unaesthetic result in the nasal reconstruction *(9–12)*.

Surgical Strategy in Nasal Reconstruction

Goals and Timing

As the nose is an extremely prominent aspect of the facial structure, even small nasal deformities may be quite noticeable. Patients want the nose restored to its original color, texture, contour, and consistency. They want a functional nose through which they can breathe, and they want all this accomplished quickly and with a minimum of inconvenience, surgical steps, and donor site deformity. Considering the foregoing, the first surgical imperative is to educate the patient and outline the necessary steps that will be required to repair the nasal defect. It is advantageous that patients visualize their nasal defects so that they fully comprehend the complexity involved and the inherent challenges of the reconstruction. A short delay until definitive repair for the patient and surgeon to appraise the deformity together is very reasonable, as closure of the wound within 4 days affords the benefits of primary wound healing as well as definitive surgical margin analysis. The surgeon must consider the individual preferences and needs of each patient and his/her particular physical, medical, and social circumstances. Patients with a high aesthetic standard will want the nose to be restored as precisely as possible, requiring the use of autologus tissue, a requisite donor site, and several operative procedures. Other patients may desire to avoid "major surgery" and accept a less aesthetic outcome. A frank discussion of the limitations of each strategy must be undertaken. The potential benefits of a nasal prosthesis should not be discounted in those patients with complex medical, surgical, or social/psychological situations or stressors. A high-quality prosthetic may be an excellent solution in patients who question the desire to proceed with the reconstruction or in whom a large surgical undertaking is impractical (Figure 10.3). Some patients, who are determined to avoid surgery initially, may return later for reconstruction. In these situations, it is important not to "burn bridges" that might be required for a subsequent reconstructive effort—such as using a forehead flap to temporarily close the wound when a skin graft or local cheek advancement flap might suffice. Despite a

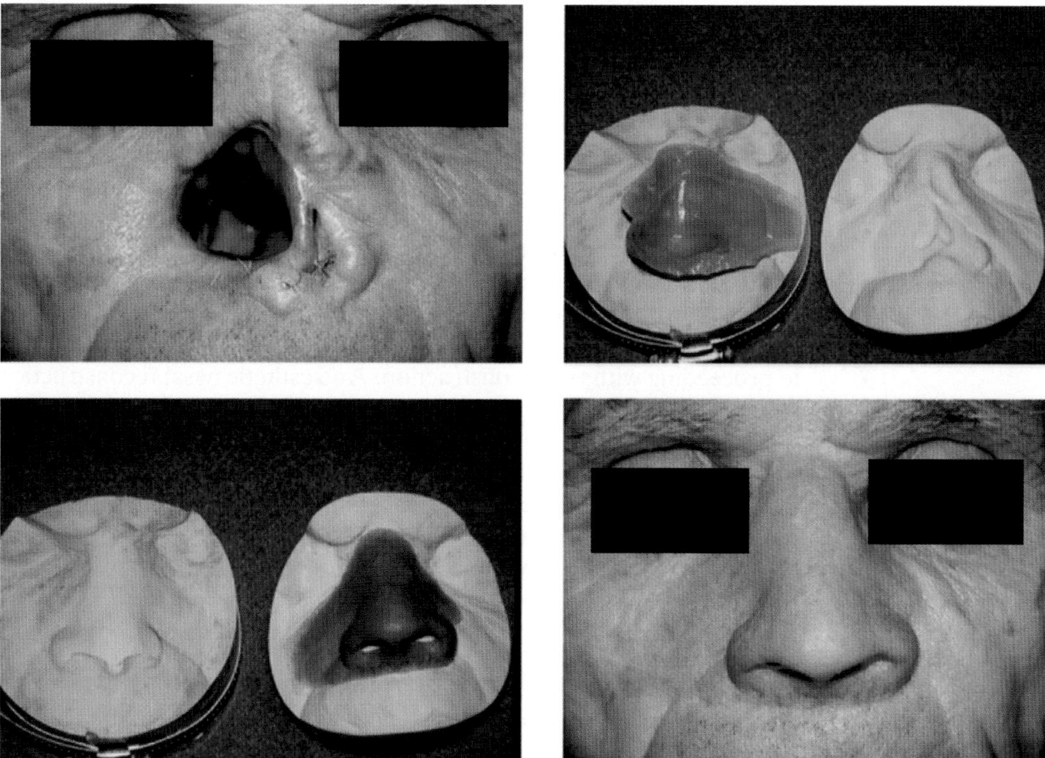

Figure 10.3. Prosthetic reconstruction of a nasal and cheek defect. A facial moulage details the dimensions and components of the facial defect, and is used as a basis for catsing and refinement of the final prosthesis. A high-quality prosthetic may be an excellent option for nasal restoration in patients who are not candidates for or unwilling to undergo autologus nasal reconstruction.

patient's desire to proceed with nasal reconstruction, there are occasional situations when reconstruction should be delayed. Following extirpation of certain cancers with a high recurrence rate or in which the histopathology suggests aggressive biologic activity, an early reconstruction may be compromised by tumor recurrence. In these cases, the reconstruction itself may require surgical removal and/or radiotherapy that could sully the reconstructive effort. There is a limited amount of available local tissues that can be used for nasal reconstruction and these should be used to their greatest effect. If there is any question as to the adequacy of the tumor resection, the potential for recurrence, or the likelihood of use of adjuvant therapies that might compromise the reconstruction, the reconstruction should be delayed. Patients with squamous cell carcinoma, melanoma, or aggressive and/or recurrent cancers are best served by an interval waiting period, usually approximately 1 year or as suggested by the surgical oncologist, before embarking on a definitive nasal reconstruction.

Assessment of the Defect

Once the decision is made to go forward with a nasal reconstruction, the surgeon should determine exactly what and how much is missing. A longstanding nasal defect will usually be distorted by contracture with reduction of the apparent size of the original defect and deviation of the normal remaining elements. Surgical release of the cicatrix and any skin graft scar and repositioning the residual nasal parts anatomically is critical for accurate assessment of the defect. Failure to do so will result in an inadequate reconstruction. The defect must be considered in terms of the missing components of lining, support and cover, as well as the location and size of the affected subunits. Attention to the integrity of the facial platform upon which the nose sits: the maxilla, cheek, and upper lip must also be addressed. Tumor extirpation of the nose often sullies the surrounding tissues, and these deficiencies must be addressed prior to proceeding with the reconstruction. An aesthetic nasal reconstruction will be rendered unaesthetic if it is malpositioned on the face or lacks the normal projection off the anterior facial plane. Defects adjacent to the nasal defect should be corrected with flaps that are separate from those used to reconstruct the nose. Using a single large flap to correct both the nasal and extranasal deformities will result in a poorly defined nose having indistinct anatomic boundaries as it relates to the face (Figure 10.4).

Formulating the Surgical Plan

A relatively simple algorithm that evaluates the nasal defect in terms of the size and extent of the missing elements and subunits can be helpful in formulating an appropriate surgical plan. The surgical plan must also consider the adverse effects of wound healing and contracture that follow reconstructive surgical injury and how these might adversely impact the final result. The missing nasal elements, therefore, must not only be restored in terms of volume and type, but also braced to withstand the

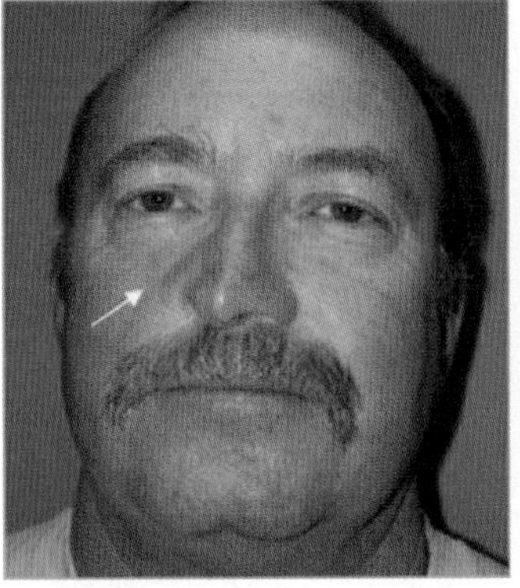
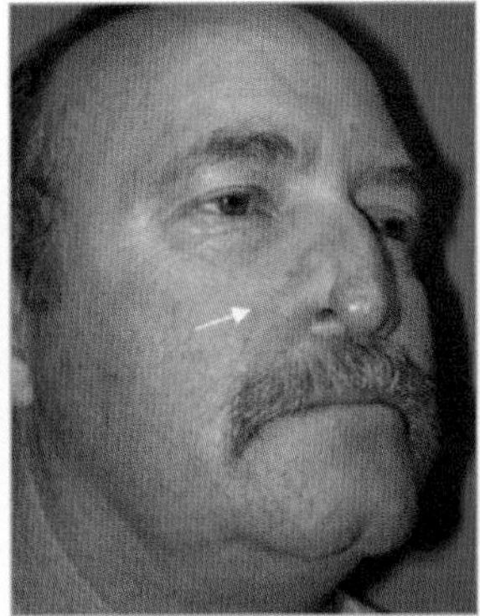
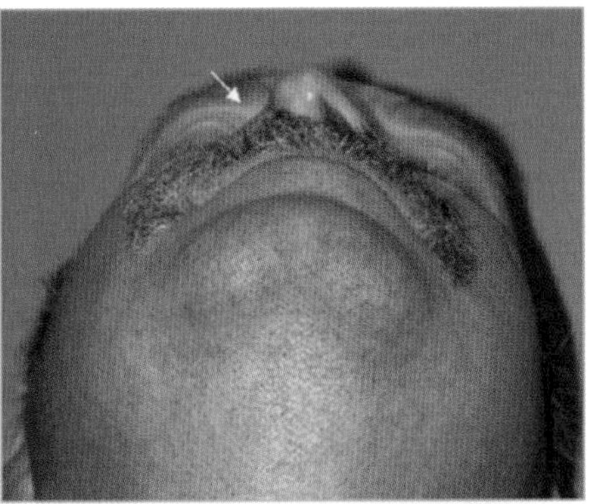

Figure 10.4. 48-year-old man with right nasal alar, sidewall, and cheek defect from melanoma initially reconstructed with a nasolabial flap. The patient presented complaining of nasal airway obstruction and a "crooked nose." Use of a single flap to reconstruct both nasal and platform elements will result in blurring of the nose into the face. Note the distortion and deviation of the nose (arrows).

anticipated scarring, contracture, and shrinkage of both the cover and lining.

Replacement of Nasal Cover

Secondary Intention

The simplest method of wound management is to leave the wound open, allowing the wound to close by secondary intention. For defects less than 5 mm in diameter, this method is quite satisfactory *(14)*. For larger defects, however, the distortion of the nose caused by wound contracture usually mitigates against this approach, especially in the ala and tip areas where distortion of the normal nasal anatomy creates asymmetry and disharmony in nasal appearance. For this reason, most surgeons prefer definitive primary wound closure with flaps or grafts as the best approach for management of acute nasal wounds.

Skin Grafts

A full-thickness graft is an excellent choice for repair of a nasal defect limited to the skin and a thin layer of subcutaneous fat provided a well-vascularized wound base is present. Full-thickness grafts are particularly suited to replacement of the thin skin of the upper one-half of the nose, but are a less ideal replacement for the nasal tip skin, because of its thickness and glandular consistency. Full-thickness skin grafts should be harvested from an area of similar color match and thickness to that of nasal skin such as the pre-auricular area or forehead. In older people, the hairless region between the sideburn and ear can provide a fairly generous graft (up to 2.5–4 cm) and is an ideal match to the skin of the upper two-thirds of the nose (Figure 10.5). Post-auricular skin is usually

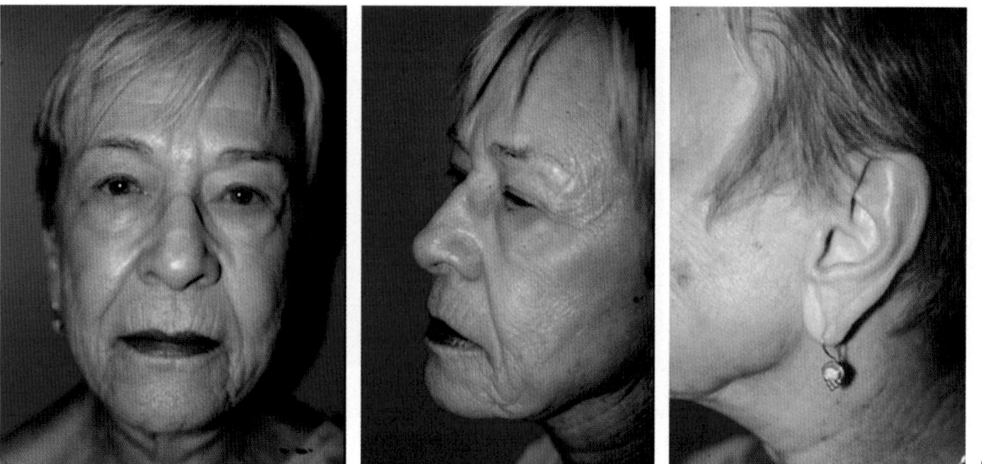

Figure 10.5. 78-year-old woman with basal cell carcinoma declined flap reconstruction and underwent reconstruction of a dorsal nasal defect with a full-thickness skin graft from the pre-auricular region **(A, B)**. A full-thickness skin graft can result in a reasonable reconstruction for the proximal two-thirds of the nose, but may result in a contour deformity in the distal nose. The pre-auricular donor site **(C)** is well healed, and favorable in elderly patients and those with some facial skin laxity.

too red and too thin for the nose. Supraclavicular skin, although plentiful, frequently takes on a shiny textured appearance, which is unlike the mat surface noted in the nasal tip. Forehead skin is an ideal color and texture match for the nose, but appears to have a higher rate of graft loss than other facial skin grafts, likely owing to its thickness. A significant part of the success of a skin graft in nasal reconstruction is meticulous preparation of the recipient site and careful application of the graft with a bolster dressing. Split-thickness skin grafts are thin, exhibit a significant degree of secondary contracture, and accordingly have very little application in primary aesthetic nasal reconstruction. Split grafts are generally reserved for temporary closure of nasal wounds when the definitive reconstruction is delayed because of planned radiotherapy or high recurrence risk.

Composite Auricular Grafts

Composite grafts of skin and cartilage from the ear possess a curvilinear shape and thin nature, which would seem ideal for nasal reconstruction, yet they have significant limitations *(15,16)*. These grafts are multi-layer composites, relying on vascular in-growth from their sides making their rate of complete survival somewhat lower than that of a regular skin graft. Classical surgical teaching has limited the use of composite grafts to a maximum size of 1–1.5 cm in diameter. Although attempts to increase the size and reliability of these grafts have included "pre-conditioning" through surgical delay, cooling, and/or windowing grafts *(17–19)*, success has been variable. The use of composite grafts in the nose is limited by their small size, a tendency for the grafts to shrink, as well as poor color match to the surrounding tissues. Composite grafts seem best used for restoration of small, full-thickness defects of the alar rims.

Local Nasal Flaps

Repair of a defect in the lower one-third of the nose is best accomplished with a flap because of the thick, sebaceous nature of the tip skin. Local flaps borrow from areas of skin laxity in the central portions and upper two-thirds of the nose or cheek, to allow flap transfer and closure of the donor site. Commonly employed local flaps include random based flaps such as the banner and bilobed flaps, which are based on the subdermal plexus, or axially patterned flaps based on a defined blood vessel. The banner flap is a simple transposition flap that uses the skin laxity in one nasal plane to derive tissue for restoration of another (Figure 10.6) *(20)*. It has been applied to defects on the nasal dorsum, but is criticized for its tendency to distort surrounding nasal landmarks, most particularly the alar margin. Modifications to this flap have included a transverse nasal design that improves the alar distortion by elevating both nostrils symmetrically (rather than just one) but the degree of donor deformity has prompted most surgeons to favor use of the bilobed flap for local nasal cover *(21)*. The bilobed flap, also a random dermal based flap, distributes the donor deficit along two separate transposition points' axis to permit primary closure of both recipient and donor sites with less distortion of the adjacent nasal landmarks. Originally described by Esser, this flap has been modified by a number of surgeons. Zitelli proposed removal of the burrows triangle that stands in path of the arc of rotation of the first element of the flap, and minimizes the "dog ear" contour deformity that results from the transposition *(22,23)*. These flaps should

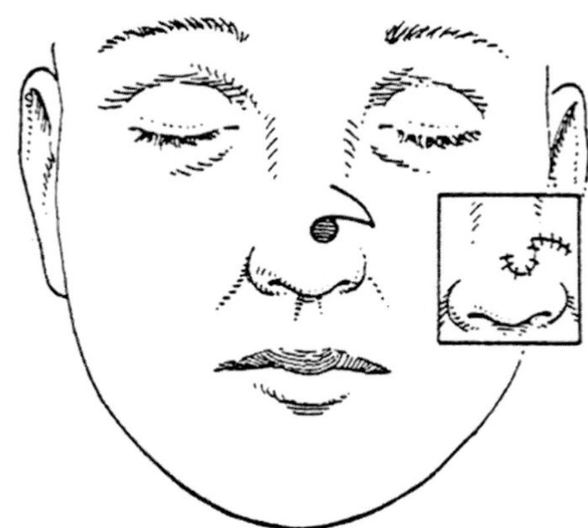

Elliott's banner flap

Figure 10.6. The banner flap is a transposition flap. Local nasal flaps, based on either a random or axial blood supply, may be used to resurface small nasal defects. The banner flap is a transposition flap. These flaps are of particular use for defects of the distal nose, where a skin graft often renders a poor aesthetic option owing to a contour deficiency. Inset demonstrates appearance of flap after transfer and closure of donor site. (Reprinted with permission from ref. *20a*).

generally be used in defects less than 1.5 cm in diameter to avoid distortion of the nose, especially in the lower one-third of the nose where the tissues are less mobile (Figure 10.7).

Slightly larger nasal defects (up to 2 cm) can be closed with axial based "dorsal nasal flaps." Rieger's dorsal nasal flap is based laterally on the angular vessels. These vessels will support a skin flap nearly the size of

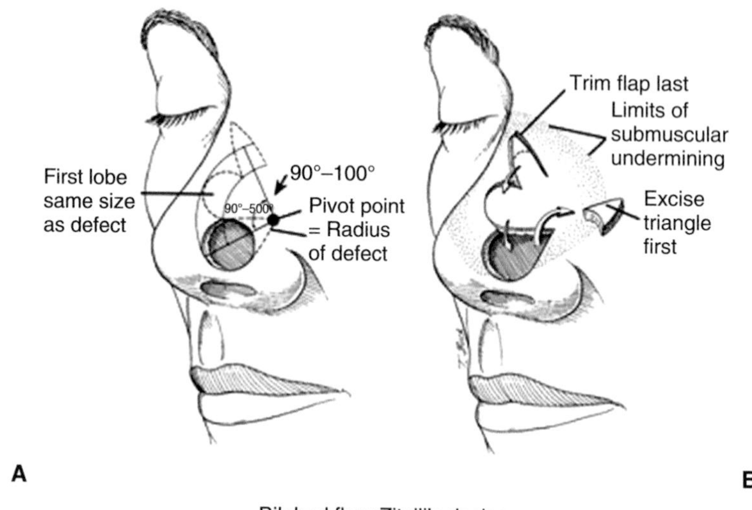

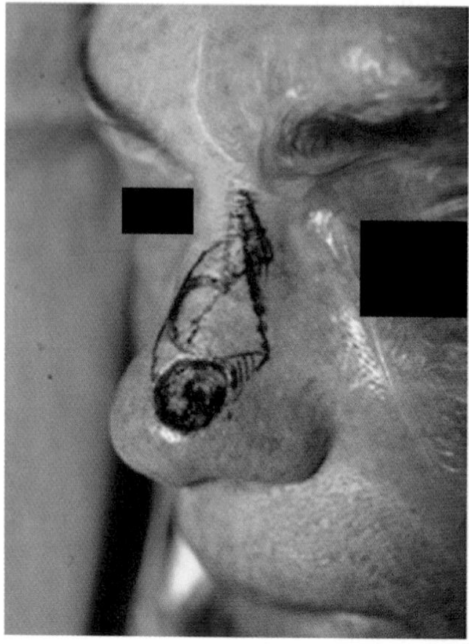

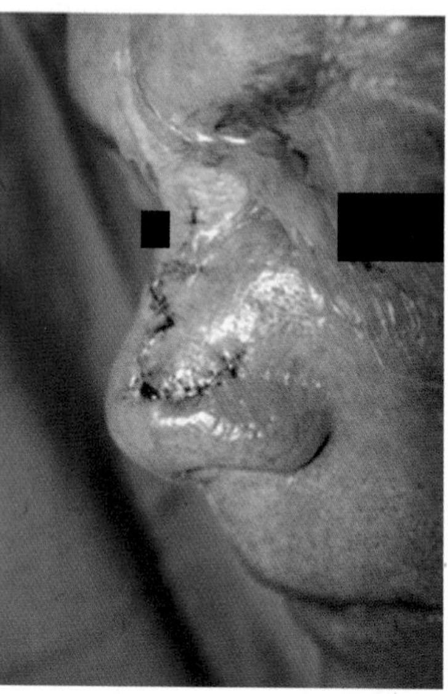

Figure 10.7. Bilobed flap. Zitelli's design **(A, B)** removes the burrows triangle initially to improve the ease of flap rotation and minimize donor-site contour deformities. The bilobed flap is best used in defects greater than 1.5 cm **(C, D)**. Precise measurement and aggressive undermining will facilitate flap rotation and inset. Design of bilobed flap for 1-cm skin defect on left nasal tip **(C)**. Appearance of flap after inset and closure of donor site **(D)**. Centripetal scar contraction may result in "pincushion" deformities of the curvilinear scars and require secondary revision. (**A, B:** Reprinted with permission from ref. *53*).

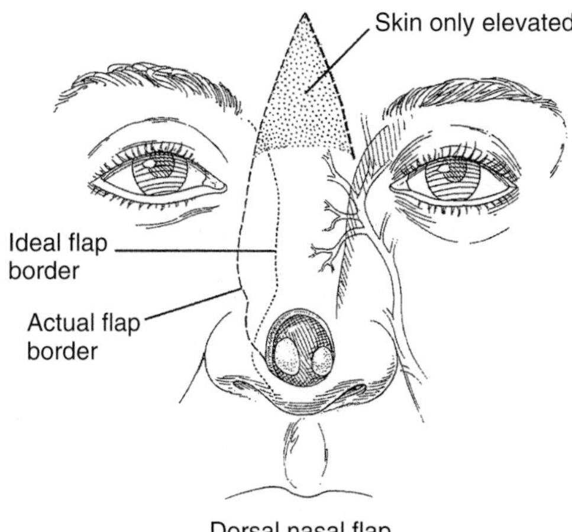

Figure 10.8. Dorsal nasal flaps are based on an axial vessel and may cover defects up to 2 cm. Donor scars will lie across critical subunits such as the nasal tip, and this may be less than ideal. (Reprinted with permission from ref. *53*).

the entire nasal dorsum, although rotation of the flap into defects inferior to the nasal tip is limited by the pedicle *(24)*. A modification of this flap, the frontonasal flap, has a similar vascular base, but is carefully backcut near the medial canthus to facilitate advancement (Figure 10.8) *(25)*. These flaps are best designed along the borders of the dorsal and tip subunits, but scars will by necessity run across the nasal tip, where they may be quite visible. (Figure 10.9). Dorsal nasal flaps are not suited to defects that extend to the columella or cross the ala because of the contour deformity they will create.

Local nasal flaps, while affording single stage closure of the defect, may distort critical nasal landmarks, such as the alar margins. Additional scars are created on the nose and there can be contraction and formation of trap-door or "pin cushion" contour deformities with these flaps, which will often require secondary debulking or geometric rearrangement to obtain an aesthetic outcome.

Regional Flaps

A regional and/or distant flap will be required for defects characterized by loss of a significant amount of subcutaneous fat, large size, or composite defects involving the nasal lining.

Cheek flaps

Nasal sidewall defects can be nicely closed with cheek advancement flaps. These flaps have been frequently used for lateral nasal defects up to 2.5 cm in the elderly patient with lax cheek skin. Care should be taken to respect the transition between the cheek and nose, and secondary procedures may be required to define the alar crease or nasal-lip-cheek interface. The cheek advancement flap can be quite effective in providing correction of an adjacent cheek or lip defect to re-establish the nasal platform, upon which the reconstruction will be based (Figure 10.10).

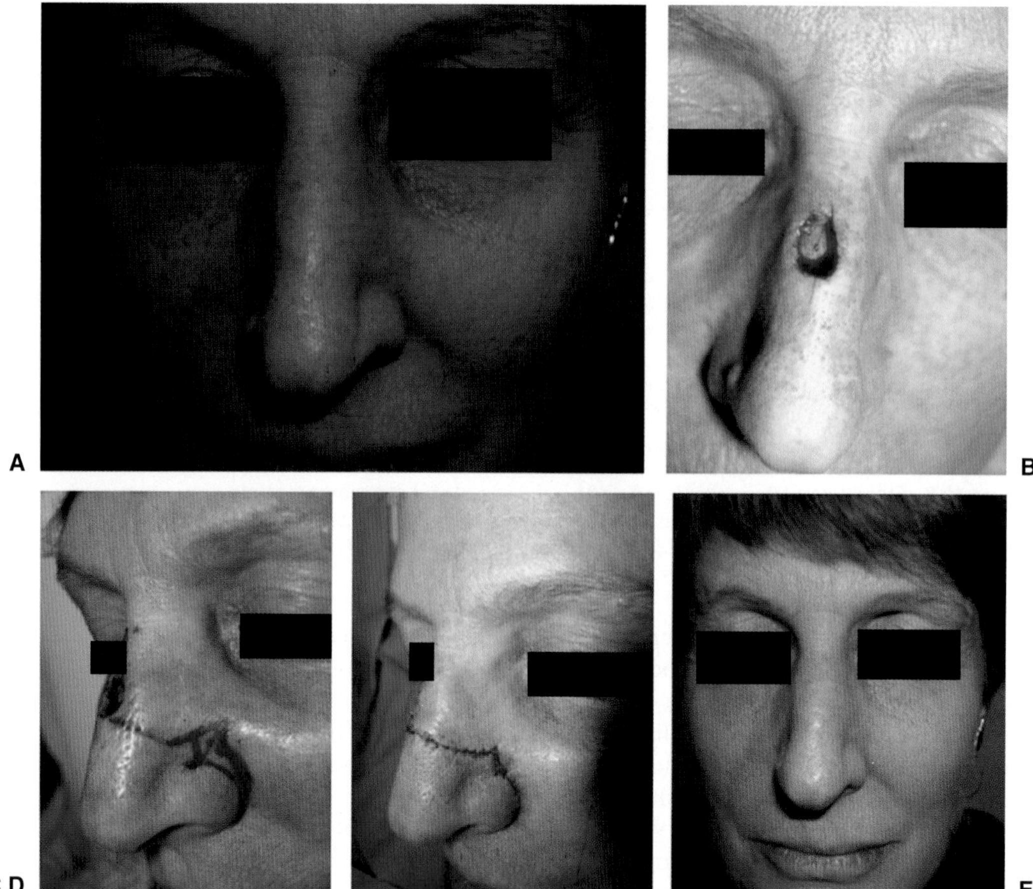

Figure 10.9. 50-year-old women with dorsal nasal defect after excision of a basal cell carcinoma. Pre-operative nasal appearance **(A)**. Defect after excision of nasal dorsal lesion **(B)**. Dorsal nasal flap design, advancing "dog ear" into alar groove **(C)**. Immediate post-operative result **(D)**. 10-month post-operative result with preservation of nasal contour **(E)**. Designing local nasal flaps with scars that lie favorably in an aesthetic unit such that the nasal dorsal lines will result in an improved post-operative appearance.

Nasolabial flaps

The nasolabial flap (also known as the melolabial flap) is a commonly used flap in nasal reconstruction. It is located in close proximity to the nasal defect, and the donor scar can be hidden in the nasolabial crease. The flap is based on perforating vessels from the facial and angular arteries that perforate the levator labia muscle near the ala and form a rich vascular plexus (Figure 10.11). Its design may be based superiorly or inferiorly and transferred as a two-stage pedicled or a single-stage island flap *(2,3,26–28)*. The superiorly based flap is more commonly used for nasal reconstruction. To maximize the appearance of the donor site, it is important to accurately identify the full extent of the nasolabial crease with the patient in the sitting position prior to the induction of anesthesia. Designing the medial edge of a superiorly based flap 1–2 mm above the nasolabial crease will precisely position the donor site scar in the

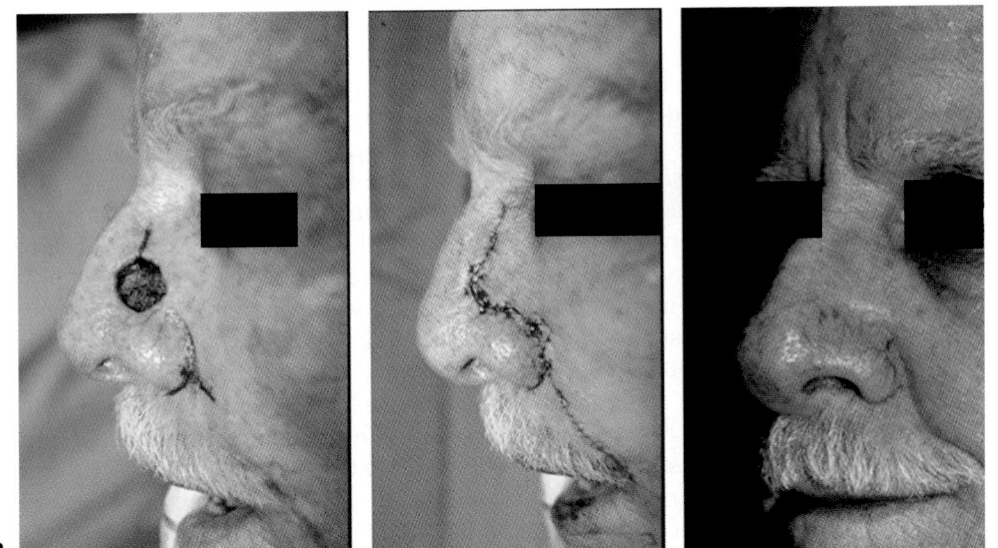

Figure 10.10. 72-year-old man nasal sidewall defect after excision of a basal cell carcinoma. Cheek advancement flaps may be used to resurface lateral nasal defects, especially in elderly patients and/or those with prominent nasaloabial folds and adequate skin laxity. Lateral nasal sidewall defect after tumor removal. Design for flap advancement with precise delineation of nasolabial fold **(A)**. Immediate post-operative result **(B)**. 24-month post-operative result **(C)**.

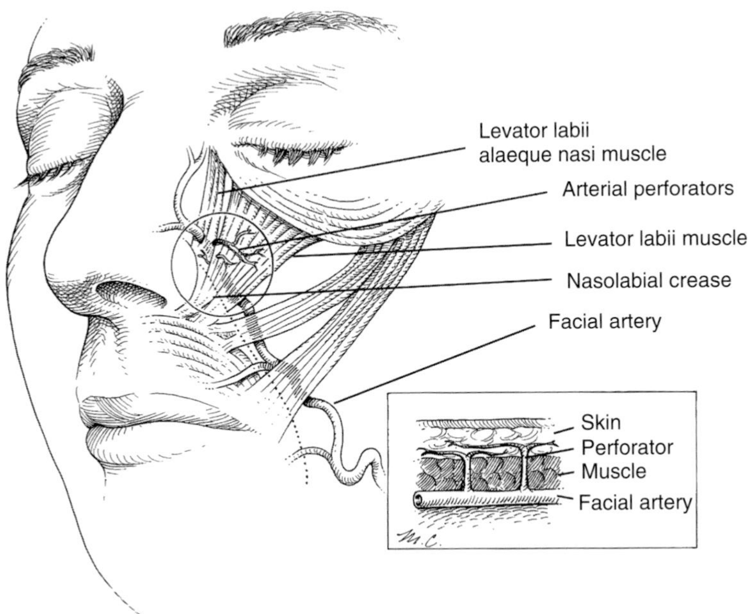

Figure 10.11. Anatomy of the nasolabial flap. Perforating vessels from the facial and angular arteries create a rich vascular plexus, allowing the nasolabial flap to be harvested as a pedicled or island flap. (Reprinted with permission from ref. *53*).

crease. In young patients, the nasolabial scar may stand out prominently on a smooth face. Conversely, older patients may exhibit flattening of a previously deep nasolabial fold after flap harvest and may request a contralateral skin/fat resection to improve the facial symmetry. The most limiting aspect of the nasolabial flap is the fleshy, soft nature of cheek tissue, which causes the flap to take on a somewhat bulbous or "biscuit" like appearance with healing and contracture particularly when used for defects of the tip or nasal side wall. This can be used to advantage in reconstruction of a rounded structure such as the ala, but it highly problematic in most other settings. The vascular supply of the flap may not be robust, especially in smokers or in patients who have undergone previous radiation. Elevation of a one-step subcutaneous-based island flap must be approached with caution, as it does often compromise the vascularity of the flap. This modification should not be attempted if there is any question as to flap reliability. Patients should generally be prepared for a series of operative intervention to achieve an aesthetic result in nasal reconstruction, and the nasolabial flap is no exception. Balancing the volume and the quality of the tissue and the donor site, the nasolabial flap is best employed in nasal reconstruction for patients with prominent nasolabial folds who have defects limited to the nasal ala. If the defect incorporates adjacent regions, such as a portion of the tip or nasal sidewall, a forehead flap is clearly a better choice (Figure 10.4). Because it demonstrates a superior reliability, greater applicability, larger tissue volume, and excellent color and texture match, the forehead flap it is the preferred donor site for most larger nasal defects and especially those involving the tip and adjacent combined subunits.

The forehead flap

Forehead flap anatomy and flap design: The forehead is a highly vascular region supplied by an interconnecting arcade of the supraorbital, supratrochlear, infratrochlear, superficial temporal, dorsal nasal, and angular vessels (Figure 10.12). The ancient Indian method of nasal reconstruction used a central forehead flap (Figure 10.1) *(29,30)* based on the vascular plexus created by these vessels. Though still used, the median forehead flap design limits pedicle length and has a less robust vascular circulation as it lacks an axial vessel *(31–33)*. The axial paramedian forehead flap incorporates a vertical arterial branch of the supratrochlear artery and is the most reliable method of transferring forehead tissue for nasal reconstruction. Accurate flap design is the most critical step in employing a forehead flap for nasal reconstruction. For hemi-nasal reconstructions, the contralateral normal side of the nose is used as a reversed template for the missing parts (Figure 10.13). If the opportunity arises, a preoperative moulage of the intact nose and face provides an excellent model upon which a template can be based. For delayed reconstructions, a moulage can be used to approximate the size and configuration of the missing parts. The rough template is then further honed following recreation of the surgical defect and returning the intact nasal elements back to their original anatomic positions. The flap template is finalized after all the necessary layers of lining and support for the nasal construct are in place. (Figures 10.14 and 10.15). Tin foil used in suture packaging

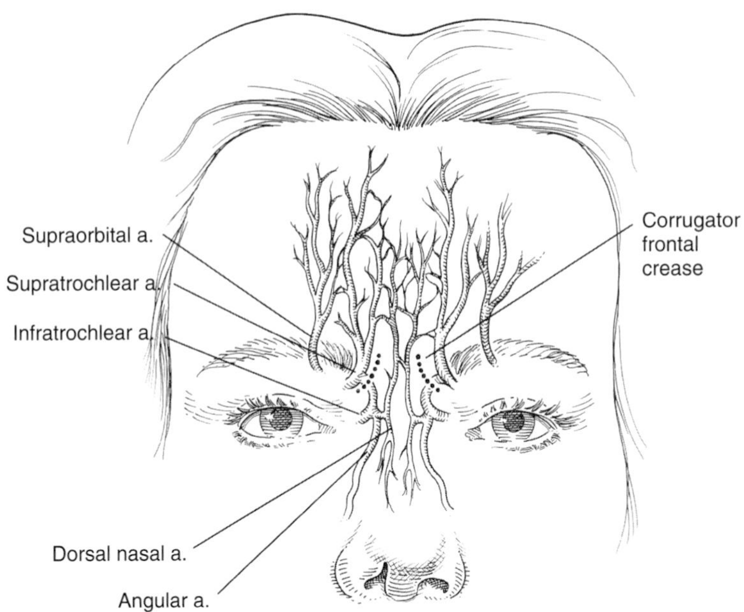

Figure 10.12. Vascular anatomy of the forehead flap. The vascular plexus created by the supraorbital, supratrochlear, infratrochlear superficial temporal, dorsal nasal, and angular vessels forms the basis for the median and paramedian forehead flaps. The paramedian flap, designed ipsilateral to the nasal defect, incorporates an axial vessel and provides the most reliable flap configuration. (Reprinted with permission from ref. *53*).

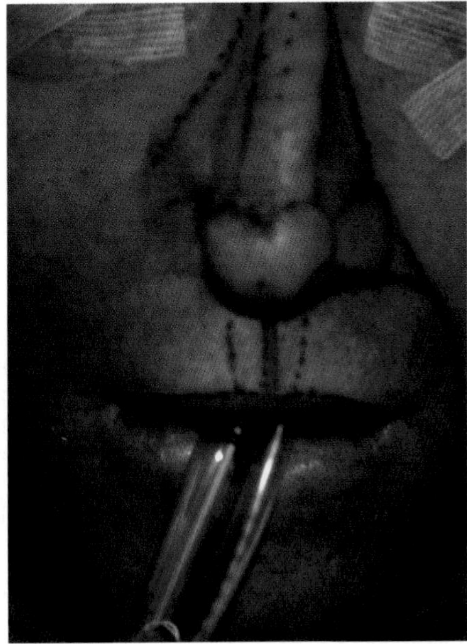

Figure 10.13. The patient in Figure 10.4 is seen prior to his forehead flap reconstruction; the nasal subunits are marked out, using the contralateral (unaffected) side as a template for the missing ala, sidewall, and cheek defects. Note that the prior nasolabial flap, which has distorted his nasal form, will be surgically released to re-establish the defect prior to forehead flap design and transfer.

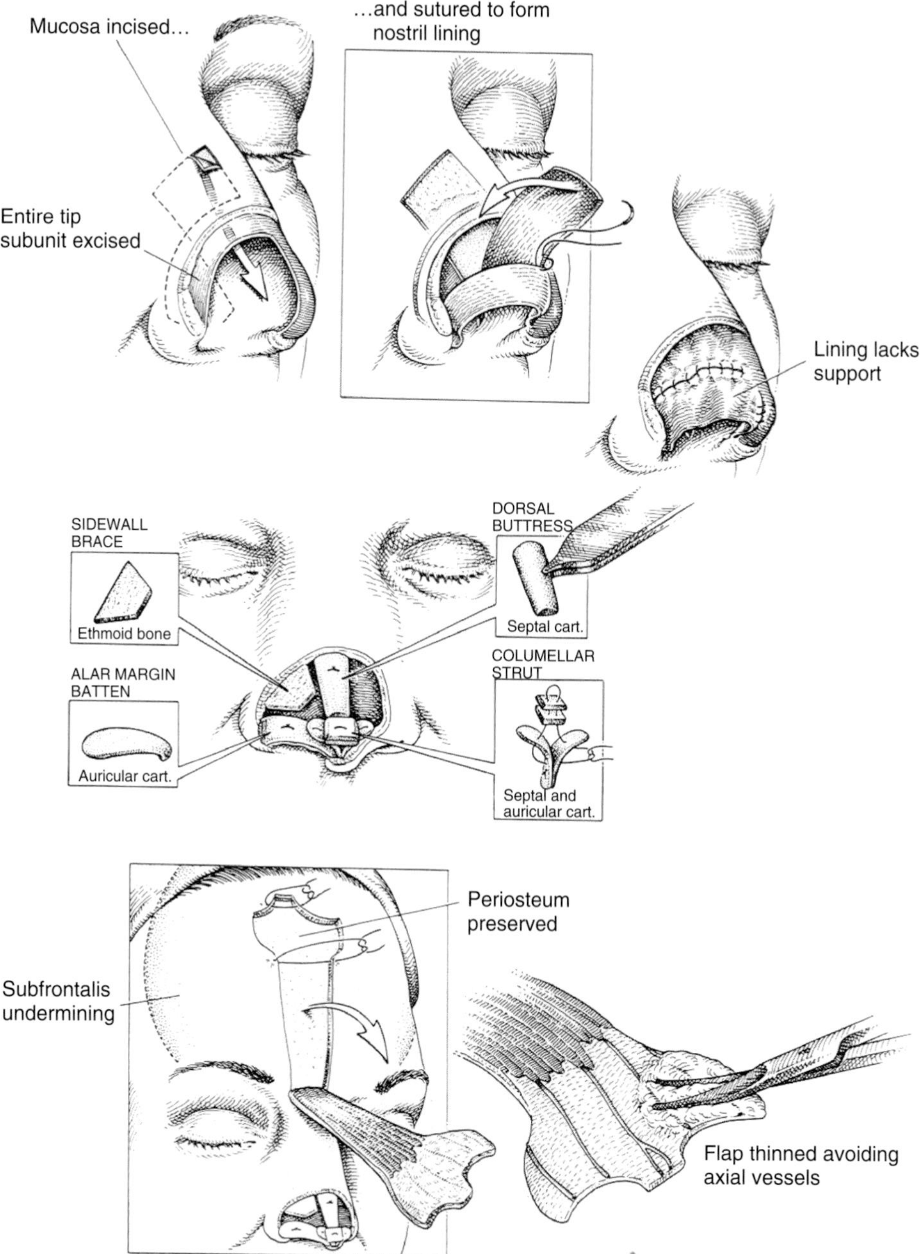

Figure 10.14. Reconstruction of a full-thickness nasal defect. Ipsilateral septal mucosal and vestibular flaps provide the lining. Sidewall, alar, dorsal, and tip cartilage grafts are fashioned for substructure support. External coverage is achieved with an ipsilateral paramedian forehead flap. The adjacent scalp may be undermined to assist in closure of the forehead. The frontal periosteum must be preserved during flap harvest to ensure aesthetic donor site closure by secondary intent in the superior forehead where primary closure may not be possible. Although the frontalis muscle should be retained with the flap proximally to maximize its vascularity, the distal 1.5 cm of the flap may be thinned in a non-smoking patient. (Reprinted with permission from ref. *39*).

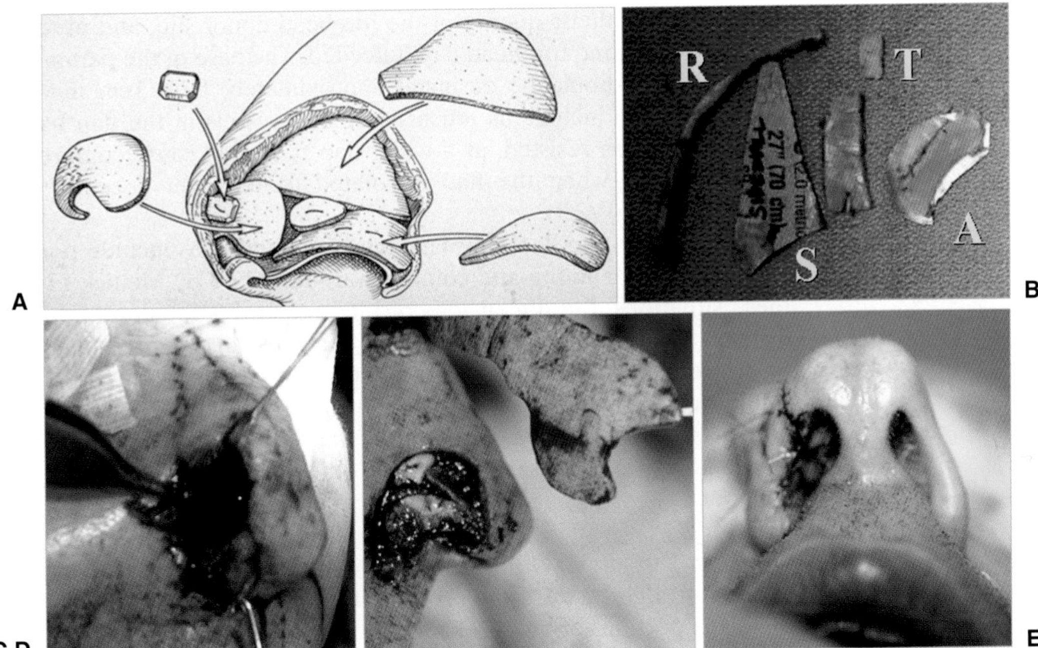

Figure 10.15. Substructure grafts are used to define the reconstruction and brace the construct against scar contracture. Diagrammatic illustration of the spectrum of substructure grafts used in the nasal tip **(A)**. Foil templates are used to precisely shape the component cartilage grafts **(B)**. Rim (R), nasal sidewall (S), alar subunit (A), and tip grafts (T) were fashioned from autologous rib. Unilateral full-thickness defect with intranasal flap for lining to support the cartilage grafts **(C)**. The ipsilateral paramedian forehead flap to cover the subunit grafts, which are secured to the underling nasal lining, restoring the nasal airway and tip position **(D)**. Intraoperative sub-mental vertex view of first stage forehead flap nasal reconstruction of defect. **(E)**. (Patient case continues from Figures 10.4 and 10.14).

works nicely as a medium for the flap template. Once created, the foil pattern is reversed, flattened into two dimensions, and oriented on the forehead overlying the central axis of the branches of the supratrochlear artery. The course of the supratrochlear artery is easily identified using a hand-held Doppler device. An ipsilateral flap permits the maximum arch of rotation. A left-sided flap should rotate clockwise, and a right-sided flap, counterclockwise. The arc of rotation of the flap should be carefully measured from the base of the flap, placed at the level of the arch of the brow. The rotation point of the flap can be extended inferiorly to gain further reach via meticulous dissection in the subperiosteal plane. Inclusion of the hair-bearing scalp with the flap is often necessary in a patient with a relatively short forehead, and/or in a distal nasal defect involving the columella. The hair can be depilated during flap harvest in a non-smoking patient by thinning the distal 1–1.5 cm of the flap or it can be removed at a later juncture (Figure 10.14). If any doubt exists, it is best to delay thinning to a subsequent revision. Attempts to gain added flap length by designing the flap obliquely on the forehead significantly increases the risk of tissue necrosis of the flap, adversely impacts the aesthetic quality of the forehead donor site, and precludes harvest of a second forehead flap if needed. The base of the paramedian forehead flap should be designed approximately 1.2–1.5 cm in width. The impulse to include as much tissue and vessels in the flap base as possible must be resisted, as a wider flap base may cause compression of the pedicle when the flap is rotated (noted over a century ago by Dieffenbach) *(2,3)*.

Occasionally, the flap template can be extended to include portions of the vestibular lining and columella as described by Menick *(34)*. In these situations, the dimensions of the missing vestibule are added as distal extensions to the alar margins of the external cover template. The lining extension is made larger than needed to accommodate a relaxed folding during inset to avoid compromising the dermal perfusion of the distal flap elements. Subsequent tailoring and debulking of the alar margins is necessary to achieve the desired dimensions of the construct.

Forehead flap farvest: Once the flap design has been finalized, flap elevation is straightforward and proceeds from distal to proximal. Although the distal portions of the forehead flap (tip, alae, and columella) may be harvested without inclusion of the frontalis muscle, this is not true for the more proximal portions of the flap, as the axial blood vessels supplying the flap course through this muscle *(34)*. The forehead flap is elevated without infiltration of epinephrine-containing solutions so as to avoid vasoconstriction of the axial vessels, which might compromise the ability to assess flap viability during inset. Marking a few transverse lines across the forehead prior to flap harvest will avoid distortion of forehead landmarks, such as the eyebrows during donor site closure. The proximal two-thirds of the forehead donor site can be easily approximated, provided that a narrow flap pedicle has been harvested. The distal portion of the donor site can be reduced in size by undermining the scalp and forehead above the level of the periostium (Figure 10.14). At this juncture, it is helpful to inject the surrounding scalp and forehead tissues with an epinephrine-containing solution to limit blood loss and facilitate visualization of the closure, but only following forehead flap elevation. It is important to avoid undue tension in the donor site closure, as this may result in tissue ischemia and necrosis. The most distal portion of the donor site cannot usually be closed primarily. Provided that periosteum has been left intact over the frontal bone and it is kept well hydrated, the residual forehead defect will close by wound contraction, forehead auto-expansion, and epithelization within 6–8 weeks, and this usually provides for an excellent aesthetic outcome. For this purpose, antibiotic ointment and petroleum gauze is packed into the wound to prevent desiccation, and this dressing is changed every several days. The importance of protecting the integrity of the periosteal covering of the frontal bone cannot be underestimated, as exposed cranium will dessicate and die, resulting in a chronic open wound with exposed bone requiring secondary intervention for closure. Tissue expansion may be used to improve the forehead donor site in such instances, but this technique requires a significant time and commitment from the patient, who must endure a rather bizarre appearance during the treatment interval.

Primary tissue expansion of the forehead and forehead flap has been promoted to permit harvest of a large forehead flap with immediate primary closure of the entire forehead donor site *(35,36)*. This approach can be problematic in that an expanded forehead flap is thickened owing to the capsule formation that occurs in response to the expander, and this may complicate flap inset and adherence. If the capsule is removed, vascularity of the flap may be compromised. Following transfer of an expanded flap, the external covering also has a proclivity to shrink, thereby distorting the reconstruction *(37)*. Most experts agree, therefore, that use of unexpanded forehead tissue is the optimal method for restoration of the external nasal covering *(9,11–13)*.

Forehead flap inset and refinement: The forehead flap must be carefully inset over the lining and cartilage framework. It is imperative to avoid compromise of the flap by too tight an inset over the rigid cartilage framework (manifested by blanching of the flap). Once inset, the underside of the forehead flap pedicle is lined with a small split skin graft to close the wound, thereby minimizing crusting, drainage, and contraction. As the skin graft is wrapped around the flap base, it is inset without tension so as to avoid flap compromise.

Reconstruction with a forehead flap necessitates multiple stages for revision and refinement of the nasal construct. The subsequent reconstructive stages are performed approximately 3–4 weeks apart, which appears to be the best balance of flap vascularity, vascular integration amongst the tissue layers, and tensile wound strength. Debulking and refining forehead flap shape/contour can be initiated distally at the level of the nasal tip, ala, and/or columella, or proximally at the level of the middle nasal vault/supra tip area. During these stages, the reconstruction is thinned and refined, elevating the forehead flap at a uniform thickness at the level of the subcutaneous fat while sculpting the underlying base of the construct. A thin layer of subcutaneous fat should be kept on the flap. Failure to do so will result in undue scarring, contracture, and distortion of the flap. Retention of the flap's vascular pedicle during the shaping stage(s) is recommended in order to enhance flap vascularity *(11,13,34)*.

The number of intermediate thinning and shaping stages can be variable, will be determined by the desired outcome, and will increase in particularly challenging cases, such as those associated with free tissue transfer. Once the construct is adequately refined, the forehead flap pedicle is divided and inset. The proximal portion of the flap is returned to the forehead, restoring any portion of the eyebrow transposed with the flap back to its anatomic position. A linear rather than a curvilinear incision is recommended at the brow and the nasal dorsum to avoid a contour deformity (Figure 10.16). After division and inset of the flap pedicle, the nasal reconstruction is allowed to settle and mature for at least 3–4 months, as there will be residual edema in the construct for a prolonged period. At this juncture, the reconstruction is critically assessed and any further refinements deemed necessary can be undertaken. Late

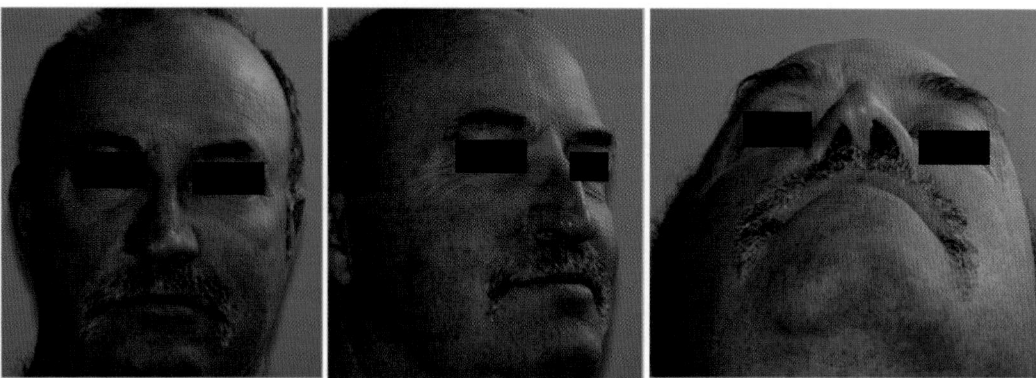

Figure 10.16. 4-year post-operative result of forehead flap reconstruction after three stages. Note the improved nasal form and airway. (Patient case continues from Figures 10.4, 10.13, and 10.15).

revisions should be conservative in order to avoid the potential of loss of a critical portion of the mature reconstruction.

Free flaps for external cover: The color match and texture of flaps harvested from sites remote to the face is poor compared to facial tissues, and this has greatly limited application of free flaps for use of the external cover in aesthetic facial and nasal reconstruction. Additionally, the robust blood supply of facial tissues compared to distant tissues enables them to endure the surgical thinning and manipulations necessary to achieve a refined and aesthetic nasal reconstruction. Remote tissues simply do not tolerate this degree of thinning without undue vascular compromise. Although we have used free flaps for external nasal reconstruction, we have limited this practice to patients in which the forehead was simply not available, such as those with extensive facial burns. The forehead flap has unsurpassed superiority for nasal cover reconstruction, affording an ideal color and textural match in a flap with a vascular supply, and we preferentially use it for this purpose.

Nasal Support

The need to introduce rigid support in nasal reconstruction has long been understood. Ollier used a piece of frontal bone attached to periosteum in a forehead flap for a nasal dorsal defect over 140 years ago *(38)*. The elements of support in nasal reconstruction should be considered in terms of their contribution to maintenance of the dimensions of dorsal height and airway as well as those necessary to effect a refined, aesthetic shape to the reconstruction.

Design of Grafts for Support

Fundamental differences exist in the skeletal requisites for support in the native nose and those necessary in nasal reconstruction. In the native nose, the nasal bones provide for rigid stability of the nasal root whereas the upper lateral and lower lateral cartilages articulate with each other allowing for considerable mobility and flexibility while retaining the three-dimensional configuration of the soft tissues they support. Once surgical trauma has been introduced, simple anatomic replacement of a missing skeletal part is inadequate for maintenance of nasal shape. The force of scar contracture is unrelenting, and a rigid skeletal framework must be introduced in both anatomic and non-anatomic fashion to render a stable nasal form. Diminished mobility of the reconstructed nose is a consequence of this necessity and is an acceptable trade off for achieving three-dimensional stability over time. In nasal reconstruction, ear and rib cartilage grafts and bone grafts are used to replace missing anatomic structural elements such as the nasal bones and alar cartilages. Non-anatomic grafts are needed to support the alar rims and to render aesthetic form, especially in the nasal tip area (Figure 10.15). Millard eloquently described the need for integral skeletal elements in the reconstructive plan in nasal surgery to maintain the shape and dimension of the soft tissues—a principle extrapolated and refined by Burget and Menick *(9,11,13,39–41)*.

Use of existing native nasal cartilages is an effective adjunct for providing skeletal support for the reconstruction. Support of the nasal midline may be nicely achieved through the use of nasal septal pivot flaps or free septal cartilage grafts for dorsal support. Pivoted nasal septal flaps are based on the septal branch of the superior labial artery, which enters the base of the septum anteriorly near the nasal spine. The composite septal/mucosal flap is back-cut posteriorly then pivoted anteriorly and secured to the remaining septum to restore the dorsal support for the middle nasal vault *(39,41,42)*. Though structurally important in the native nose, the septum proper is not generally considered a major element of the reconstructive effort. If the septum is compromised, dorsal grafts configured as "L" strut and cantilever grafts are used for midline nasal support *(30,42,43)*. The cantilever graft is articulated with and supported by the remaining nasal bone at the radix. They extend to the nasal tip without columellar support. These grafts are usually derived from calvarial bone because of its resiliency, hardness, and resistance to resorption. Despite the advantages of the calvarial graft, however, cantilever grafts are inherently unstable and may collapse at the level of the nasal tip because of lack of columellar support. To provide more stability to the reconstruction, an integrated dorsal and columellar support is essential. This can be achieved through articulation of a nasal dorsal graft with a columellar strut or by using an integrated "L" configured graft of cartilage or bone.

Missing anatomic support structures such as the lower lateral cartilages are replaced as nasal sidewall grafts made from templates rendered in the surgical setting. Non-anatomic supportive grafts such as a columellar strut and/or nasal tip grafts are used to provide support and affect certain desired nuances of tip shape. Small, match-stick-thin rim cartilage grafts provide support for the alar rims to maintain their shape and prevent collapse during inspiration *(9,39)*.

Materials for Support

The materials used to provide rigid support in nasal reconstruction are primarily autogeneous cartilage and bone. Prosthetic materials carry an unacceptably high complication rate in the nose. Bone grafts, either from the iliac crest or calvarium, may be used for the nasal dorsum and/or sidewall, but these are difficult to shape. Cartilage is a far more versatile graft material. Auricular cartilage, harvested from the conchal bowl, provides elastic cartilage that nicely replicates the curved lower lateral cartilages, but the small volume and weak, pliable nature of the cartilage limits its application in nasal reconstruction. The nasal septum provides high-quality, strong cartilage, but the septum may be unusable in cases of nasal reconstruction, and/or provide inadequate volume of graft material for the reconstruction. Rib cartilage is the favored graft material in nasal reconstruction and complex secondary rhinoplasty because of the quality and volume of graft available. The "floating" 12th rib is commonly selected because of its ease of harvest and adequacy in length for use in restoring the alar cartilages, columella, and nasal tip. This cartilage graft is harvested through with a small incision using a muscle splitting approach. Patients should be admonished that the donor site may be painful.

Following harvest, the cartilage must be carved with care, as it has a unique tendency to warp. Cartilage will warp away from the edge on which it is cut, especially if the uncut side is the outermost layer of the graft with or without attached perichondrium. To avoid warping of the graft, the concept of carving the graft with a balanced, cross-sectional area has been introduced. To understand this concept, it is useful to consider the cartilage graft as having a pressurized stromal core that is restrained by an outer cortex and perichondrial lining. Removal of the restraining forces (cortex and lining) on one side of the graft will result in expansion of the unrestrained core with bending or warping of the graft. To avoid this problem, the graft, to be straight, must be carved so that the core and restraining forces are equal on all sides. Alternatively, costal cartilage graft warping can be stifled by the placement of selected permanent mattress sutures as described by Gunter *(44)*. These sutures can also be used to effect a desired curvature to a graft that is stable over time and have proved utility in all types of nasal surgery.

In elderly patients, autogenous rib cartilage may be calcified and brittle and crack when manipulated. These grafts are frequently inadequate for use in nasal reconstruction. As an alternative to autologous cartilage grafts in elderly patients, cadaver rib cartilage grafts can be used. The utility of these grafts appears to relate to the method in which they are preserved following harvest. We have found that lyophylized, irradiated cartilage grafts are prone to softening and resorption over time and are generally unsuitable for use in nasal reconstruction. When irradiated and preserved in saline, however, cadaver rib cartilage allografts are excellent alternatives to autologous cartilage grafts in patients over 50 years of age. This cartilage is rendered acellular with radiation and has been successfully used in rhinoplasty *(45)*. Although concerns for infectious sequela from the donor and increased resorption compared to autologus cartilage have not been manifest in most studies, the long-term stability over time remains unproven.

All non-vascularized bone and cartilage grafts have the potential for resorption. The small size and generally high success rate of non-vascularized grafts in nasal reconstruction renders the need for a microsurgically augmented graft rare. Vascularized bone and/or cartilage grafts have been used in problematic cases such as repeated infection of non-vascularized grafts in a heavily irradiated setting *(46)*.

Reconstruction of Nasal Lining

Nasal lining should be considered the cornerstone of a successful nasal reconstruction. It was recognized early that unlined flaps for nasal reconstruction did not permit stability of nasal shape and form over time and nasal airway function was dismal. Historically, the majority of techniques used to create lining in a nasal reconstruction have focused on transfer of available local tissues. Application of free tissue transfer for restoration of the nasal lining, using precisely designed and fabricated flaps, has been increasing.

Facial Flaps

For small nasal lining defects, the turning in of flaps of local nasal tissue along the wound margins has been successful. A nasolabial flap, a second forehead flap, or the incorporation of extensions to a forehead flap used for nasal cover have also been used for larger nasal lining defects *(8,41,42)*. Facial flaps are generally too bulky for use in restoration of the nasal lining, as they may crowd the nasal airway and comprise the appearance of the reconstruction.

Skin Grafts for Nasal Lining

A skin graft for nasal lining is easy to harvest, avoids the bulk of a vascularized flap, but has some inherent disadvantages *(34,43,47)*. The avascular skin graft cannot support primary cartilage grafts, and must first be approximated to the undersurface of the external cover flap, usually the paramedian forehead flap, with placement of the cartilage grafts delegated to a subsequent procedure. Full-thickness skin grafts are preferred over split-thickness skin grafts for lining restoration because they result in less contraction, and, over time, can be dissected to a variable degree for the placement of cartilage graft support. Cartilage grafts, in this instance, are best inserted into the substance of the frontalis muscle of a forehead flap, deep to the skin-grafted lining. Timely placement of the cartilage grafts, usually approximately 3 weeks after the initial skin graft placement, is critical to allow for adequate time for initial skin graft take without compromising graft vascularity. Though successful in some applications, in complex or compromised defects, the skin graft may provide inadequate support of the cartilage or bone grafts, resulting in unacceptable nasal form and/or airway compromise or infection *(34,43)*.

Intranasal Flaps

Intranasal flaps from the vestibule or middle vault and septum have proven utility in subtotal nasal reconstruction *(39,46)*. These flaps are thin, do not distort the shape of the nasal construct, and have sufficient vascularity to support placement of primary cartilage grafts. These flaps may be designed axially or as random flaps, nourished by the rich vascular network of the mucosa. Nasal septal mucosal flaps can be either unilateral or bilateral, and may incorporate a cartilage component as well. A contralateral, septal cartilage/mucosal flap, based dorsally, may be passed through a cartilage window in the dorsal septum to line the middle or upper nasal vault. A unilateral septal mucosal flap can be transposed laterally to provide lining for the ipsilateral vestibule or lateral nasal sidewall alone or in combination with a bipedicled flap of vestibular skin, based medially on the nasal septum and laterally on the nasal floor (Figure 10.15). The reliability of these flaps relates to the surgical injury, prior radiotherapy, and smoking, all of which may compromise flap vascularity. Use of the nasal septum or adjacent nasal airway lining tissues for reconstruction of the missing nasal lining carries risk for compromise of the nasal airway and for destabilization and loss of support for the central nose. These issues limit the application of intranasal flaps in large and complex defects.

Free Tissue Transfer for Restoration of the Nasal Lining

Techniques for the use of distant tissues for nasal lining have recently been refined through the use of carefully designed free flaps. Free tissue transfer can permit successful nasal reconstruction in patients with compromise or absence of surrounding local tissues, who might otherwise be impossible to reconstruct. There are very few reports in the literature describing the use of free tissue transfer for restoration of the nose or nasal lining *(48–54)*. In general, the use of free flaps in nasal reconstruction has led to a poor aesthetic outcome when the flaps are used for external cover, and a poor functional outcome when they are used as lining. The limitations of flap design coupled with the poor color match and bulk of remote tissues applied for facial reconstruction largely influence these results. In our experience, precisely designed and fabricated free flaps are ideal for restoration of the nasal lining in total and subtotal nasal defects. The paramedian forehead flap, however, remains the gold standard for nasal cover.

Free flap lining design

The radial forearm flap possesses a number of characteristics that make it well suited for microvascular reconstruction of the nose and, particularly, the nasal lining. The flap has a long vascular pedicle with large caliber vessels, reliable anatomy, and it is relatively thin. The radial forearm flap is well vascularized and can be divided into multiple cutaneous islands, each based on a separate perforating vessel. The drawbacks of the flap include the relative thickness of the flap compared to the native nasal lining, the visible donor site and the relatively poor color match of the forearm skin to the facial tissues. Harvest of the flap in the suprafascial plane base results in a thinner flap, which retains excellent vascular perfusion. Careful dissection is employed to avoid injury to the sensory branches of the radial nerve. Preservation of the deep fascia on the forearm during flap harvest, and closure of the defect with a meticulously placed full-thickness skin graft from the inguinal region, have helped to maximize the aesthetic and the functional outcomes of the radial forearm donor site. Other free flaps, including the anterior lateral thigh, dorsalis pedis, scapular, and composite rib, serratus, and latissimus perforator flaps have been used for restoration of the nasal lining. Although these flaps have allowed successful restoration of the nasal lining defect, none has matched the utility of the radial forearm flap.

Prelamination of free flaps, as initially proposed by Pribaz and Fine, permits the addition of bone, cartilage, skin, and/or the mucosa to the fabrication of a composite tissue construct *(55)*. This approach has allowed for rendering of the nasal construct on the forearm, thereby minimizing the period of time in which the patient has an unsightly "surgical effort" in progress on the face, where it is difficult to camouflage. Although prelamination may increase the number of operative interventions, it appears to provide for more precise control over the reconstruction. Further documentation is required to verify the long-term effects of this technique (Figure 10.17).

Free tissue transfer for nasal lining may use a staged, pre-laminated construct or a geometrically configured, defatted free flap *(46)*. The optimal flap design depends on the components of the defect, the urgency of reconstruction, as well as the available donor site anatomy. Each patient must be individualized. The ultimate goal in these endeavors is to provide a means for creating a nasal base upon which the remaining nasal reconstruction can progress.

Free tissue transfer has proved to be an extraordinary addition to nasal reconstructive surgery. Free flaps in nasal reconstruction are most applicable to the reconstruction of the nasal lining and nasal platform. The poor color match and the limited ability to manipulate, refine, and shape microvascular flaps compared to the forehead flap suggests that tissues remote to the face must be considered a second-line for external nasal cover. The design of the free flaps for nasal lining, a distillation of our anatomic dissections and longitudinal clinical experience, is a critical adjunct in the successful application of this technology. Microsurgical reconstruction of the nose and nasal lining is a demanding and challenging intervention that continues to evolve.

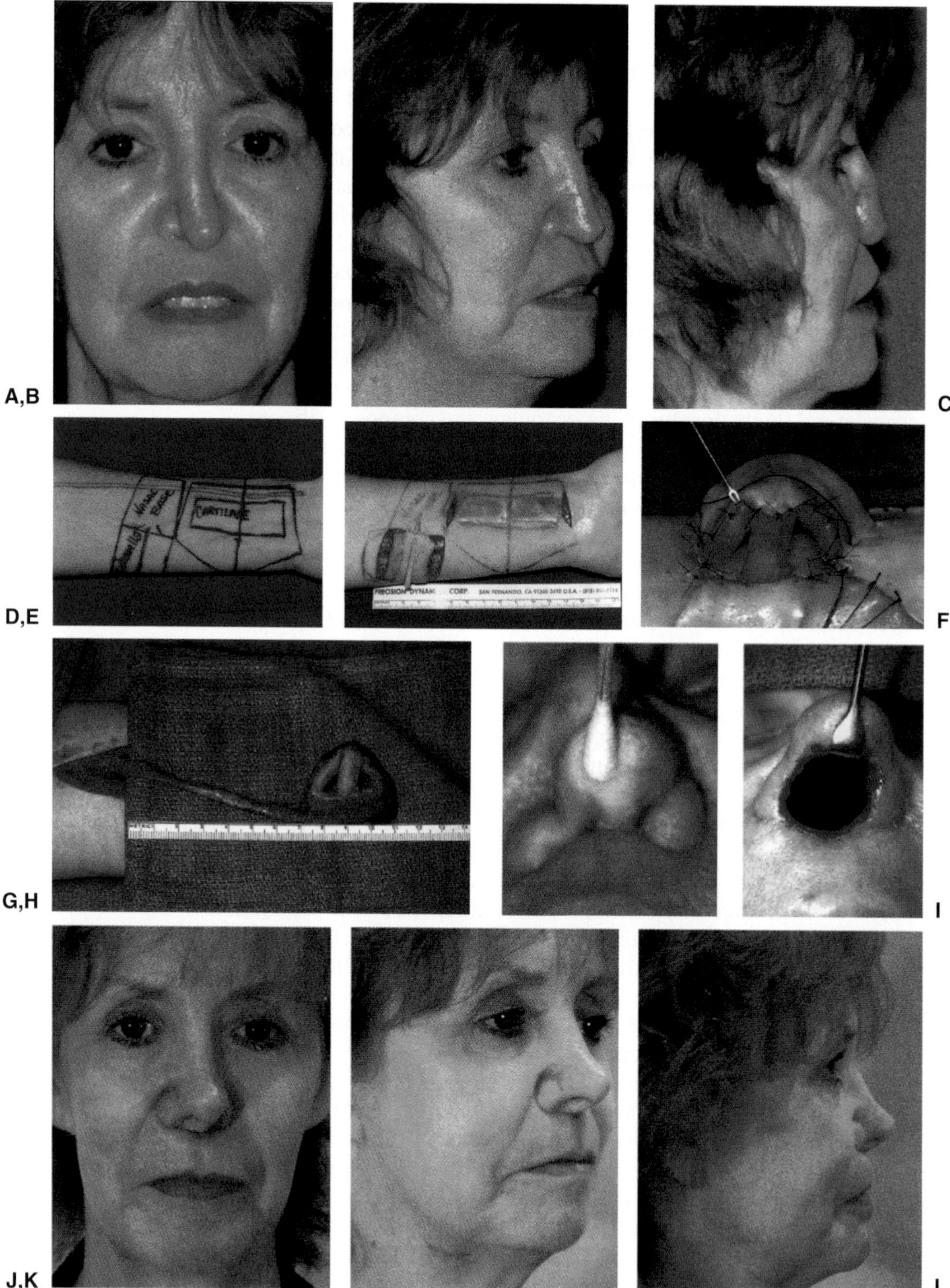

Figure 10.17. Free tissue transfer for nasal lining. A 56-year-old woman with complete nasal airway obstruction from pemphigous, failed attempted reconstruction with local flaps and grafts **(A, B, C)**. A pre-laminated radial forearm skin/cartilage flap was used to reconstruct the nasal lining, requiring several surgical delays on the forearm **(D, E, F)**. The pre-laminated flap isolated on the radial vascular pedicle before transfer to the nasal defect. **(G)**. The constricted nasal lining was released and excised **(H, I)**, and the flap inset and revascularized to the facial vessels. The patient demonstrates a patent nasal airway and improved nasal form 2.5 years post-operatively. Post-operative views **(J, K, L)**. (Figure reprinted in part with permission from ref. *48*).

References

1. Sushruta S. In: Bhishagratna KKL (ed.), *Sushruta samhita*. Calcutta: Bose; 1907–1916.
2. Dieffenback JF. *Chirurgische erfahrungen, besonders euber die viderherstellung zerstoerter theile des menschlichen coerpers nach neuen methoden*. Berlin: TCF Enslin; 1829.
3. Dieffenbach JF. *Die operative chirurgie*. Leipzig FA: Brockhaus, 1845.
4. Milstein S, Joseph J (translator). *Rhinoplasty and facial plastic surgery with a supplement on mammaplasty*. Phoenix: Columella Press; 1987.
5. Rogers, BO. The development of aesthetic plastic surgery: a history. Aesth Plast Surg 1976;1:3.
6. Mazzola RF, Marcus S. History of total nasal reconstruction with particular emphasis on the folded forehead flap technique. Plast Reconstr Surg 1983;72:408–414.
7. Carpue J. *An account of two successful operations for restoring a lost nose*. London: Longman, Hurst, Rees, Orme, and Brown; 1816.
8. Blair VP. Total and subtotal restoration of the nose. JAMA 1925;85:1931.
9. Burget GC, Menick FJ. In: Reilly T (ed), *Restoration of the nose after skin cancer. Plastic surgery educational foundation: instructional courses, volume one*. St. Louis: Mosby—Year Book; 1988.
10. Burget GC, Menick FJ. Subunit principle in nasal reconstruction. Plast Reconstr Surg 1985;76:239.
11. Burget GC. Aesthetic restoration of the nose. Clin Plast Surg 1985;12:463–480.
12. Burget GC, Menick FJ. Nasal reconstruction: Seeking a fourth dimension. Plast Reconstr Surg 1986;78:145.
13. Singh DJ, Bartlett SP. Aesthetic considerations in nasal reconstruction and the role of modified subunits. Plast Recon Surg 2003;111(2):639–648.
14. Becker CD, Adams LA, Levin BC. Non surgical repair of perinasal nasal skin defects. Plast Reconstr Surg 1991;88:768–776.
15. Konig F. On filling defects of the nostril wall. Berl Klin Woch 1902;39:137.
16. Brown JB, Cannon B. Composite free grafts of skin and cartilage from the ear. Surg Gynecol Obstet 1946;82:253.
17. Avelar JM, Psillakis JM, Viterbo F. Use of large composite grafts in the reconstruction of deformities of the nose and ear. Br J Plast Surg 1984;37:55.
18. Walton RL, Beahm EK. Use of extended composite grafts in facial reconstruction. Abstract and presentation, American Association of Plastic Surgeons 76th Annual Meeting, Microsurgical reconstruction of the nasal lining, May 1997.
19. Conley JJ, VonFraenkel PH. The principle of cooling as applied to the composite graft in the nose. Plast Reconstr Surg 1956;17:444.
20. Elliot RA. Rotation flaps of the nose. Plast Reconstr Surg 1969;44:147.

20a. Burget CG, Menick FJ. Reconstruction of the nose. In: Jurkiewicz MJ, Krizek TJ, Mathes SJ, Ariyan S (eds.), *Plastic surgery principles and practice, volume two*. St. Louis: CV Mosby; 1990:1463–1506.

21. Masson JK, Mendelson BC. The banner flap. Am J Surg 1977;13:419.
22. Esser JFS. Gestiele locale nasenplastik mit zweizipfligen lappen, decking des secundaren defeks vom ersten zipfel udrch den zweiten. Dtsch Z Chir 1918;143:385.
23. Zitelli JA. The bilobed flap for nasal reconstruction. Arch Dermatol 1989;125:957.
24. Rieger RA. A local flap for repair of the nasal tip. Plast Reconstr Surg 1967;40:147.

25. Marchac D, Toth B. The axial frontonasal flap revisited. Plast Reconstr Surg 1985;76:686.
26. Herbert DC, Harrison RG. Nasolabial subcutaneous pedicle flaps: 1. Observations on their blood supply. Br J Plast Surg 1975;28:85.
27. Heller N. Subcutaneous pedicle flaps in facial repair. Ann Plast Surg 1991;27:421.
28. Cameron RR, Latham WD, Dowling JA. Reconstruction of the nose and upper lip with nasolabial flaps. Plast Reconstr Surg 1973;52:145.
29. Gillies HD. The development and scope of plastic surgery. The Charles H. May Lectureship in Surgery, 45th Lecture. Q Bull Northwest Univ Med Sch 1985;35:1.
30. Gillies HD, Millard DR. *The principles and art of plastic surgery*. Boston: Little Brown; 1957.
31. Kazanjian VH. The repair of nasal defects with the median forehead flap: primary closure of the forehead wound. Surg Gynecol Obstet 1946; 83:37.
32. Antia NH, Daver BM. Reconstructive surgery for nasal defects. Clin Plast Surg 1981;8:535–563.
33. Converse JM, McCarthy JG. The scalping flap revisited. Clin Plast Surg 1981;8:413.
34. Menick FJ. A 10-year experience in nasal reconstruction with the three-stage forehead flap. Plast Reconstr Surg 2002;109(6):1839–1855.
35. Adamson JE. Nasal reconstruction with the expanded forehead flap. Plast Reconstr Surg 1988;81:12.
36. Kroll SS, Rosenfield L. Delayed pedicle separation in forehead flap nasal reconstruction. Ann Plast Surg 1989;23:327.
37. Bolton LL, Chandraseker B, Gottlieb ME. Forehead expansion and total nasal reconstruction. Ann Plast Surg 1988;21:210.
38. Ollier L. Application de l'osteoplastie a la restauration du nez; transplantation du perioste frontal. Bull Gen Therapeut 1861;61:510.
39. Burget GC, Menick FJ. Nasal support and lining: the marriage of beauty and blood supply. Plast Reconstr Surg 1989;84:189.
40. Millard DR Jr. Reconstructive rhinoplasty for the lower half of a nose. Plast Reconstr Surg 1974;53:133.
41. Millard DR Jr. Reconstructive rhinoplasty for the lower two-thirds of the nose. Plast Reconstr Surg 1976;57:722.
42. Gilles HD. Plastic surgery of the face. London: Oxford Medical Publishers; 1920.
43. Millard DR Jr. Total reconstructive rhinoplasty for and a missing link. Plast Reconstr Surg 1966;37:167.
44. Gunter JP, Clark CP, Friedman RM. Internal stabilization of autogenous rib cartilage grafts in rhinoplasty: a barrier to cartilage warping. Plast Reconstr Surg 1997;100:161–169.
45. Strauch B, Sharzer LA, Petro J, et al. Replantation of amputated parts of the penis, nose, ear, and scalp. Clin Plast Surg 1983;10(1):115–124.
46. Menick FJ. The use of skin grafts for nasal lining. Clin Plast Surg 2001;28:311–321.
47. Kazanjian VH. Plastic repair of deformities about the lower part of the nose resulting from loss of tissue. Trans Am Acad Ophthal Otolaryngal 1937;42:338.
48. Walton RL, Burget GC, Beahm EK. Microsurgical reconstruction of the nasal lining. Plast Reconstr Surg 2005;115(7):1813–1829.
49. Shenaq SM, Dinh TA, Spira M. Nasal alar reconstruction with an ear helix free flap. J Reconstr Microsurg 1989;5(1):63–67.

50. Upton J, Ferraro N, Healy G, et al. The use of prefabricated fascial flaps for lining of the oral and nasal cavities. Plast Reconstr Surg 1994;94(5):573–579.
51. Costa H, Cunha C, Guimaraes I, Comba S, Malta A, Lopes A. Prefabricated flaps for the head and neck: a preliminary report. Br J Plast Surg 1993;46:223.
52. Marshall DM, Wolf AI. Use of the radial forearm flap for deep, central mid-facial defects. Plast Reconstr Surg 2003;111(1):56.
53. Burget GC, Menick FJ. *Aesthetic reconstruction of the nose.* St. Louis: CV Mosby; 1994.
54. Winslow CP, Cook TA, Burke A, Wax MK. Total nasal reconstruction: utility of the free radial forearm fascila flap. Arch Facial Plast Surg 2003;5:159.
55. Pribaz JJ, Fine NA. Prelamination: defining the prefabricated flap. A case report and review. Microsurgery 1994;15:618.

11

Extremity Reconstruction

S. Baumeister, H. Levinson, M. Zenn, and L. Scott Levin

Extremity tumors are predominantly of musculoskeletal origin. Of these, soft-tissue sarcomas (STS) are more common than the bone sarcomas. STS comprise approximately 1% of all adult malignancies and 15% of all pediatric malignancies *(1)*. There are approximately 8700 new cases of STS diagnosed in the United States per year compared to 2900 cases of bone cancers (predominantly osteosarcoma and chondrosarcoma) *(2)*. The deficits that result from resection of these tumors are often large and need extensive reconstructive surgery.

Planning for extremity reconstruction begins prior to tumor extirpation. Pre-operative planning involves a multi-disciplinary team approach including medical oncologists, surgical oncologists, plastic surgeons, orthopedic surgeons, radiologists, and pathologists who determine disease staging and a treatment plan. This inlcudes pre-operative therapy, resection, reconstruction, chemotherapy, radiation, and rehabilitation. Team coordination is usually directed by a medical oncologist or oncological surgeon. The role of the plastic and reconstructive surgeon consists of the restoration of soft tissue, bony defects, and functional deficits. The most effective reconstructive plan takes into consideration the extent of disease, tumor size, and the management plan. Furthermore, prognosis, patient's desires and functional expectations need to be considered as well.

Diagnostic Work-Up

The treatment plan is determined by the extent of disease and tumor biology. The staging evaluation involves delineation of local disease and exclusion of systemic disease, usually with contrast-enhanced computed tomography (CT) scan or magnetic resonance imaging (MRI). A multi-institutional study by the Radiology Diagnostic Oncology Group (RDOG) has not shown any statistical difference between CT and MRI in accuracy of local disease staging *(3)*. Most surgeons, however, recommend MRI as the method of choice for delineating soft tissue involvement. Diagnostic

Table 11.1. Enneking Classification for the Surgical Staging of Musculoskeletal Sarcoma

Stage	Grade	Site
IA	Low (G_1)	Intracompartmental (T_1)
IB	Low (G_1)	Extracompartmental (T_2)
IIA	High (G_2)	Intracompartmental (T_1)
IIB	High (G_2)	Extracompartmental (T_2)
III	Any (G) Regional or distant metastasis	Any T

imaging should precede diagnostic biopsy to avoid confounding soft-tissue distortion that may even accompany a needle biopsy.

The technique of biopsy is critical. Mankin et al. compared pathological diagnosis of the biopsy with the final diagnosis in 597 bone sarcomas and STSs. The error rate of a varying diagnosis of biopsy and final tumor pathology was 17.8% *(4)*. The biopsy should be performed by the resecting surgeon. The principles to consider when taking a biopsy in the extremity include: (1) make a small, longitudinal incision directly over the tumor to prevent tumor spread to adjacent tissue compartments; (2) achieve meticulous hemostasis; (3) avoid placing suction drains in the wound to prevent spread of tumor cells (drains may be placed in an area that will later be resected); (4) take a biopsy sample from the tumor periphery where the tumor is most actively growing. When a pathological diagnoses is uncertain, a second opinion by a reference pathologist is recommended *(1)*.

The diagnostic work-up determines type of tumor and stage of disease. Enneking developed a classification system of musculoskeletal sarcomas in 1980 *(5,6)*. The three stages (IA/B, IIA/B, III) of his classification system consider surgical grade (histological differentiation, roentgenographic, and clinical aggressiveness), extent of local disease (extra versus intracompartmental) and the presence or absence of distant metastases (Table 11.1). His classification system is used to outline a treatment plan with surgery as the cornerstone of treatment for STS.

Tumor Extirpation

Tumor extirpation in North America is usually performed by an oncologic surgeon, and reconstruction is usually performed by a plastic or orthopedic reconstructive microsurgeon. In some centers, tumor removal may be performed by a reconstructive surgeon. In either scenario, the reconstructive surgeon must be involved in pre-operative planning to assess the extent of the planned resection, discuss the role of pre- or post-operative radiation, determine the expected functional loss, and discuss reconstructive options. Pre-operative evaluation often determines whether limb salvage is possible. At times, amputation is recommended when the salvaged extremity would be painful or non-functional.

On rare occasion, the decision between reconstruction or amputation may need to be determined intra-operatively.

Limb Salvage Versus Amputation

Tumor resection aims for complete tumor excision by radical resection. However, radical resection does not exclude limb salvage. Several questions are raised in deciding whether to preserve a limb. Is it easier to obtain a wide margin of resection with an amputation? Is it ethical to provide limb salvage? What margins are adequate to prevent local recurrence and maximize long-term survival?

Resection Margins

Resection margins should be free of tumor to prevent local recurrence *(7–11)*. The optimal "negative"-sized margin for local control is unclear. Some authors found that local recurrence was not affected by the extent of negative margins (≤1 mm or >1 mm) *(7,12)*. McKee et al. on the other hand showed that resection margins of 10 mm or larger independently predict a lower rate of local recurrence *(13)*. Other authors recommend 2-, 3- or 5-cm negative margins for adequate resection *(14,15)*.

Factors that determine the required resection margin are the positioning within the compartment, involved natural barriers, concomitant radiation or chemotherapy, and tumor grading *(14)*. It is well known that sarcoma within a compartment spreads more rapidly along the longitudinal border of the fascia than the transverse border, bridging the fascia. Therefore, the absolute distance of healthy tissue around the tumor in millimeters does not give adequate information to ensure adequate resection. A 1- to 2-mm resection margin transversally, including the fascia, may be better than a 5-mm longitudinal margin within the fascia or bone marrow space. If a resection is performed outside the compartment, and an intact fascia is between tumor and healthy tissue, this is considered an adequate resection despite the absolute "short" distance from the tumor. If the resection is performed within a compartment or extracompartmental (subcutaneous or cutaneous) area, resection margins of up to 3–5 cm are recommended *(15)*.

Natural barriers such as fascia, joint capsule, tendon sheath, epineurium, vascular sheath, or peritoneum were classified by Kawaguchi et al. into "thick" and "thin" barriers and converted into absolute distances in millimeters (e.g., "thick" barrier equivalent to 3 cm) *(14)*. Thereby, in resecting a tumor that is adjacent to a thick barrier such as the iliotibial band, it may be adequate to have less than a 3-cm margin. Kawaguchi also differentiates between high-grade and low-grade sarcoma and advocates larger resection margins in sarcomas that do not react to pre-operative chemotherapy (3-cm resection margin) compared to those that do react to chemotherapy (2-cm resection margin). Kawaguchi thereby describes commonly accepted principles, but the distances of resection he recommends have not been confirmed by evidence-based data.

For intra-articular tumors, is it generally accepted that whole joint resection is necessary. It is further agreed upon that tumors reactive to neoadjuvant chemotherapy or radiotherapy might need narrower margins. Routine lymphadenectomy is not usually performed, as sarcoma predominantly metastasizes hematogenously. Following these guidelines, classical compartment resections are rarely performed and the compartmental border is more important in the transverse direction than in the longitudinal direction. The lack of a consensus defining an adequate negative resection margin in millimeters becomes appearent by Enneking's differentiation into four types of resection *(5,6)*. Although published in 1980, it is still valid today and considers a wide or radical excision as sufficient. Resection margins are defined as: (1) intralesional, in which the dissection passes within the lesion; (2) marginal, in which the plane of dissection continues through the pseudocapsule or reactive tissue about the lesion; 3) wide, in which a surrounding cuff of normal tissue is removed but within the diseased compartment; and 4) radical, in which normal tissue outside the involved compartment is removed.

Several studies have highlighted that limb-sparing surgery is associated with a higher rate of local tumor recurrence than with amputation *(16,17)*. It is controversial, however, whether local recurrence affects survival. Some authors believe local recurrence predicts metastatic disease and therefore survival *(18–20)*, in which case amputation would be preferable to limb salvation. On the other hand, most authors agree that systemic disease and survival is independent of local recurrence *(8,17,21–23)*. Ramanathan et al. reported that local recurrence is not a direct cause of distant metastases, but that it is a marker of a higher risk group to develop metastases. Gaynor et al. reported that tumor size (<5 cm, 5–10 cm, or >10 cm), histologic grade (low, intermediate, or high), and time to local recurrence (>36 months, 6–36 months, or <6 months), but not local recurrence, predicts distant metastases and overall prognosis *(24,25)*. Therefore, limb salvage surgery has a higher rate of local recurrence, but not a negative effect on overall survival *(8,16,17)*. Thus, the most important consideration in deciding between limb salvage versus amputation is the comparison of functional outcomes and quality of life. In the upper extremity, limb salvage achieves a far better functional outcome than does amputation. However, in the lower extremity the comparison between limb salvage and amputation is more complex.

Renard used the rating system of the American Musculoskeletal Tumor Society (MSTS) to compare functional outcomes in patients with amputation versus limb preservation for extremity bone sarcoma *(26)*. He found there was a significantly better function in the limb salvage group compared to the ablative group. However, other authors dispute the benefits of limb salvage, showing comparable functional outcome after limb salvage or amputation *(27)* or only minimal functional improvement in the limb salvage group *(28,29)*. Postma et al. showed patients with limb preservation had more physical complaints than amputees *(30)*.

Quality of life can be measured by multi-dimensional factors including social, psychological, physical function, and disease- and treatment-related symptomatology *(29)*. These factors involve assessment of health, employment, finances, recreation, partnership, peer relations, self-perception, sexuality, social relations, housing, pain, level of activity, emotional acceptance, walking ability, gait, and use of orthopedic devices. Questionnaires that can be used for this complex assessment are the EORTC QLQ-C30 questionnaire *(28,31)*, the Life Satisfaction Questionnaire (FLZ) the Musculoskeletal Tumour Society Score (MSTS) *(28,33)*, the Toronto Extremity Salvage Score (TESS) *(34)*, the Short-form-36 (SF36), or the Reintegration to Normal Living (RNL) *(34)*. In general, quality of life measurements have shown similar outcomes between limb salvage and traumatic amputation *(27,28,34–37)*.

There are several confounders in comparing limb salvage with amputation. Most studies enroll limited numbers of patients, and limb salvage procedures vary significantly in their complexities. For example, there is a significant difference between a complex soft- and bone-tissue defect including a resected ischial nerve or a joint reconstruction using an endoprosthesis. Furthermore, newer free microsurgical reconstruction techniques have improved reconstruction substantially over the last several decades and older studies need to be re-evaluated.

In summary, multiple factors need to be considered before deciding whether to proceed with limb salvage or amputation. Resection margins need to be sufficiently wide to prevent disease recurrence and to optimize prognosis. Post-operative limb function and quality of life is considered and discussed with the patient. Age, activity level, and social support network help guide the decision process. Most patients prefer to keep their extremity. The evolution of microsurgery, enhanced imaging techniques, and the expanded use of adjuvant radiation and chemotherapy has enabled surgeons to offer patients much better outcomes. Limb salvage is, therefore, the method of choice in the treatment of STS and osteosarcomas of the extremities *(16,38)*.

Limb Reconstruction

Reconstructive Goals

The goals of reconstruction are restoration of form and function. In extremity reconstruction, particularly the upper extremity, functional aspects predominate over form and appearance. The upper extremity performs delicate and gross movements and provides sensibility to interact with our surrounding. It provides means for independent self-care, work, and recreational activities. Restoring function is a challenge because of the complex interaction of bone, joints, tendons, and nerves. The lower extremity, on the other hand, is primarily used for walking and standing but not fine movements or tactile gnosis. Reconstruction in the lower extremity is commonly required for soft-tissue defects, bone, or joint replacements. The most challenging aspect of lower extremity reconstruction is repair of the weight-bearing surface of the foot because of its unique anatomic structure. Aesthetic restoration is important, albeit less so than with the arm, because visible deformities can be highly disturbing during social interactions, when shaking hands, or wearing shorts.

Reconstructive Principles

When choosing the best reconstructive technique, it is helpful to analyze the defect by outlining the specific tissue components that are missing such as skin, muscle, nerve, tendon, subcutaneous tissue, bone, or joint. In general, it is best to "replace like with like;" a principle stated by the modern father of plastic and reconstructive surgery, Sir Harold Gilles. One way to learn about extremity reconstruction is to divide the extremities into specific sites. In the upper extremity, there is the upper arm, elbow, forearm, wrist, and hand. The lower extremity consists of the thigh, knee, lower leg, and foot.

Soft-Tissue Reconstruction

Soft-tissue reconstruction includes soft-tissue coverage for restoration of surface continuity and functional restoration, including nerve and vascular reconstruction or tendon or muscle free transplants or transpositions.

Soft-tissue defects can be closed by simple primary suture or by more complex means, such as split- or full-thickness skin grafts, local flaps, regional flaps, or microsurgical free flaps. The reconstructive tree outlines some of the ways to reconstruct a wound (Figure 11.1). In choosing which method to use to close a wound, the least complex procedure that covers the defect and replaces the missing tissue is often the best choice. In many patients, however, the ideal approach requires ascending the reconstructive ladder and using a more complex operation. Free tissue transfer, termed "free flap," is the autologous transplantation of composite tissue and its arterial and venous blood supply to a distant site. Although complex, free flaps may be the easiest technique to reconstruct a wound. Experience has confirmed that the complication rate of local flaps is similar to that of free flaps. Microsurgery, therefore, has become the standard and mainstay of reconstructive extremity surgery *(39)*.

Because reconstructive surgeons are comfortable with performing microsurgery and handling large complex wounds, one does not have to limit the resection margins to make reconstruction possible. Lohman et al. confirmed that resection margins of STSs are smaller in cases when the defect was closed primarily and margins were larger when a flap was employed for reconstruction *(40)*. It can therefore not be overemphazised that for any surgical tumor treatment, a reconstructive microsurgeon needs to be available to provide reconstruction.

Free Tissue Transfer

The list of microsurgical reconstructive options is immense and complex. One way to categorize free flaps is to arrange them according to the type of tissue that they contain, such as muscle, musculocutaneous, fasciocutaneous, fascial, or bony. Tissue composition is essential to determining which type of free flap to use. Cutaneous flaps, such as the radial forearm, scapular, or anterolateral thigh flap, provide pliability, and good

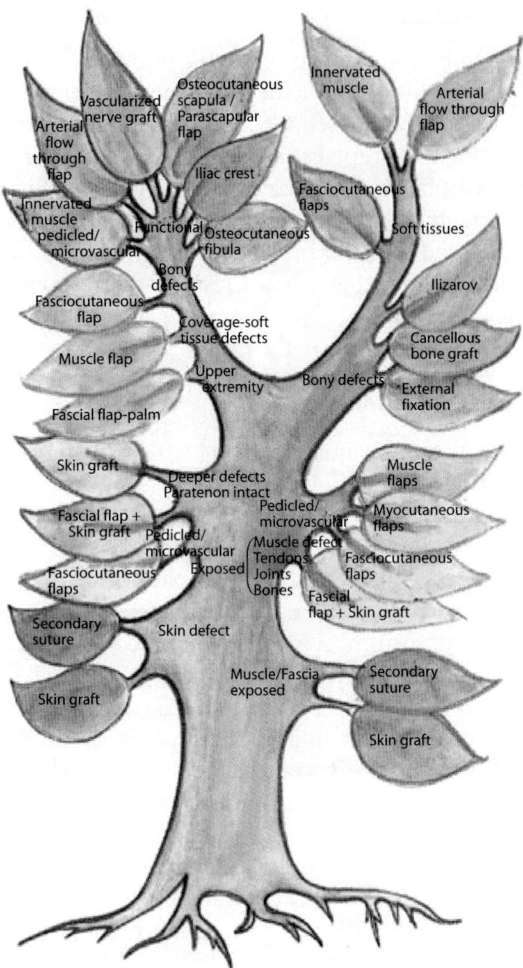

Figure 11.1. Reconstructive options represented in the "reconstructive tree." (With permission of G. Germann.)

aesthetics. Muscle flaps are well perfused and the commonly used latissimus dorsi flap provides a large surface area. Fascial flaps, including the temporalis fascia flap, are thin and pliable.

Defect size, donor site morbidity, and intra-operative patient positioning also influence the choice of free flap for reconstruction. Repositioning a patient in the middle of a case prolongs operative times and limits the number of surgeons who can work together. Careful pre-operative planning and positioning of the patient is necessary to allow for this simultaneous two-team approach.

With the evolution of microsurgery, more sophisticated procedures such as sensate flaps, composite free flaps containing bone, skin, fat, muscle or nerves, transplantation of amputated limbs, flow-through free flaps with proximal and distal arterial anastomosis, and tissue transplantation in the young (e.g., premature newborns) are now possible *(41)*.

Essentially, any wound can be reconstructed, the only limitation is the surgeon's creativity.

Functional Reconstruction

Functional reconstruction involves nerve, tendon, muscle and vascular transplantation and is predominantely used in upper extremity reconstruction. Generally, neural defects can be reconstructed by primary suture, nerve graft, or vascularized free nerve transfers. The most common donor nerve is the sural nerve. Free nerve grafts are indicated when a wound bed is poorly perfused, scarred, or irradiated, and they can be incorporated as a sensory component in a free flap. Nerve reconstructions have the best outcome in the young patient. In the elderly, a complex nerve reconstruction of a proximal nerve defect is often not indicated.

Tendon transfers can also be used to restore function for extremity reconstruction and are most commonly performed in the upper extremity. Like free nerve grafts, tendon grafts can be incorporated into composite free flaps. Similarly, muscle reconstruction can be achieved by functional muscle transposition. The latissimus dorsi flap can be used as a pedicled flap to replace a resected biceps *(42,43)* or triceps muscle, or as a free muscle transplant. In a free functional muscle transplant, the motor nerve needs to be coapted by neurorraphy to a recipient motor nerve to regain reinnervation *(44–47)*.

Bone Defects

Defects in the long bones without articular involvement can be bridged with vascularized or non-vascularized autologous bone graft, distraction osteogenesis (Ilizarov), allograft, or tumor endoprosthesis.

Microsurgical transfer of a vascularized bone graft involves transforming a segment of bone with its intrinsic blood vessels to a recipient site and anastomosing the artery and vein *(48,49)*. The fibula is the most common bone donor, but the iliac crest, rib, radius, and scapula grafts are also options *(50)*. Vascularized transplants with their native blood supply survive longer and healing is optimal. Vascularized bone grafts have the highest union rate when compared to other means of bone reconstruction. Furthermore, the graft can increase in structural strength by hypertrophy *(51,52)*. In general, vascularized bone grafting is indicated for bony defects measuring more than 5–6 cm, or when there is insufficent soft-tissue coverage, or impaired perfusion of the recipient bed, such as after irradiation.

Distraction osteogenesis is another method of bone reconstruction (technique of Ilizarov) *(53–55)*. Distraction osteogenesis induces bone and soft-tissue regeneration through tractional forces applied by a minimally invasive external fixation device. Slow distraction is performed in a controlled fashion at a rate of approximately 1 mm/day in an axial direction. The distracted tissue gap closes by bone regeneration, thereby lengthening the limb *(56)*. The soft tissue surrounding the distracting bone lengthens in conjunction with the bone. One disadvantage of the

Ilizarov technique is a long-lasting distraction time, which can last up to several months.

Non-vascularized allograft bone obtained from deceased donors has no vital and immunogenic cells and therefore serves as an extracellular matrix scaffolding for cellular regrowth. Transplant rejection is not a concern. Allografts have a high complication rate, including non-union, infection, and fracture, and often require revision; yet, overall allograft survival is good (60–80%) *(57–59)*. These grafts particularly require good soft-tissue cover and are used in conjunction with free tissue transfer.

Lastly, tumor endoprostheses can be used to reconstruct bony defects. Proponents of endoprostheses emphasize the advantages of immediate weight bearing, early rehabilitation, and a low complication rate. Ward et al. demonstrated that the most frequent serious early complication is infection (5%), which is exacerbated by post-operative radiation (9%) *(60)*. Most prosthetic failures, however, occur late. The most concerning long-term problems include cement loosening and particulate wear debris-induced osteolysis. Mechanical fatigue fracture failures through the endoprosthesis are uncommon *(60)*.

If joints are resected, reconstructive options include osteoarticular allografts, endoprosthetic implants, rotationplasty, or arthrodesis *(59)*.

Lower Extremity Reconstruction

Thigh

The upper leg has an abundance of soft tissue; thus, soft-tissue defects from tumor resection are often closed primarily or by local muscle flaps including rectus abdominis, rectus femoris, vastus lateralis, tensor fasciae lata, or biceps femoris *(61)*. Indications for free tissue transfer are rare but may be necessary for coverage of a tumor prosthesis or structural allograft, filling a dead space prior to radiation therapy, or secondary salvage of a complicated wound secondary to irradiation. Mastorakos et al. have shown that additional flap coverage after allograft reconstruction reduces infection and enhances bony healing *(62)*.

Tumor resections of the femur can be reconstructed by a tumor prosthesis or a vascularized bone graft such as a free fibula. Free fibula grafts to the femur provide stability for lower-extremity weight bearing. They can be harvested from the ipsilateral or contralateral leg, as a double barrel, or in combination with an allograft to increase stability *(39,48,63,64)*. Ceruso and Innocenti provide an overview of various surgical reconstructive options using the free vascularized fibula graft *(65)*.

Reconstruction of major vessels of the leg can be achieved using synthetic (e.g., polytetrafluoroethylene) or autologous vein bypass grafts *(66)*. Defects of the ischial nerve can be reconstructed using nerve grafts, such as a sural nerve graft, which is desirable in the young patient. Interestingly however, Fuchs et al. has demonstrated that even without sciatic nerve reconstruction, good functional results can be achieved *(67)*.

Knee

Unlike the upper leg, the knee has little soft-tissue coverage. For soft-tissue reconstruction, there are only a few local flaps, such as the lateral or medial gastrocnemius flap, the biceps femoris flap or the reversed anterolateral thigh flap that will provide sufficient coverage. As these flaps are limited in their volume, surface area, and arc of rotation, a free flap may be required.

Reconstruction of bony defects may require knee joint replacement or alternatively, arthrodesis, amputation, or rotationplasty.

Knee joint replacement can be achieved by conventional knee arthroplasty, a custom-made tumor endoprosthesis, or a composite endoprothetic allograft. All of these joint replacement methods require superimposed well-vascularized, durable soft-tissue coverage. Free flap reconstruction may be necessary to achieve these goals if local flaps are not sufficient in size. An arthrodesis requires extensive bone grafting. Conventional autologeous bone grafts from the iliac crest do usually not provide enough bone. Allografts may show a slow or inadequate healing particularly in the elderly or irradiated patient with a high complication rate *(68)*. A vascularized bone graft represents a perfect reconstructive option in these cases. The osteocutaneous fibula graft, supplied by the peroneal artery, can be used as an ipsilateral pedicled flap or a contralateral free flap *(69)*. The ends of the free fibula should be dowelled into the recipient bone to increase stability, and post-operative rigid external fixation or an intramedullary rod is necessary to ensure healing. An intramedullary rod is much easier to work around than an external fixator when microsurgery is required.

Preservation of length is important with amputation to optimize limb function and improve prosthetic rehabilitation. Prosthetic devices are more easily applied if there is sufficient length distal to a joint and energy expenditure required for walking is decreased. Thus, even with amputation, reconstructive surgery may be required *(70)*. Free microvascular flaps may be used to provide durable soft-tissue coverage to avoid unnecessary shortening of the bone or to lengthen an amputation stump.

An important concept in limb amputation is the use of tumor-free "spare parts" from the distal amputated limb for reconstruction. One example is the fillet of the foot for proximal stump coverage *(70–72)*. It contains the soft tissues of the foot after removal of the bones. Another example is the rotationplasty. In rotationplasty, the distal portion of the limb and the foot are maintained during tumor removal *(73–75)*. The ankle and foot are rotated 180°, then attached to the remaining proximal femur so that the transposed ankle is at the height of the contralateral knee. The ankle joint replaces the resected knee joint so that extension of the ankle bends the new knee joint. Rotationplasty is beneficial because it provides a functional "knee" joint, is a stable reconstruction, and ultimately it requires less energy for walking. The major disadvantage of rotationplasty is the resultant disfigurement, particularly in females and adolescents *(29)*.

Lower leg

The thickness of the soft-tissue envelope of the lower leg is much less than on the upper leg. Therefore, distal tumors are more difficult to completely resect and limb salvage is more challenging. Vital structures, such as vessels and nerves, are likely to be involved by the tumor or surgery, reducing the likelihood for an optimal functional outcome. Furthermore, there are only a few local options that can be used for defect coverage. The distal leg is a site of end perfusion and often has impaired blood flow, particularly in high-risk patients with diabetes, peripheral vascular disease, venous insufficiency, advanced age, or a smoking history. Vascular compromise may impair healing and limit the availability of recipient vessels for free flap transfer. If the patient has a history of vascular disease, claudication, rest pain, or if pulses are not palpable, a pre-operative vascular work-up is necessary. In the compromised patient, free flap transfer can be performed in conjunction with a vascular bypass *(76,77)*, subsequent to a vascular bypass *(78)* or the flap artery itself can act as a bypass graft, termed a "flow-through" flap *(77,79)*. A free flap can be nourished by retrograde flow through a distally based recipient vessel.

The main goals in lower leg reconstruction are skin resurfacing and bony stability. Free flap coverage is commonly applied for soft-tissue reconstruction because of a lack of local options. Both fasciocutaneous and muscular free flaps are equally successful in defect coverage. Functional reconstruction, such as transfer of the posterior tibial tendon to the anterior tibial and peroneal tendons to reconstruct a dropped foot, is rarely required. These reconstructions, however, are more commonly seen in the trauma setting.

For bone reconstruction, a vascularized fibula graft is the first choice for larger defects (Figure 11.2). Small defects may be bridged by conventional corticocancellous grafts (autologeous or allogeneic) or the Ilizarov technique *(80)*.

Foot and ankle

Foot reconstruction is challenging, particularly when it involves functional restoration of the weight bearing area. Knowledge of normal foot function including gait patterns, stabilizing regions, and weight bearing areas, as well as an intimate knowledge of regional anatomy is mandatory to develop the best reconstructive strategy *(81)*.

Amputation has often been recommended as the method of choice for ablative surgery in the foot because there is low morbidity of an amputation with good functional results after prosthetic rehabilitation *(69,82)*. However, foot salvage may, at times, provide better outcomes. Sophisticated free flap reconstructions have been performed to preserve the weight-bearing area and to optimize aesthetic outcomes *(69,83,84)*.

There are two different approaches for reconstruction of the weight-bearing foot. Many microsurgeons advocate the use of muscle flaps with split-thickness skin grafts (e.g., latissimus dorsi, gracilis, rectus abdominis free flap), whereas other authors favor fasciocutaneous flaps (e.g., scapular, radial forearm flap, anterolateral thigh flap) *(85,86)*. Comparative studies have not demonstrated superiority of one technique over another *(87,88)*. A third alternative is the use of fascial flaps with split-thickness skin grafts. In foot reconstruction, there is ongoing debate about the usefulness of sensory re-innervation of the sole. Sensate flap reconstruc-

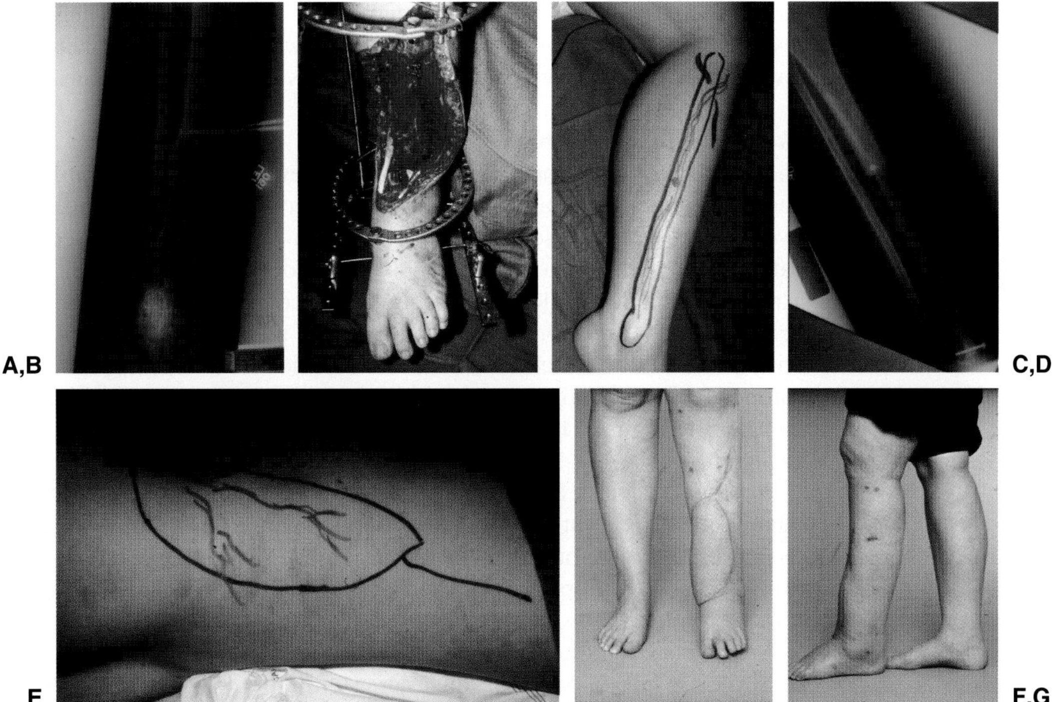

Figure 11.2. **(A)** Radiographic view of a osteogenic sarcoma of the distal tibia in a 25-year-old female patient. **(B)** Intraoperative defect of bone and soft tissue after tumor resection in the distal leg. **(C)** Contralateral lower leg outlining the harvest of a free fibula bone flap. **(D)** Radiographic post-operative view with the free fibula flap replacing the tibial defect. **(E)** Donor site of the right shoulder/back for harvest of a musculocutaneous latissimus dorsi flap; the patient is lying in the left lateral position. **(F, G)** Post-operative view after soft-tissue reconstruction with a free musculocutaneous latissimus dorsi flap.

tion can be performed by connecting a sensory nerve in the free flap to a recipient sensory nerve. Numerous studies investigated the re-innervation of free flaps to the foot and found improved sensibility of the free flap in comparison to insensate reconstruction *(85–87,89–92)*. None of these studies however demonstrated a correlation between sensory recovery and ulcer formation. A direct comparison of re-innervated versus non-innervated free flaps to the weight-bearing foot showed no difference in the incidence of complications *(93)*.

Whichever reconstructive option is chosen for the weight-bearing foot, special footwear should be considered and patients should be educated about meticulous foot care, involving frequent inspection and early problem identification. Lifelong vigilance is mandatory for a long-lasting successful result.

Reconstruction of the Upper Extremity

Upper limb salvage is even more critical than lower limb salvage because the arm and hand maximize a patient`s activities and life styles. Reconstruction of the upper extremity is more challenging than the lower extremity because of functional and anatomical complexities. Nerves, tendons, muscles, or joints frequently need to be replaced, and they are responsible for finer sensation than in the lower extremity. As with the lower limb, the reconstructive site determines the surgical options.

Shoulder and upper arm

Shoulder reconstruction is difficult to achieve, given the complexity of the shoulder joint and surrounding structures. Again, the restorative procedure is chosen based on location and extent of resection, patient age, and functional demands placed on the new shoulder *(94)*. The most reliable predictor of functional outcome is the degree of bony resection, and preservation of rotator cuff and deltoid. Methods of bony reconstitution include a prosthetic device, an allograft-prosthetic composite, a prosthetic spacer, flail shoulder, arthrodesis, or vascularized bone graft (Figure 11.3) *(94,95)*. Each method has its advantages and disadvantages.

Prosthetic devices are best used in low to moderately active people but are insufficient for children. Prosthetic spacers and flail shoulders are the easiest to create but have the least mobility. Overall, more than 50% of prostheses develop complications, of which glenohumeral instability is most common.

Arthrodesis is indicated in deltoid and rotator cuff insufficiency, brachial plexus injury, paralytic disorders, failed primary reconstructions, severe refractory instability, and for bone deficiencies after tumor resection. It is particularly good in young patients with strenuous activity demands. In a retrospective review of 21 patients followed over 11 years, Fuchs et al. found that arthrodesis led to good functional results. Nonetheless, there were significant complications in 43% of patients ranging from infection allografts, to post-operative fractures and Volkmann's contracture *(94)*. When the rotator cuff, axillary nerve, or deltoid are removed, Kassab et al. advocate using a scapulohumeral arthrodesis or a massive humerus prosthesis for reconstruction *(95)*. If the rotator cuff or deltoid is preserved then they recommend reconstruction with composite prosthesis including suturing of the cuff tendons. Scapulohumeral arthrodesis can also be selectively used. It is performed using autogenous or allogeneic bone grafts. Alternatively, Amin et al. used a vascularized scapula based on the circumflex scapular artery as a pedicled flap *(96)*.

The traditional method of managing a shoulder girdle tumor historically was a forequarter amputation with coverage provided by the biceps, triceps, and deltoid, but this is seldom necessary nor oncologically required. The Tikhoff-Linberg procedure is an interscapulothoracic amputation of the arm that was first described in 1928. It can be used for tumors of the shoulder or scapula and can be combined with soft-tissue reconstruction by a latissimus dorsi, serratus anterior, and pectoralis major flaps or a fillet of the arm *(97,98)*.

Reconstruction of humeral defects without articular involvement is less demanding. Reconstruction can be performed using a free vascularized fibular graft or other vascularized bone transfers *(99,100)*, a humeral allograft, or a tumor endoprosthesis *(101,102)*.

Soft-tissue reconstruction of the shoulder or in the upper arm serves two goals: defect coverage and functional restoration. Defect coverage

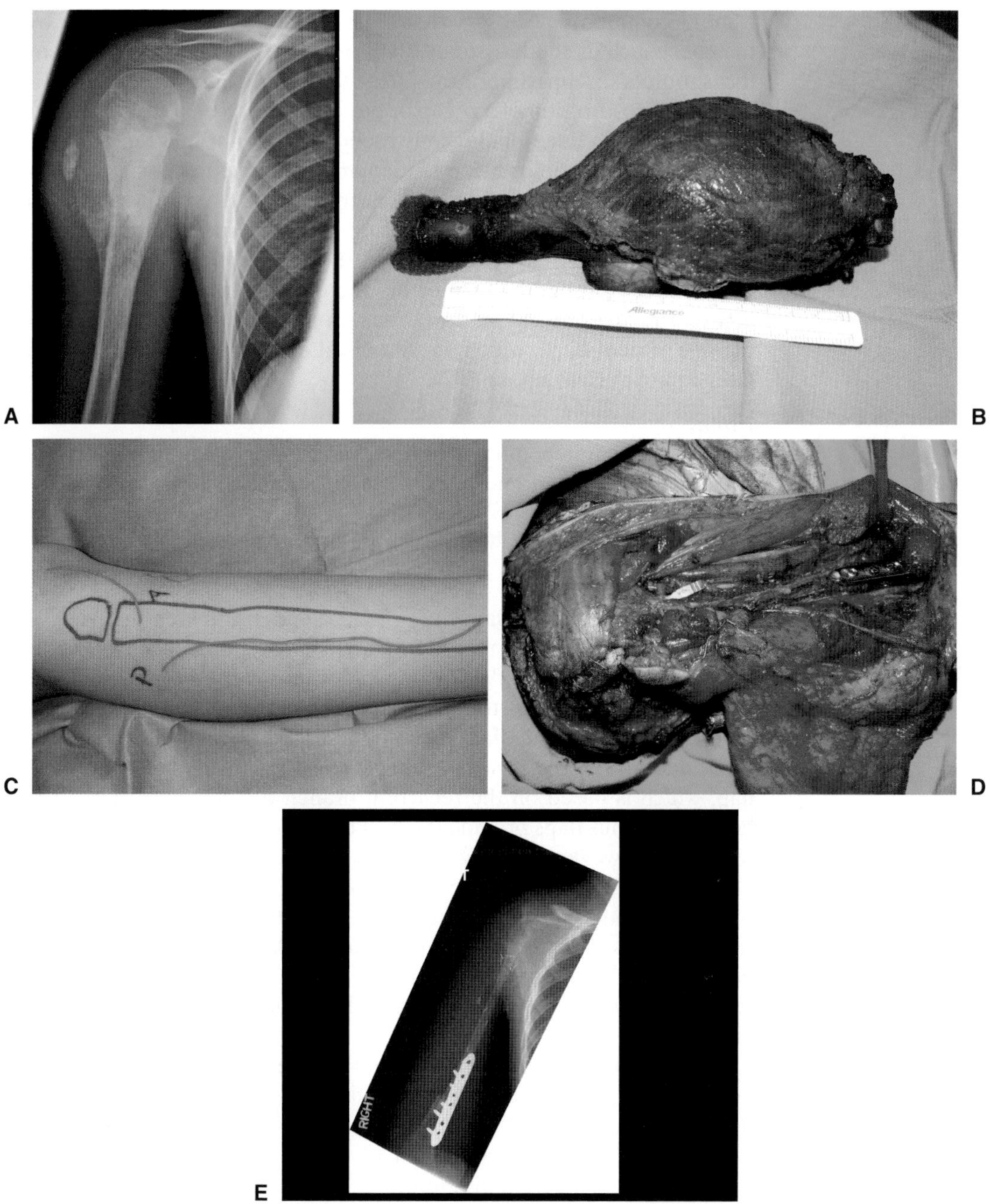

Figure 11.3. A 10-year-old boy presented with an osteosarcoma of the right proximal humerus. **(A)** Preoperative radiographic view of the osteosarcoma in the proximal humerus. **(B)** Resection of the tumor. **(C)** Markings at the donor site for harvest of a free vascularized epiphyseal fibula flap. **(D)** Intraoperative view after transplantation and insetting of the fibula. **(E)** Post-operative X-ray of the reconstructed humerus with free fibula flap.

is more commonly necessary than return of function. Pedicle flaps from the chest such as the latissimus dorsi or pectoralis major flap can cover the shoulder or proximal arm *(103–107)*. Both flaps can be used for functional restoration of a tricep or bicep muscle to enable elbow flexion or extension. In functional reconstruction, the donor muscle is fixated to the end of the tricep or bicep tendon and its native nerve supplies function. For larger or more distal defects, free flaps are required and numerous options are available including fasciocutaneous, muscular, or musculocutaneous flaps. Again, free functional muscle reconstruction can be accomplished by connecting the donor motor nerve of the free flap to a recipient local motor nerve. An alternative for large defects is the use of fillet flaps, which use the distal extremity as a soft-tissue flap after removal of the bone *(72)*.

Elbow

The elbow is an uncommon site for primary or metastatic tumors but if the elbow is affected and resected, joint reconstruction can be accomplished using total elbow arthroplasty or allograft-prosthetic composite reconstruction (Figure 11.4) *(108,109)*.

Forearm

The forearm contains numerous muscles, tendons, nerves, and vessels in close proximity. Tumor resection frequently requires removal of these structures. The type of flap or transplant that is used for repair largely depends on the type of tissue missing, the defect size, and the location *(110)*. Local soft-tissue flaps include the radial forearm flap supplied by the radial artery, the posterior interosseus flap, or the so-called Becker flap, which is based on the recurrent branch of the ulnar artery. These fasciocutaneous flaps provide the best tissue consistency and replace like with like; however, their size and arc of rotation limit their usefulness. Cutaneous flaps such as the radial forearm, lateral arm, anterolateral thigh, or scapular flap provide the best aesthetic result. For large defects, the latissimus dorsi flap is commonly used. The latissimus dorsi flap can be harvested with the scapular flap, serratus anterior flap, or parts of the scapula; all flaps are based on the subscapular vessels (so-called "chimeric" flaps).

Tendon transfers are used to rebuild muscle and tendon units, and free neurovascular muscle transfers have been described for replacement of flexor or extensor tendons in the forearm *(111)*. Isolated nerve reconstruction requires transplantation of nerve grafts, of which the sural nerve is the most common donor.

For composite tissue defects involving tendons, nerves, bone, or skin, a composite free tissue transfer is the best reconstructive option. One example is the radial forearm free flap from the contralateral arm including the palmaris longus tendon, the antebrachial cutaneous sensory nerve and a part of the radius. Similarly, the lateral cutaneous arm flap can be harvested along with the posterior cutaneous forearm nerve and part of the humerus.

For bone reconstruction, the same modes of treatment can be applied as described for the lower extremity or humerus. Vascularized grafts as well as allografts have been used for replacement of the radius *(112)*.

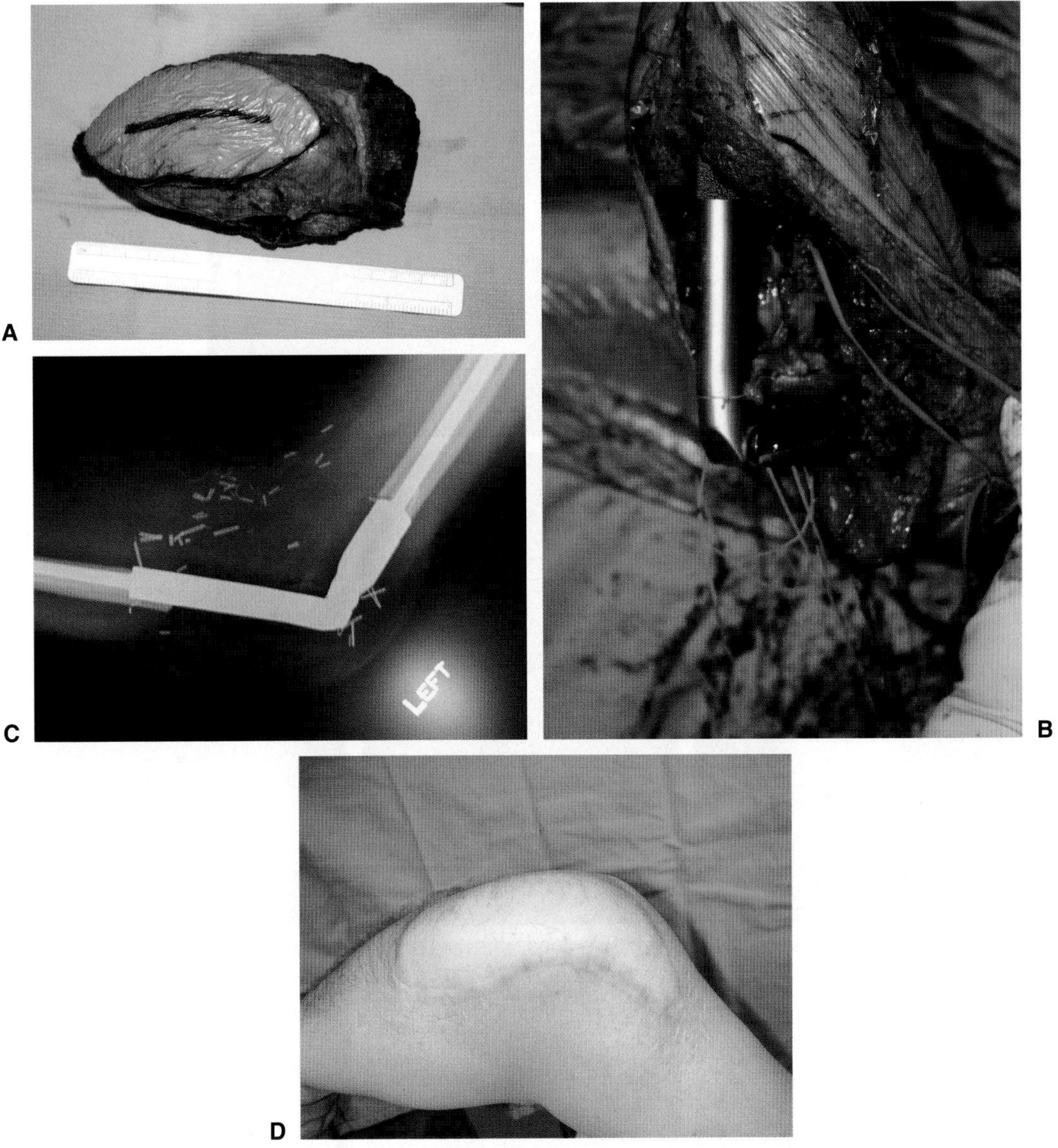

Figure 11.4. A 49-year-old male patient presented with an osteosarcoma of his right elbow. **(A)** Resected tumor including the elbow joint and overlying skin. **(B)** Joint reconstruction with an elbow-tumor prosthesis. **(C)** Radiographic view of elbow prosthesis. **(D)** Post-operative view of soft-tissue reconstruction using an anterolateral thigh flap.

Hand

Reconstruction becomes more difficult the further distally reconstruction takes place and the more complex the function becomes. Local options for tissue coverage and reconstruction are limited; thus, free flaps are frequently used. Some authors advocate fascia flaps with skin grafts *(113,114)* to rebuild the thin, pliable soft-tissue of the native hand, whereas others prefer thin cutaneous flaps *(115,116)*. However, to achieve radical resection, fingers, ray-, and partial hand amputation are still commonly required to achieve complete tumor resection (Figure 11.5).

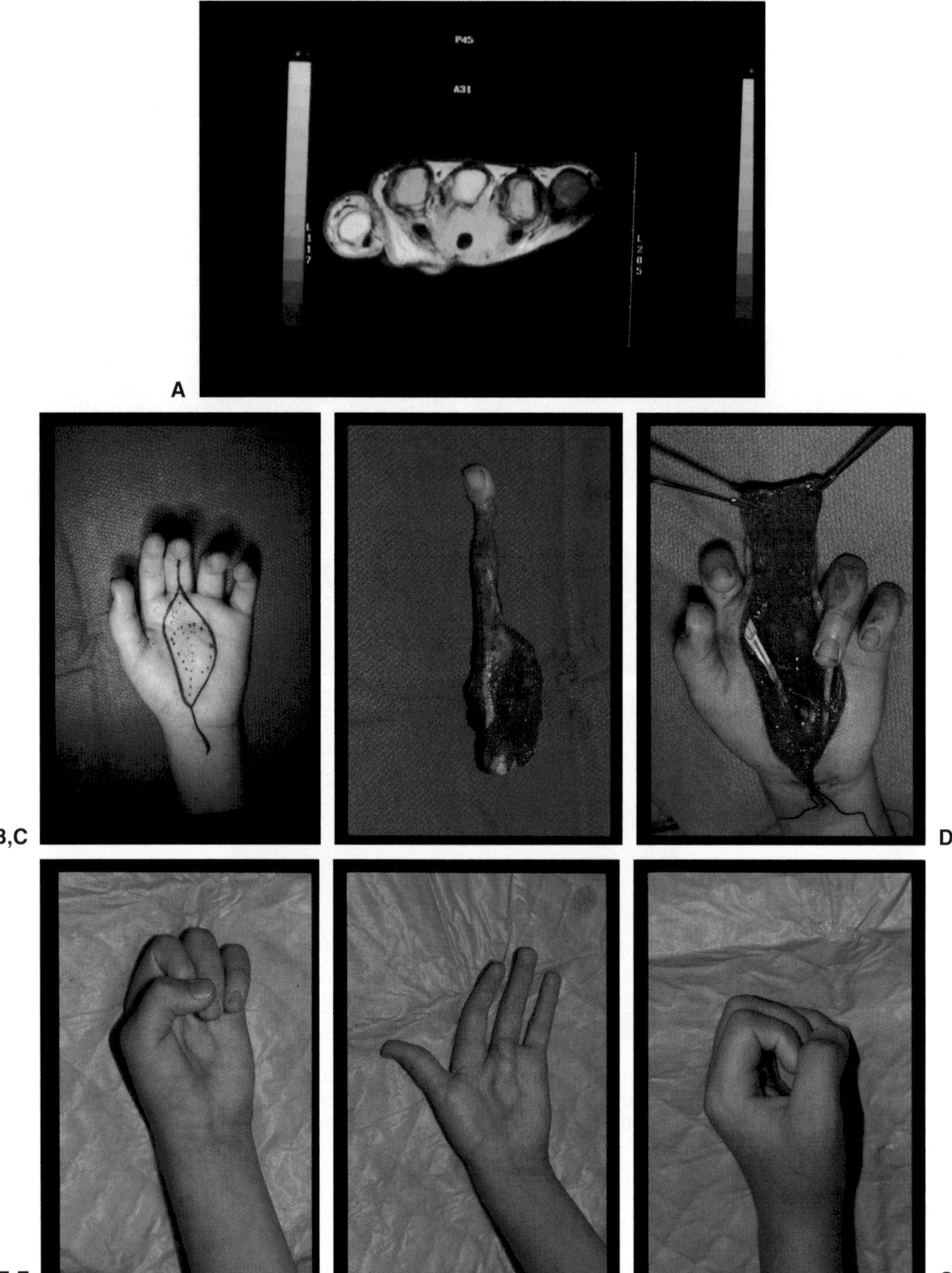

Figure 11.5. **(A)** Coronal MRI of the metacarpus of a 10-year-old boy showing a tenosynovial sarcoma on the palmar site of the third metacarpal bone. **(B)** Intraoperative marking outlining the resection of the tumor. **(C)** Tumor resection by means of a ray amputation of the third ray. **(D)** The dorsal filet of the third finger is preserved and used for defect coverage. **(E, F, G)** Post-operative outcome with good flexion and extension of the remaining fingers.

Pediatric Consideration

Tumor reconstruction is challenging in the pediatric population as children are more active and have a long life span. The reconstructive surgeon needs to consider the skeletal and psychological immaturity of the young patients as well as the long-term durability of any procedure. The growth potential of the child should be taken into account when one or more growth plates are resected or irradiated. Reconstructed soft and bony tissue usually adapts and stretches with the child's growth. Exceptions include skin grafts, which might contract, and non-vascularized bone, which does not grow adequately. Custom-made prostheses for bone or joint replacement, as well as a vascularized bone graft, might fit well in the younger patient, but are temporary in the growing child. Even functional amputations may become dysfunctionally short. Length discrepancies that result are less of a functional problem in the upper extremity than in the lower extremity.

Solutions to these child specific-problems include using an expandable prosthetic device *(117)* or transplanting a vascularized bone graft with an epiphyseal plate, such as a fibula flap with the fibula head *(65)*. This specific fibula flap has its blood supply from the anterior tibial artery *(118)*.

Considerations in the Elderly

There is no age limit for performing a free flap in the elderly or any other complex reconstructive procedure apart from general anesthetic and medical restrictions. A two-team approach to limit operative time is particularly important in these cases.

When discussing reconstructive options with the patient, the preoperative activity level needs to be taken into account. The patient may not want to undergo a lengthy operative procedure or a long rehabilitation, but rather prefer a less optimal reconstruction or even an amputation in exchange for a quicker recovery. Refaat et al. showed that the elderly are more satisfied with an amputation in comparison to the young *(27)*.

References

1. Khatri VP, Goodnight JE Jr. Extremity soft tissue sarcoma: controversial management issues. Surg Oncol 2005;14:1–9.
2. Greenlee RT, Hill-Harmon MB, Murray T, Thun M. Cancer statistics, 2001. CA Cancer J Clin 2001;51:15–36.
3. Panicek DM, Gatsonis C, Rosenthal DI, et al. CT and MR imaging in the local staging of primary malignant musculoskeletal neoplasms: report of the Radiology Diagnostic Oncology Group Radiology. 1997;202:237–246.
4. Mankin HJ, Mankin CJ, Simon MA. The hazards of the biopsy, revisited. Members of the Musculoskeletal Tumor Society. J Bone Joint Surg Am 1996;78:656–663.
5. Enneking WF, Spanier SS, Goodman MA. A system for the surgical staging of musculoskeletal sarcoma. Clin Orthop Relat Res 1980;153: 106–120.

6. Enneking WF, Spanier SS, Goodman MA. Current concepts review. The surgical staging of musculoskeletal sarcoma. J Bone Joint Surg Am 1980;62:1027–1030.
7. Sadoski C, Suit HD, Rosenberg A, Mankin H, Efird J. Preoperative radiation, surgical margins, and local control of extremity sarcomas of soft tissues. J Surg Oncol 1993;52:223–230.
8. Rosenberg SA, Tepper J, Glatstein E, et al. The treatment of soft-tissue sarcomas of the extremities: prospective randomized evaluations of (1) limb-sparing sur gery plus radiation therapy compared with amputation and (2) the role of adjuvant chemotherapy. Ann Surg 1982;196:305–315.
9. Fagundes HM, Lai PP, Dehner LP, et al. Postoperative radiotherapy for malignant fibrous histiocytoma. Int J Radiat Oncol Biol Phys 1992;23: 615–619.
10. LeVay J, O'Sullivan B, Catton C, et al. Outcome and prognostic factors in soft tissue sarcoma in the adult. Int J Radiat Oncol Biol Phys 1993; 27:1091–1099.
11. Tanabe KK, Pollock RE, Ellis LM, Murphy A, Sherman N, Romsdahl MM. Influence of surgical margins on outcome in patients with preoperatively irradiated extremity soft tissue sarcomas. Cancer 1994;73:1652–1659.
12. Potter DA, Kinsella T, Glatstein E, et al. High-grade soft tissue sarcomas of the extremities. Cancer 1986;58:190–205.
13. McKee MD, Liu DF, Brooks JJ, Gibbs JF, Driscoll DL, Kraybill WG. The prognostic significance of margin width for extremity and trunk sarcoma. J Surg Oncol 2004;85:68–76.
14. Kawaguchi N, Ahmed AR, Matsumoto S, Manabe J, Matsushita Y. The concept of curative margin in surgery for bone and soft tissue sarcoma. Clin Orthop Relat Res 2004;419:165–172.
15. Dürr HR, Jansson V, Jauch KW, et al. Operative Therapie Von Knochen- Und Weichteiltumoren. In: Tumorzentrum München (ed.), *Manual: Knochentumoren und Weichteilsarkome, fourth edition*. München: W. Zuckschwerdt Verlag; 2004.
16. Williard WC, Hajdu SI, Casper ES, Brennan MF. Comparison of amputation with limb-sparing operations for adult soft tissue sarcoma of the extremity. Ann Surg 1992;215:269–275.
17. Grimer RJ, Taminiau AM, Cannon SR. Surgical outcomes in osteosarcoma. J Bone Joint Surg Br 2002;84:395–400.
18. Collin C, Godbold J, Hajdu S, Brennan M. Localized extremity soft tissue sarcoma: an analysis of factors affecting survival. J Clin Oncol 1987; 5:601–612.
19. Lewis JJ, Leung D, Heslin M, Woodruff JM, Brennan MF. Association of local recurrence with subsequent survival in extremity soft tissue sarcoma. J Clin Oncol 1997;15:646–652.
20. Markhede G, Angervall L, Stener B. A multivariate analysis of the prognosis after surgical treatment of malignant soft-tissue tumors. Cancer 1982;49: 1721–1733.
21. Brennan MF, Hilaris B, Shiu MH, et al. Local recurrence in adult soft-tissue sarcoma. A randomized trial of brachytherapy. Arch Surg 1987;122: 1289–1293.
22. Trovik CS, Bauer HC, Alvegard TA, et al. Surgical margins, local recurrence and metastasis in soft tissue sarcomas: 559 surgically-treated patients from the Scandinavian Sarcoma Group Register. Eur J Cancer 2000;36:710–716.
23. Ueda T, Yoshikawa H, Mori S, et al. Influence of local recurrence on the prognosis of soft-tissue sarcomas. J Bone Joint Surg Br 1997;79: 553–557.

24. Gaynor JJ, Tan CC, Casper ES, et al. Refinement of clinicopathologic staging for localized soft tissue sarcoma of the extremity: a study of 423 adults. J Clin Oncol 1992;10:1317–1329.
25. Ramanathan RC, A'Hern R, Fisher C, Thomas JM. Prognostic index for extremity soft tissue sarcomas with isolated local recurrence. Ann Surg Oncol 2001;8:278–289.
26. Renard AJ, Veth RP, Schreuder HW, van Loon CJ, Koops HS, van Horn JR. Function and complications after ablative and limb-salvage therapy in lower extremity sarcoma of bone. J Surg Oncol 2000;73:198–205.
27. Refaat Y, Gunnoe J, Hornicek FJ, Mankin HJ. Comparison of quality of life after amputation or limb salvage. Clin Orthop Relat Res 2002;397:298–305.
28. Zahlten-Hinguranage A, Bernd L, Ewerbeck V, Sabo D. Equal quality of life after limb-sparing or ablative surgery for lower extremity sarcomas. Br J Cancer 2004;91:1012–1014.
29. Nagarajan R, Neglia JP, Clohisy DR, Robison LL. Limb salvage and amputation in survivors of pediatric lower-extremity bone tumors: what are the long-term implications? J Clin Oncol 2002;20:4493–4501.
30. Postma A, Kingma A, De Ruiter JH, et al. Quality of life in bone tumor patients comparing limb salvage and amputation of the lower extremity. J Surg Oncol 1992;51:47–51.
31. Fayers PM, Aaronson NK, Bjordal K, et al. The EORTC QLQ-C30 Scoring Manual, third edition. Brussels: 2001.
32. Fahrenberg J, Myrtek M, Schumacher J, Brähler E. Fragebogen zur Lebenszufriedenheit (FLZ)- Handanweisung. Göttingen: 2000.
33. Enneking WF, Dunham W, Gebhardt MC, Malawar M, Pritchard DJ. A system for the functional evaluation of reconstructive procedures after surgical treatment of tumors of the musculoskeletal system. Clin Orthop Relat Res 1993;286:241–246.
34. Davis AM, Devlin M, Griffin AM, Wunder JS, Bell RS. Functional outcome in amputation versus limb sparing of patients with lower extremity sarcoma: a matched case-control study. Arch Phys Med Rehabil 1999; 80:615–618.
35. Sugarbaker PH, Barofsky I, Rosenberg SA, Gianola FJ. Quality of life assessment of patients in extremity sarcoma clinical trials. Surgery 1982;91: 17–23.
36. Hudson MM, Tyc VL, Cremer LK, et al. Patient satisfaction after limb-sparing surgery and amputation for pediatric malignant bone tumors. J Pediatr Oncol Nurs 1998;15:60–69.
37. Weddington WW Jr, Segraves KB, Simon MA. Psychological outcome of extremity sarcoma survivors undergoing amputation or limb salvage. J Clin Oncol 1985;3:1393–1399.
38. Ghert MA, Abudu A, Driver N, et al. The indications for and the prognostic significance of amputation as the primary surgical procedure for localized soft tissue sarcoma of the extremity. Ann Surg Oncol 2005;12:10–17.
39. Cordeiro PG, Neves RI, Hidalgo DA. The role of free tissue transfer following oncologic resection in the lower extremity. Ann Plast Surg 1994; 33:9–16.
40. Lohman RF, Nabawi AS, Reece GP, Pollock RE, Evans GR. Soft tissue sarcoma of the upper extremity: a 5-year experience at two institutions emphasizing the role of soft tissue flap reconstruction. Cancer 2002; 94:2256–2264.
41. Van Landuyt K, Hamdi M, Blondeel P, Tonnard P, Verpaele A, Monstrey S. Free perforator flaps in children. Plast Reconstr Surg 2005;116:159–169.

42. Haninec P, Smrcka V. Reconstruction of paralyzed biceps brachii muscle by transposition of pedicled latissimus dorsi muscle: report of two cases. Acta Chir Plast 1998;40:41–44.
43. Mailander P, Machens HG, Rieck B, Wittig K, Berger A. [Bilateral biceps replacement-plasty by transposition of the latissimus dorsi muscle in arthrogryposis multiplex congenita. A case report]. Handchir Mikrochir Plast Chir 1996;28:59–63.
44. Willcox TM, Smith AA, Beauchamp C, Meland NB. Functional free latissimus dorsi muscle flap to the proximal lower extremity. Clin Orthop Relat Res 2003;410:285–288.
45. Park C, Shin KS. Functioning free latissimus dorsi muscle transplantation: anterogradely positioned usage in reconstruction of extensive forearm defect. Ann Plast Surg 1991;27:87–91.
46. Uhm KI, Shin KS, Lee YH, Lew JD. Restoration of finger extension and forearm contour utilizing a neurovascular latissimus dorsi free flap. Ann Plast Surg 1988;21:74–76.
47. Krimmer H, Hahn P, Lanz U. Free gracilis muscle transplantation for hand reconstruction. Clin Orthop Relat Res 1995;314:13–18.
48. Erdmann D, Bergquist GE, Levin LS. Ipsilateral free fibula transfer for reconstruction of a segmental femoral-shaft defect. Br J Plast Surg 2002;55:675–677.
49. Erdmann D, Giessler GA, Bergquist GE, et al. [Free fibula transfer. Analysis of 76 consecutive microsurgical procedures and review of the literature]. Chirurg 2004;75:799–809.
50. Georgescu AV, Ivan O. Serratus anterior-rib free flap in limb bone reconstruction Microsurgery 2003;23:217–225.
51. de Boer HH, Wood MB. Bone changes in the vascularised fibular graft. J Bone Joint Surg Br 1989;71:374–378.
52. Heitmann C, Erdmann D, Levin LS. Treatment of segmental defects of the humerus with an osteoseptocutaneous fibular transplant. J Bone Joint Surg Am 2002;84-A:2216–2223.
53. Park S, Lee TJ. Strategic considerations on the configuration of free flaps and their vascular pedicles combined with Ilizarov distraction in the lower extremity. Plast Reconstr Surg 2000;105:1680–1686.
54. Carrington NC, Smith RM, Knight SL, Matthews SJ. Ilizarov bone transport over a primary tibial nail and free flap: a new technique for treating Gustilo grade 3b fractures with large segmental defects. Injury 2000;31:112–115.
55. Gugenheim JJ Jr. The Ilizarov method. Orthopedic and soft tissue applications. Clin Plast Surg 1998;25:567–578.
56. Levin LS. The ilizarov method and microsurgery: the best of both worlds. Am Soc Reconstr Microsurg Newsl 1995;2:23–24.
57. Ortiz-Cruz E, Gebhardt MC, Jennings LC, Springfield DS, Mankin HJ. The results of transplantation of intercalary allografts after resection of tumors. A long-term follow-up study. J Bone Joint Surg Am 1997;79:97–106.
58. Mankin HJ, Springfield DS, Gebhardt MC, Tomford WW. Current status of allografting for bone tumors. Orthopedics 1992;15:1147–1154.
59. Sim FH, Beauchamp CP, Chao EY. Reconstruction of musculoskeletal defects about the knee for tumor. Clin Orthop Relat Res 1987;221:188–201.
60. Ward WG, Yang R-S, Eckardt JJ. Endoprosthetic bone reconstruction following malignant tumor resection in skeletally immature patients. Orthop Clin North Am 1996;27:493–502.
61. Bunkis J, Walton RL, Mathes SJ. The rectus abdominis free flap for lower extremity reconstruction. Ann Plast Surg 1983;11:373–380.

62. Mastorakos DP, Disa JJ, Athanasian E, Boland P, Healey JH, Cordeiro PG. Soft-tissue flap coverage maximizes limb salvage after allograft bone extremity reconstruction. Plast Reconstr Surg 2002;109:1567–1573.
63. Chang DW, Weber KL. Segmental femur reconstruction using an intercalary allograft with an intramedullary vascularized fibula bone flap. J Reconstr Microsurg 2004;20:195–199.
64. Hou SM, Liu TK. Reconstruction of skeletal defects in the femur with "two-strut" free vascularized fibular grafts. J Trauma 1992;33: 840–845.
65. Ceruso M, Falcone C, Innocenti M, Delcroix L, Capanna R, Manfrini M. Skeletal reconstruction with a free vascularized fibula graft associated to bone allograft after resection of malignant bone tumor of limbs. Handchir Mikrochir Plast Chir 2001;33:277–282.
66. Schwarzbach MH, Hormann Y, Hinz U, et al. Results of limb-sparing surgery with vascular replacement for soft tissue sarcoma in the lower extremity. J Vasc Surg 2005;42:88–97.
67. Fuchs B, Davis AM, Wunder JS, et al. Sciatic nerve resection in the thigh: a functional evaluation. Clin Orthop Relat Res 2001;382:34–41.
68. Donati D, Giacomini S, Gozzi E, et al. Allograft arthrodesis treatment of bone tumors: a two-center study. Clin Orthop Relat Res 2002;400: 217–224.
69. Zenn MR, Levin LS. Microvascular reconstruction of the lower extremity. Semin Surg Oncol 2000;19:272–281.
70. Erdmann D, Sundin BM, Yasui K, Wong MS, Levin LS. Microsurgical free flap transfer to amputation sites: indications and results. Ann Plast Surg 2002;48:167–172.
71. Kuntscher MV, Erdmann D, Homann HH, Steinau HU, Levin SL, Germann G. The concept of fillet flaps: classification, indications, and analysis of their clinical value. Plast Reconstr Surg 2001;108:885–896.
72. Kuntscher MV, Erdmann D, Strametz S, Sauerbier M, Germann G, Levin LS. [The use of fillet flaps in upper extremity and shoulder reconstruction] Chirurg 2002;73:1019–1024.
73. Wang HC, Lu YM, Chien SH, Lin GT, Lu CC. Rotationplasty for limb salvage in the treatment of malignant tumors: a report of two cases. Kaohsiung J Med Sci 2003;19:628–634.
74. Hardes J, Gebert C, Hillmann A, Winkelmann W, Gosheger G. [Rotationplasty in the surgical treatment plan of primary malignant bone tumors. Possibilities and limits]. Orthopade 2003;32:965–970.
75. Rodl RW, Pohlmann U, Gosheger G, Lindner NJ, Winkelmann W. Rotationplasty—quality of life after 10 years in 22 patients. Acta Orthop Scand 2002;73:85–88.
76. Tukiainen E, Biancari F, Lepantalo M. Lower limb revascularization and free flap transfer for major ischemic tissue loss. World J Surg 2000;24: 1531–1536.
77. Quinones-Baldrich WJ, Kashyap VS, Taw MB, et al. Combined revascularization and microvascular free tissue transfer for limb salvage: a six-year experience. Ann Vasc Surg 2000;14:99–104.
78. Lorenzetti F, Tukiainen E, Alback A, Kallio M, Asko-Seljavaara S, Lepantalo M. Blood flow in a pedal bypass combined with a free muscle flap. Eur J Vasc Endovasc Surg 2001;22:161–164.
79. Tseng WS, Chen HC, Hung J, Tasi TR, Chen HH, Wei FC. "Flow-through" type free flap for revascularization and simultaneous coverage of a nearly complete amputation of the foot: case report and literature review. J Trauma 2000;48:773–776.

80. Ceruso M, Falcone C, Innocenti M, Delcroix L, Capanna R, Manfrini M. Skeletal reconstruction with a free vascularized fibula graft associated to bone allograft after resection of malignant bone tumor of limbs. Handchir Mikrochir Plast Chir 2001;33:277–282.
81. Baumeister S, Germann G. Soft tissue coverage of the extremely traumatized foot and ankle. Foot Ankle Clin 2001;6:867–903, ix.
82. Lange RH. Limb reconstruction versus amputation decision making in massive lower extremity trauma. Clin Orthop Relat Res 1989;243:92–99.
83. Heller L, Levin LS. Lower extremity microsurgical reconstruction. Plast Reconstr Surg 2001;108:1029–1041.
84. Langstein HN, Chang DW, Miller MJ, et al. Limb salvage for soft-tissue malignancies of the foot: an evaluation of free-tissue transfer. Plast Reconstr Surg 2002;109:152–159.
85. Gaulke R, Partecke B-D. Nachuntersuchung und Gandstudie bei Patienten mit plastisch-chirurgisch gedeckten Fubsohlendefekten Unfallchirurg 1994; 97:47–53.
86. Noever G, Bruser P, Kohler L. Reconstruction of heel and sole defects by free flaps. Plast Reconstr Surg 1986;78:345–352.
87. Goldberg JA, Adkins P, Tsai TM. Microvascular reconstruction of the foot: weight-bearing patterns, gait analysis, and long-term follow-up. Plast Reconstr Surg 1993;92:904–911.
88. Santanelli F, Tenna S, Pace A, Scuderi N. Free flap reconstruction of the sole of the foot with or without sensory nerve coaptation. Plast Reconstr Surg 2002;109:2314–2322.
89. Sommerlad BC, McGrouther DA. Resurfacing the sole: long-term follow-up and comparison of techniques. Br J Plast Surg 1978;31:107–116.
90. Rautio J, Kekoni J, Hamalainen H, Harma M, Asko-Seljavaara S. Mechanical sensibility in free and island flaps of the foot. J Reconstr Microsurg 1989;5:119–125.
91. Lahteenmaki T, Waris T, Asko-Seljavaara S, Sundell B. Recovery of sensation in free flaps. Scand J Plast Reconstr Surg Hand Surg 1989;23: 217–222.
92. Sinha AK, Wood MB, Irons GB. Free tissue transfer for reconstruction of the weight-bearing portion of the foot. Clin Orthop Relat Res 1989;242:269–271.
93. Potparic Z, Rajacic N. Long-term results of weight-bearing foot reconstruction with non-innervated and reinnervated free flaps. Br J Plast Surg 1997;50:176–181.
94. Fuchs B, O'Connor MI, Padgett DJ, Kaufman KR, Sim FH. Arthrodesis of the shoulder after tumor resection. Clin Orthop Relat Res 2005;436: 202–207.
95. Kassab M, Dumaine V, Babinet A, Ouaknine M, Tomeno B, Anract P. [Twenty nine shoulder reconstructions after resection of the proximal humerus for neoplasm with mean 7-year follow-up]. Rev Chir Orthop Reparatrice Appar Mot 2005;91:15–23.
96. Amin SN, Ebeid WA. Shoulder reconstruction after tumor resection by pedicled scapular crest graft. Clin Orthop Relat Res 2002;397:133–142.
97. Sandy G, Shores J, Reeves M. Tikhoff-Linberg procedure and chest wall resection for recurrent sarcoma of the shoulder girdle involving the chest wall. J Surg Oncol 2005;89:91–94.
98. Hidalgo DA, Zenn MR, Marcove RC. Aesthetic reconstruction of Tikhoff-Linberg shoulder defects with a dual-pedicle TRAM free flap. Plast Reconstr Surg 1993;91:1340–1343.

99. Yajima H, Tamai S, Ono H, Kizaki K, Yamauchi T. Free vascularized fibula grafts in surgery of the upper limb. J Reconstr Microsurg 1999;15: 515–521.
100. Jupiter JB, Kour AK. Reconstruction of the humerus by soft tissue distraction and vascularized fibula transfer. J Hand Surg [Am] 1991;16:940–943.
101. Lukin AV, Kiss EE, Grishkin VA, Chernova VI. [Individual endoprosthesis in a malignant tumor of the humerus]. Vestn Khir Im I I Grek 1987;139: 65–66.
102. Grzesik M. [Endoprosthesis of the humerus in osteochondroma] Chir Narzadow Ruchu Ortop Pol 1966;31:763–767.
103. D'Aniello C, Grimaldi L, Bosi B, Brandi C. Shoulder reconstruction by latissimus dorsi myocutaneous flap based on the serratus branch after advanced soft-tissue sarcoma excision. Plast Reconstr Surg 2000;105: 2082–2085.
104. Capanna R, Manfrini M, Briccoli A, Gherlinzoni F, Lauri G, Caldora P. Latissimus dorsi pedicled flap applications in shoulder and chest wall reconstructions after extracompartimental sarcoma resections. Tumori 1995; 81:56–62.
105. Ihara K, Shigetomi M, Muramatsu K, et al. Pedicle or free musculocutaneous flaps for shoulder defects after oncological resection. Ann Plast Surg 2003;50:361–366.
106. Auba C, Yeste L, Herreros J, Hontanilla B. Upper-third arm and shoulder reconstruction with the island latissimus dorsi flap. J Shoulder Elbow Surg 2004;13:676–679.
107. Shigehara T, Tsukagoshi T, Satoh K, Tatezaki S, Ishii, T. A reversed-flow latissimus dorsi musculocutaneous flap based on the serratus branch in primary shoulder reconstruction. Plast Reconstr Surg 1997;99: 566–569.
108. Sperling JW, Pritchard DJ, Morrey BF. Total elbow arthroplasty after resection of tumors at the elbow. Clin Orthop Relat Res 1999;367:256–261.
109. Weber KL, Lin PP, Yasko AW. Complex segmental elbow reconstruction after tumor resection. Clin Orthop Relat Res 2003;415:31–44.
110. Ceruso M, Angeloni R, Innocenti M, Lauri G, Capanna R, Bufalini C. [Reconstruction with free vascularized or island flaps of soft tissue loss in the upper limb after tumor resection. 16 cases]. Ann Chir Main Memb Super 1995;14:21–27.
111. Innocenti M, Ceruso M, Angeloni R, et al. Reinnervated free gracilis muscle transplantation in the treatment of Volkmann's syndrome of the forearm. Chir Organi Mov 1996;81:287–293.
112. Yu GR, Yuan F, Chang SM, Lineaweaver WC, Zhang F. Microsurgical fibular graft for full-length radius reconstruction after giant-cell tumor resection: a case report. Microsurgery 2005;25:121–125.
113. Fotopoulos P, Holmer P, Leicht P, Elberg JJ. Dorsal hand coverage with free serratus fascia flap. J Reconstr Microsurg 2003;19:555–559.
114. Buehler MJ, Pacelli L, Wilson KM. Serratus fascia "sandwich" free-tissue transfer for complex dorsal hand and wrist avulsion injuries. J Reconstr Microsurg 1990;15:315–320.
115. Javaid M, Cormack GC. Anterolateral thigh free flap for complex soft tissue hand reconstructions. J Hand Surg [Br] 2003;28:21–27.
116. Muneuchi G, Suzuki S, Ito O, Kawazoe T. Free anterolateral thigh fasciocutaneous flap with a fat/fascia extension for reconstruction of tendon gliding surface in severe bursitis of the dorsal hand. Ann Plast Surg 2002;49: 312–316.

117. Eckardt JJ, Kabo JM, Kelley CM, et al. Expandable endoprosthesis reconstruction in skeletally immature patients with tumors. Clin Orthop Relat Res 2000;373:51–61.
118. Innocenti M, Delcroix L, Manfrini M, Ceruso M, Capanna R. Vascularized proximal fibular epiphyseal transfer for distal radial reconstruction. J Bone Joint Surg Am 2005;87 (Suppl 1):237–246.

12

Abdominal Wall Tumors and Their Reconstruction

Gregory A. Dumanian

Introduction

Abdominal Wall Tumor Resection and Reconstruction

The abdominal wall protects and contains the abdominal viscera, and serves to position and stabilize the thorax and upper body in space during movement. Components of the abdominal wall may be completely replaced if needed. The internal protective function of the abdominal wall can be replaced with synthetic meshes, fascial flaps, or grafts. External skin can usually be replaced with advancement of adjacent skin or regional thigh flaps. The loss of muscle function of the abdominal wall is generally well tolerated and can be adjusted to with time.

Repair of abdominal wall defects is limited only by the creativity of the reconstructive surgeon. One approach to abdominal wall reconstruction after tumor resection is to separate the two independent but related problems—how to reconstruct the internal abdominal wall, and how to replace the overlying skin.

This chapter begins with a discussion of tumor types that can involve the abdominal wall. The anatomy and physiology of the abdominal wall as it relates to abdominal wall reconstruction is then discussed. In the final section of the chapter, an algorithm for abdominal wall reconstruction is proposed, based on the need to replace the internal abdominal wall, the abdominal skin, or both following tumor removal.

Neoplasms of the Abdominal Wall

A wide variety of neoplasms can involve the abdominal wall. The abdominal wall is defined as the soft tissues and bony structures that contain the abdominal viscera, excluding the retroperitoneal structures and the musculature of the back. Various skin tumors including basal cell carcinoma, squamous cell carcinoma, and melanoma can occur in the abdominal skin. These tumors tend to be easily managed, superficial, and without involvement of deeper structures. Within the abdominal wall, sarcomas such as rhabdomyosarcoma, malignant fibrous histiocytoma (pleomorphic sarcoma), leiomyosarcoma, malignant nerve tumors, and liposarcomas can occur *(1)*. Masses found on physical examination are confirmed radiographically, usually with a contrast-enhanced computed tomography (CT) scan or magnetic resonance imaging (MRI). Needle biopsy often yields the diagnosis of the tumor type, though the lack of a definitive tissue diagnosis may not obviate the need for surgical excision. Intra-abdominal tumors such as colon and cervical cancer can invade the abdominal wall by direct extension, sometimes requiring a full-thickness abdominal wall resection. A more recently recognized cause of abdominal wall neoplasms is direct tumor implantation at the time of laparoscopy *(2)*, needle aspirations of the viscera *(3)*, and percutaneous gastrostomy tube placement for patients with head and neck cancer *(4)*. Finally, urachal carcinoma represents the neoplastic transformation of embryologic remnants within the abdominal wall *(5)*.

One tumor that is relatively common in the abdominal wall compared to other sites in the body is the desmoid tumor, or deep fibromatosis *(6)*. This is in contradistinction to the superficial fibromatoses, including Dupuytren's disease of the hand and Peyronie's disease of the penis, which share some properties such as local recurrence, but with a markedly decreased intensity of disease. The desmoid tumors are considered to be low-grade malignancies, roughly one-half occur in the abdominal wall, but they can occur elsewhere in the body, including the shoulder girdle and the chest wall. The tumors generally do not metastasize, but frequently re-occur locally and cause significant morbidity from their mass effect or their infiltration into adjacent normal tissues and viscera. During tumor resection, desmoid tumors grossly have poorly defined margins without a pseudocapsule. Histologically, the mass is comprised predominately of bland-appearing fibroblasts. Secondary pathologic criteria of mitotic figures or nuclear pleomorphism are rare. The tumors are associated with increased estrogen levels of pregnancy and the tumors in women occur during or following pregnancy. Abdominal wall desmoids are also a part of the clinical diagnosis of Gardner's intestinal polyposis syndrome. Finally, trauma, including the tissue injury of surgery, is associated with the development of desmoid tumors. Patients undergoing laparotomy for intestinal polyposis have also been known to develop desmoid tumors at their incision sites.

Treatment of desmoid tumors is initially surgical, and based on the local growth characteristics and symptoms caused by the mass. Resection to microscopic tumor-free margins is the goal *(7)*, with gross surgical margins of several centimeters recommended. Patients with negative microscopic margins have tumor recurrence rates of 33% at 10 years. Functional outcome of the abdominal wall should be preserved whenever possible, because negative histologic margins have not been shown to be a guarantee for local tumor control. Some studies have even shown no association between negative margins and recurrence rates *(8)*. Tumor recurrences typically occur within 2 years of the initial desmoid excision.

Non-surgical treatments including radiation therapy, chemotherapy, and estrogen deprivation have occasionally been effective at controlling the increase in tumor size. Radiation is occasionally used to help control tumors that would be difficult to resect or for recurrent tumor. The association of desmoids with pregnancy has led to trials of anti-estrogens for patients with these neoplasms. Non-steroidal anti-inflammatory drugs (NSAIDs) have also occasionally been effective in reducing the size of tumors. Patients who have failed surgery, radiation, anti-estrogens, and NSAIDS often have been treated with chemotherapy such as doxorubicin. One issue that must be factored into the long-term studies of desmoid tumors is the occasional occurrence of "growth arrest," whereby the tumor spontaneously stops enlarging and becomes more quiescent.

Anatomy and Physiology of the Abdominal Wall

The abdomen can be viewed as a pressurized closed cylinder. The top of the cylinder represents the diaphragm, the bottom of the cylinder is the bony pelvis, and the sidewalls consist of the retroperitoneum posteriorly and the abdominal wall muscles laterally and anteriorly. Neoplastic processes that involve the posterior aspect of the abdominal wall are better characterized as retroperitoneal tumors and will not be discussed in this chapter.

The layers of the abdominal wall are consistent and important in the planning of tumor excisions. Adjacent to the intestines and abdominal viscera is the peritoneum, a thin filmy piece of tissue that lines the inner aspect of the abdominal wall. The next layers to be found laterally and anterolaterally on the abdominal wall are the transversalis fascia and the transversus abdominis muscle. The transversus abdominis muscle is typically tightly attached to the next most superficial muscle of the lateral and anterolateral abdominal wall, the internal oblique muscle. The fibers of the internal oblique are classically described as running in the same orientation as if one's fingers were placed fully extended into one's back pants pockets. The internal oblique muscle is thinnest as it follows the curves of the rib cage as the fibers approach the anterior rectus fascia, whereas the muscle is thickest near the iliac crest. The motor and sensory nerves to the abdominal wall run in the plane between the transversus abdominis and internal oblique muscles.

A natural dissection plane exists between the internal oblique and the external oblique muscles. The external oblique muscle and fascia, in contradistinction to the internal oblique, has fibers running in an orientation as if one's extended fingers are in one's front pants pockets. Like the internal oblique muscle, the external oblique acts to rotate the upper trunk around a fixed pelvis. The muscle has its blood flow entering segmentally along the imaginary mid-axillary line. Multiple small perforating blood vessels enter the muscle via the rib segmental vessels, and much larger blood vessels enter near the superolateral aspect of the iliac crest. A lack of connections between the external oblique and internal oblique muscles therefore allows for a surgical plane of dissection along the abdominal wall, from the semilunar line anteriorly (the insertion of the lateral abdominal wall musculature into the rectus abdominis fascia) to the mid-axillary line posteriorly. The external oblique muscle and fascia can act as an excellent surgical plane for excisions of tumors of the subcutaneous tissues. The three lateral abdominal muscles insert onto the lateral aspect of the paired rectus abdominis muscles. These two muscles, joined in the midline at the linea alba, are trunk flexors, with origins on the symphisis pubis and insertions along the rib cage and xyphoid. The segmental innervation by the intercostal nerves runs between the transversus abdominis and the internal oblique muscles. The blood supply to the rectus abdominis muscle is from the superior epigastric artery, the deep inferior epigastric artery, and laterally from smaller segmental vessels, which run with the motor nerves to the muscle.

The abdominal wall is important for movement and the prevention of hernias, but it is expendable. Logically, the less of the abdominal wall is lost, the less is the functional deficit. Loss of one entire rectus muscle is common for breast reconstruction, and is generally well tolerated. At 6 months, compensation for the loss of the muscle occurs, and women have similar exercise tolerances after surgery as they did before surgery *(9)*. Many women undergo removal of BOTH rectus muscles for bilateral breast reconstruction. These women often have functional alterations in their torsos, frequently not being able to perform a leg lift or sit up from a lying position without the use of their arms. However, the remaining abdominal muscles tend to compensate over time, rendering the muscle loss more tolerable. Tumor excisions of the flank have more variable outcomes. Loss of the full-thickness abdominal wall laterally by necessity also removes the nerves that run to more anterior musculature including the rectus muscle on that side. Generalized abdominal wall bulges can occur after flank tumor excisions. These bulges are almost impossible to restore to a mirror contour image of the unaffected side.

Reconstruction of the Abdominal Wall

Good communication between the surgical oncologist and the reconstructive surgeon is the first step in the reconstructive plan for the patient. Anticipation as to the size and depth of the surgical defect is critical for patient expectations as to the magnitude of the procedure, prepping and draping of the patient to include possible flap harvest sites, and the existence in the operating room of bioprosthetic and prosthetic meshes of adequate size and quantity. The reconstructive surgeon must devise strategies for solving two independent but related questions: How to close the internal abdominal wall, and how to close the skin.

The Planning of How to Close the Internal Abdominal Wall

Closure of the abdominal wall is critical to prevent evisceration, and needs to be performed whenever the abdominal cavity is entered. After tumor removal, the abdominal wall defects usually cannot be primarily sutured together. Rather, a replacement of the abdominal wall is needed, and the easiest manner to repair the abdominal wall is with a bioprosthetic or a synthetic mesh. Mesh selection is based on an analysis of the quality of the tissues both above and below the mesh. A strategy for abdominal wall reconstruction and choice of mesh will be presented in the next sections based on the quality of the local tissues.

Adequate soft tissues above and below the mesh

Prosthetic meshes are commonly used for abdominal wall reconstruction. They are durable, flexible, and available in numerous sizes. Polypropylene mesh is porous, allows for the egress of fluid collections and the ingrowth of fibrous tissue for improved incorporation into the tissues. Several studies have advocated intraperitoneal placement of polypropylene mesh, stating that bowel adhesions are minimized if the mesh is placed under tension to avoid wrinkles. There are generalized concerns by many surgeons, however, that adhesions between the synthetic mesh and the bowel can lead to bowel injury, fistulae, and bowel obstructions. For this reason, polypropylene mesh is placed intra-abdominally in clean surgical cases (those without bacterial contamination), when the viscera are not swollen (allowing the mesh to be placed tight and flat without wrinkles), and when there is a adequate vascularized tissue (such as greater omentum) to interpose between the mesh and the viscera to prevent direct contact of the mesh to bowel.

Adequate soft tissues above the mesh, clean wound, but inadequate soft tissues below

Patients who have undergone tumor excision with extensive bowel manipulation and with little or no available greater omentum to interpose between the mesh and the bowel have a greater risk of mesh-related bowel adhesions. For these patients, a less adhesogenic mesh is commonly chosen. Expanded polytetrafloroethylene mesh (ePTFE) can be placed against the bowel, and this smooth non-porous mesh does not tend to cause significant bowel adhesions. The lack of adhesions to the mesh is both its most favorable characteristic and its major drawback. The lack of incorporation to surrounding tissues (fascia, muscle, and subcutaneous fat) contributes to an extremely unlikely ability to salvage the mesh reconstruction without surgical removal in the event of an infection, and prevents its use in contaminated cases. Bioprosthetic mesh materials (derived from decellularized human or animal tissues) are also an option in these situations because they generally result in low adhesion formation and do incorporate into the surrounding tissues.

Inadequate soft tissues above and adequate soft tissues below the mesh

Thin atrophic skin above a tumor typically is resected, so patients with poor-quality tissues overlying the tumor can be reconstructed with synthetic meshes if local skin or tissue flaps from remote areas can be used to cover the mesh reconstruction site. Treatment of the skin in abdominal wall reconstruction surgery will be discussed in a subsequent section.

Inadequate soft tissues above and below the mesh, or a contaminated surgical field

Various biologic tissue or bioprosthetic mesh options exist for placement into a surgical field contaminated by a pre-existing wound or bowel surgery. Bioprosthetic mesh material including human acellular dermis are ideal for reconstruction of the fascia in a contaminated surgical site, because of their ability to become quickly vascularized, resist infection, and prevent adhesions to bowel *(10,11)*. Acellular dermis may result in a bulge at the surgical site in these contaminated cases, but allows for fascial closure in challenging wounds. Other bioprosthetic meshes include porcine submucosa and decellularized xenogenic dermis. Another option in these cases is the use of autologous fascia lata harvested from the patient's own lateral leg. A section of fascia lata $22 \times 12\,cm^2$ in size can be harvested from a linear thigh incision. The local wound complications from taking the fascia lata from an ambulatory patient are common, including hematoma and seroma, but not overly problematic or functionally debilitating. The fascia lata is most easily used as a tissue graft, detaching the tissue, and transferring it to the abdominal wall for repair of the defect. For infra-umbilical defects, the fascia lata can remain attached to its blood supply (as a pedicled flap) attached the tensor fascia lata and/or rectus femoris muscle *(12)*. The use of vascularized tissue may improve the ability of the wound site to resist infection, but greatly increases the difficulty in transferring the tissue and insetting it into the abdominal wound defect (Figures 12.1 and 12.2).

The Planning of How to Close the Skin

Tumor resection often involves the creation of sizeable skin defects. The blood flow reaches the abdominal skin through numerous sites. The most important source is the peri-umbilical perforating blood vessel system that originates from the deep inferior epigastric artery and runs through the rectus abdominous muscle. Numerous other segmental vessels reach the abdominal skin from the superior epigastric, intercoastal, femoral, and superficial inferior epigastric arteries. The natural direction of blood to flow in the skin of the abdominal wall is along the nerve dermatomes—roughly parallel to a line drawn from the tip of the scapula to the umbilicus.

There is no substitute for close communication between the oncologic and reconstructive teams for the planning of the dimensions and orientation of these defects. When possible, incisions should be aligned along the dermatomes for two reasons. First, this allows for the undermining of skin above and below the defect, without compromising the skin blood flow (which enters the skin as described previously). Second, oblique skin incisions along dermatome lines cut the fewest peripheral skin nerves, and potentially limit nerve pain morbidity after the procedure. Finally, the patient can be placed with the center of the defect at the "break" of the operating room table. Skin closure for oblique and transverse incisions can be aided by flexing the patient on the operating room table, thereby taking tension off of the skin closure. The abdominal skin

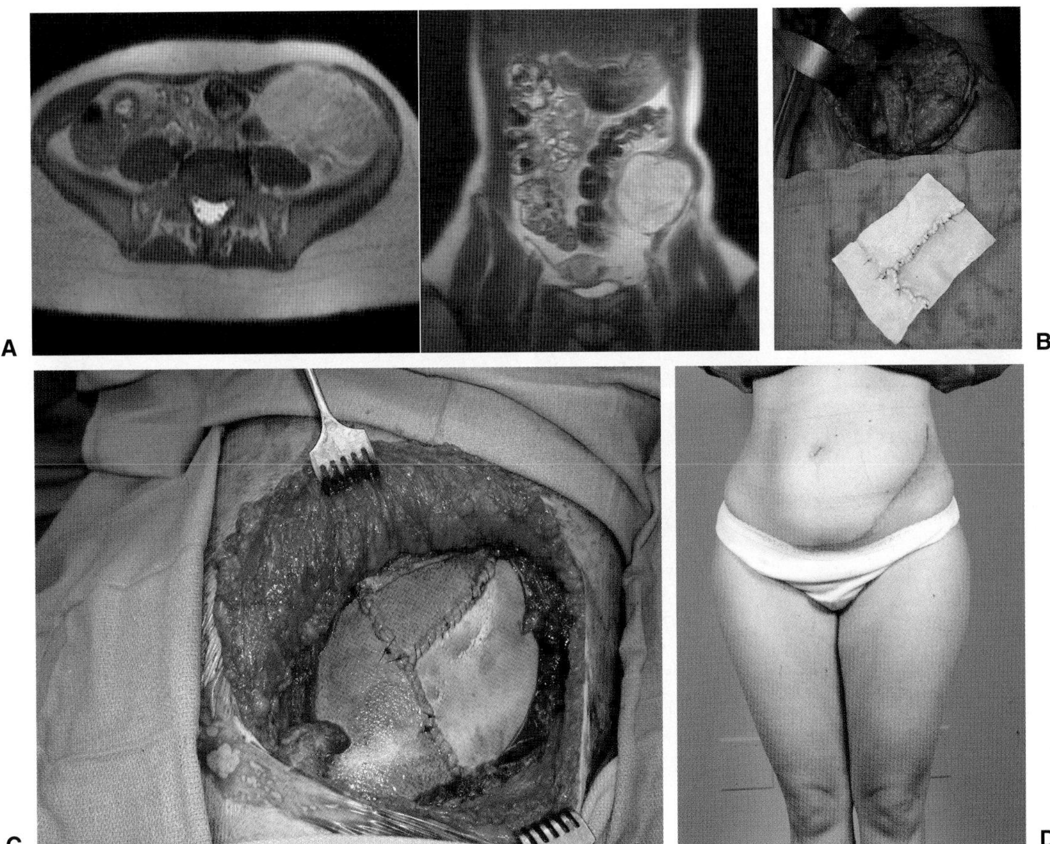

Figure 12.1. A 34-year-old woman with a desmoid tumor of left lower quadrant. There was adequate skin coverage, but without adequate greater omentum to interpose between synthetic prosthetic mesh and the bowel. (Case courtesy of Dr. Jeff Wayne). **(A)** CT scan shows the large tumor is attached to the left iliac crest. **(B)** Intraoperative photograph of the defect, with three sheets of acellular human dermis joined together with polypropylene sutures, which were used to reconstruct the muscle/fascia defect. **(C)** Intraoperative photograph of muscle/fascia reconstruction using human acellular dermis. **(D)** Appearance of reconstructed abdominal wall at 2-years follow-up.

stretches slowly in the post-operative period so the patient can eventually stand straight.

An example of good communication between the services is exemplified by the use of panniculectomy incisions for infra-umbilical abdominal wall tumors. Vertical incisions are problematic in obese patients, and performance of a panniculectomy for access to the abdominal wall has been shown to be efficacious in morbidly obese gynecology patients. The resulting incision is straightforward in its closure *(13)*.

All patients undergo the "pinch test" to assess the mobility of abdominal wall skin pre-operatively by the reconstructive team. This assessment of skin mobility is critical in planning if a direct skin closure over the defect is possible. Patient-specific factors such as obesity, previous incisions, previous weight loss, open wounds, stomas, and prior radiation therapy all are important factors in assessing pre-operatively if a patient can be closed with local tissue confidently. Cases exist when local tissues

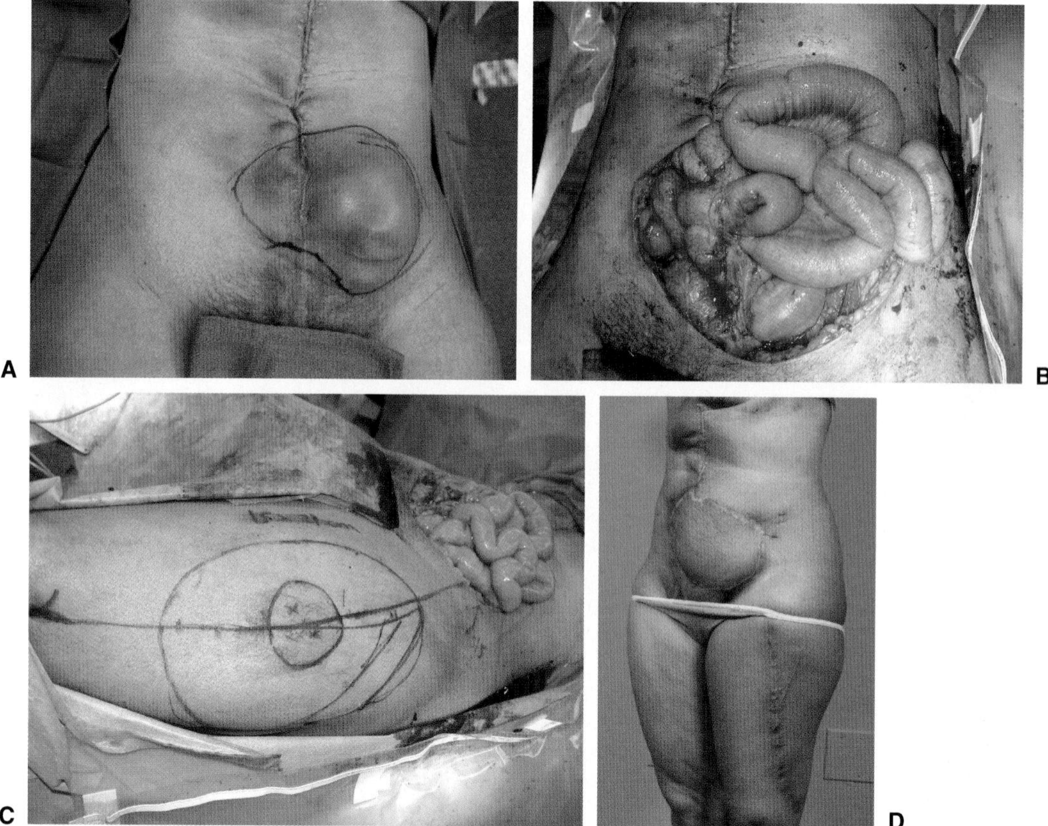

Figure 12.2. A 28-year-old woman with a multiply recurrent abdominal wall desmoid tumor with previous radiation therapy. (Case courtesy of Dr. Kevin Bethke). **(A)** Pre-operative view of tumor outlined in pen. There was poor-quality soft-tissue cover and inadequate greater omentum for interposition between mesh and the bowel. **(B)** Appearance of defect after tumor excision. **(C)** Design of an anterolateral thigh free flap for reconstruction of soft tissues. The lateral thigh fascia included in the flap was used to replace the muscle/fascia defect and the skin of the flap replaced the overlying skin defect. The left femoral vessels with vein graft interposition were used as recipient vessels for vascular anastomoses. **(D)** Oblique view of flap donor site on leg after abdominal wall reconstruction.

do not suffice for closure. If the abdominal wall is intact and only a skin defect exists, then a simple skin graft can be used for closure. However, if the abdominal cavity has been entered and mesh is used for reconstruction and would be exposed, then a soft-tissue flap with vascularized tissue must be transferred to cover the defect. Several groups have devised algorithms for flap reconstruction of soft-tissue defects of the abdomen, based on the location of the defect *(14,15)*. The most useful soft-tissue flaps come from the abdominal wall itself or the thigh. The tensor fascia lata flap can be used to provide soft-tissue cover to the lower abdomen; however, the distal tip of the flap may be unreliable owing to inconsistent vascular perfusion to the distal skin. A "delay" of the skin flap—outlining and elevating the flap without actually transferring it—is helpful to improve the flap's reliability several days to weeks prior to transfer to the abdomen. For the upper abdomen, the latissimus myocutaneous flap can be transferred from the back to the upper, lateral abdominal wall to provide soft-tissue coverage. Larger defects may require a free tissue transfer, in which the soft tissue is transferred and revascularized by reattaching the flap blood vessels recipient vessels near the defect. These free tissue transfers to the abdominal wall often require vein grafts from the leg to extend the reach of the transferred tissue because adequate recipient vessels may not be available close to the defect (Figure 12.2).

Midline Defects

A special situation exists for midline tumors. For these tumors, especially in the supra-umbilical location, skin mobilization for a superior-inferior closure is difficult. For these patients, a closure of BOTH the abdominal wall and the skin can be aided by the creation of bilateral rectus abdominis myocutaneous flaps (Figure 12.3) This technique referred to as "component

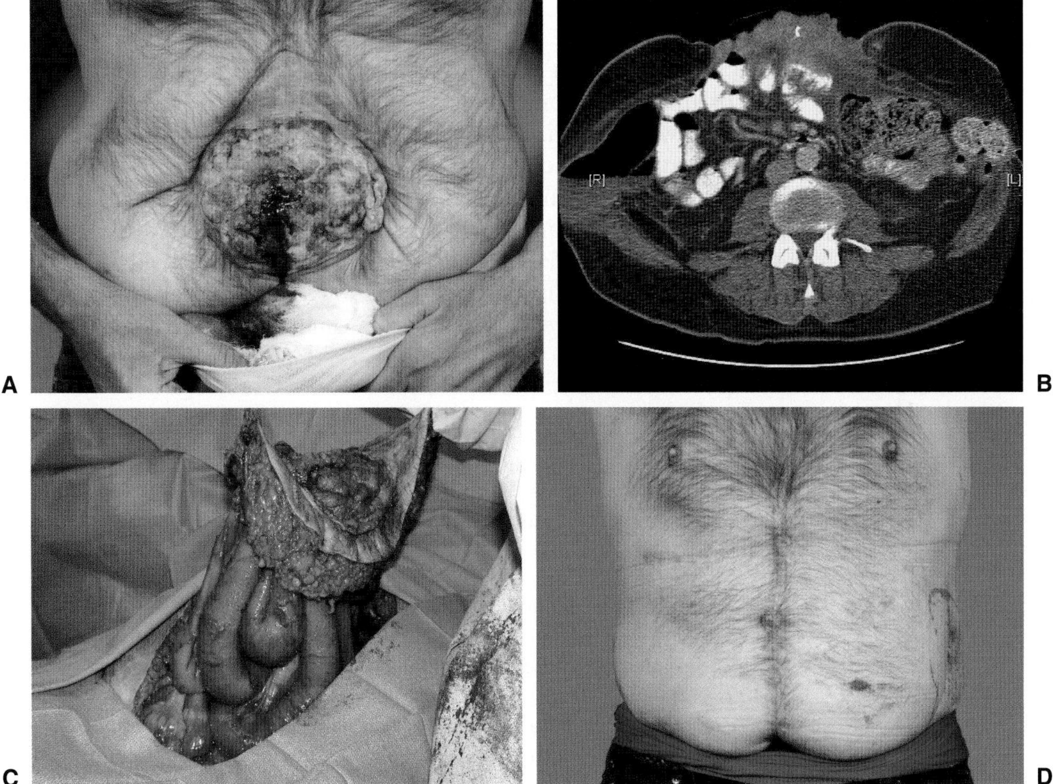

Figure 12.3. A 47-year-old male with a 14 × 16 cm^2 Marjolin's ulcer (squamous cell carcinoma) of the abdominal wall, invading into the bowel. An open abdominal wall wound with exposed polypropylene mesh for 11 years was believed to contribute to the development of this carcinoma. **(A)** Pre-operative appearance of abdomen prior to resection. **(B)** CT scan demonstrating involvement of the small bowel. **(C)** The entire cancer and contaminated abdominal wall wound was resected, en bloc, including loops of small and large bowel, which required small and large bowel resections. **(D)** Post-operative appearance of the abdominal wall after reconstruction with component separation and fascia lata graft.

separation" or the "separation of parts" involves releases of the external oblique muscle tendon as it inserts onto the anterior rectus fascia, which allows for a tremendous mobilization and medial transportation of lateral skin and abdominal wall muscle fascia towards the midline. The external oblique is the least elastic of the three lateral abdominal wall muscles. A disinsertion of the external oblique as it joins with the rectus abdominis sheath allows for 6–10 cm of movement of the medial-most tissue towards the midline. Previously, this procedure had been associated with a high post-operative wound complication rate owing to the wide elevation of skin flaps in order to perform the release of the external oblique. The post-operative wound complication rate has been shown to be markedly reduced when the skin is left attached to the abdominal wall. This maintains skin vascularity and reduces dead space. The releases of the external oblique muscle at the semilunar line can be performed through tunnels created through separate transverse incisions placed at the inferior aspect of the rib cage *(16)*.

Conclusion

The abdominal wall is essentially an expendable organ, used for movement of the upper torso and for containment and protection of the abdominal wall viscera. Tumor excision of the abdominal wall is limited only by what can be reconstructed. A straightforward analysis of the two related but independent questions of how to repair the internal or structural abdominal wall and how to close the skin leads to a decision tree involving mesh or fascial flap selection and the possible need for a simultaneous skin flap. With proper planning and coordination with the oncologic surgeon the reconstruction can be simplified and patient outcomes improved.

References

1. Stojadinovic A, Hoos A, Karpoff HM, et al. Soft tissue tumors of the abdominal wall: analysis of disease patterns and treatment. Arch Surg 2001;136: 70–79.
2. Camignani CP, Sugarbaker PH. Regional lymph node metastasis from port site implants after laparoscopic surgery. Surg Endosc 2004;18:2828.
3. Aldahham A, Boodai S, Alfuderi A, Almosawi A, Asfer S. Abdominal wall implantation of hepatocellular carcinoma. World J Surg Oncol 2006; 4:72.
4. Cruz I, Mamel JJ, Brady PG, Cass-Garcia M. Incidence of abdominal wall metastasis complicating PEG tube placement in untreated head and neck cancer. Gastrointest Endosc 2005;62:708–711.
5. Siefker-Radtke AO, Gee J, Shen Y, et al. Multimodality management of urachal carcinoma: the M.D. Anderson Cancer Center Experience. J Urol 2003;169:1295–1298.
6. Schlemmer M. Desmoid tumors and deep fibromatoses. Hematol Oncol Clin N Am 2005;19:565–571.
7. Ballo MT, Zagars G, Gunar K, Pollack A, Pisters PW, Pollock RA. Desmoid tumor: Prognostic factors and outcome after surgery, radiation therapy,

or combined surgery and radiation therapy. J Clin Oncol 1999;17: 158–167.
8. Phillips SR, A'Hern RA, Thomas JM. Aggressive fibromatosis of the abdominal wall, limbs and limb girdles. Br J Surg 2004;91:1624–1629.
9. Kind GM, Rademaker AW, Mustoe TA. Abdominal wall recovery following TRAM flap: a functional outcome study. Plast Reconstr Surg 1997;99:417–428.
10. Butler CE, Langstein HN, Kronowitz SJ. Pelvic, abdominal, and chest wall reconstruction with Alloderm in patients at increased risk for mesh-related complications. Plast Reconstr Surg 2005;116:1263–1275.
11. Butler CE, Prieto VG. Reduction of adhesions with composite Alloderm/ polypropylene mesh implants for abdominal wall reconstruction. Plast Reconstr Surg 2004;114:464.
12. Kozlowski JM, Dumanian GA, Fine NA, Cohn EB. Utility of the "Mutton-Chop" flap for reconstruction of large defects involving the lower abdominal wall and groin. Contemp Urol 1997;9:85–96.
13. Reid RR, Dumanian GA. Pannniculectomy and the separation of parts hernia repair: a solution for the large infraumbilical hernia in the obese patient. Plast Reconstr Surg 2005;116:1006–1012.
14. Mathes SJ, Steinwald PM, Foster RD, Hoffman WY, Anthony JP. Complex abdominal wall reconstruction: a comparison of flap and mesh closure. Ann Surg 2000;232:586–596.
15. Rohrich RJ, Lowe JB, Hackney FL, Bowman JL, Hobar P. An algorithm for abdominal wall reconstruction. Plast Reconstr Surg 2000;105:202–216.
16. Saulis AS, Dumanian GA. Periumbilical rectus abdominis perforator preservation significantly reduces superficial wound complications in "separation of parts" hernia repairs. Plast Reconstr Surg 2002;109:2275–2280.

13

Reconstruction of the Intra-Abdominal Pelvis and the Perineum

Gregory A. Dumanian

Introduction

Reconstruction following excision of cancers involving the pelvis, perineum, or vagina is complex for many reasons. First, the perineum is the exit site for three separate epithelialized structures—the rectum and gastrointestinal tract, the urethra and urologic tract, and in women, the vagina and gynecologic tract. Second, the deep location of the pelvis is difficult to access, and the perineum and vaginal areas are relatively remote from common flap donor sites. Third, the unyielding nature of the bony pelvis acts to block wound contracture as a means of wound healing. And fourth, the pelvis, perineum, and vagina are associated with multiple sexual, reproductive, and body image issues of variable importance to each patient. This chapter will elucidate some of the reconstructive options unique to the intra-abdominal pelvis, the perineum, the vagina, and the buttocks.

Reconstruction of the Intra-Abdominal Pelvis

The intra-abdominal pelvis is defined as the space below the pelvic inlet, and above the peritoneal reflections between the bladder, uterus, and rectum. Abdominoperineal resections (APR) of the distal colon/rectum/anus and anterior pelvic exenterations of the bladder and uterus/vagina for bladder and uterine cancer, posterior exenterations of the uterus/vagina and rectum for locally invasive rectal cancer, and total pelvic extenterations for a variety of locally advanced tumors all create soft-tissue defects within the intra-abdominal pelvis. Left untreated, the pelvis can become filled with fluid, and cause problems including drainage, infection (abscess), and perineal wound breakdown. This space may also be filled by the small intestine, resulting occasionally in bowel obstructions and/or herniation through the perineal wound. Therefore, reconstruction of the intra-abdominal pelvis is performed in order to fill the space created by tumor excision, as well as in certain instances to reconstruct the vagina.

Rectal Cancer

The rectum is a tubular structure of the alimentary tract, located within a bony cavity. The bony cavity of the pelvis renders the rectum difficult to reach for the cancer surgeon. Resection of the rectum results in a contaminated surgical field, increasing the risk of early infections and wound breakdowns. Reconstructive flaps are often able to help prevent and or treat wound-healing problems associated with rectal cancer surgery, particularly APRs.

The closer the lesion is to the anus, the less likely the surgeon can remove the tumor and anastomose the proximal transected bowel segment to the distal segment deep in the pelvis near the anal sphincter. This procedure, called a low anterior resection (LAR), is the most common surgery for cancer of the rectum for tumors more than 7 cm from the anus. When the tumor is less than 5 cm from the anus, it is frequently impossible for the surgeon to remove the tumor and preserve a functional sphincter mechanism. Patients with cancer of the rectum located near the anus usually undergo the APR procedure, which includes removal of the rectum and anus and placement of a permanent colostomy through the abdominal wall. The APR is problematic for several reasons. The contaminated nature of the procedure (owing to the transection of the colon) and the removal of the tumor from within the confines of the bony pelvis have already been mentioned. An added difficulty is the dead space caused by removal of the rectum and the inability of local soft tissues to collapse the space in the bony pelvis. With LAR, the space previously occupied by the rectum is replaced by a segment of left colon (similar in diameter and bulk) mobilized and brought inferiorly to anastomose to the rectal remnant. APR, in contrast, does not replace the rectal space with a similarly sized segment of colon. Rather, the distal colon is brought out through the abdominal wall as a permanent colostomy. Thus, the pelvic space formerly occupied by the rectum is empty, and if it is left unmanaged fills with fluid or small bowel. The fluid can become infected, and small bowel adherent within the pelvis can become obstructed. The possibility of these complications may be reduced if a flap is placed into the pelvic defect.

When APR was devised almost 100 years ago, surgeons would close the peritoneum to hold the intestines within the abdominal cavity and leave the pelvic space packed open with dressings to help prevent infection *(1)*. Management of the deep pelvic space in this manner was difficult, because open dressings of the perineum would require months for the soft tissues to contract and allow for secondary intention wound closure. The bony confines of the pelvic ring act to slow the wound contracture process dramatically. A completely different treatment of the pelvic dead space was adopted in the 1970s, when Silen and Glotzer reported on a technique that allowed the space to be filled by the intestines *(2)*. Filling the pelvis with vascularized tissue (the intestines) decreased fluid collection and subsequent abscess formation within the pelvis, and consequently, there was a decrease in wound breakdown rates. Unfortunately, the tight confines of the pelvis occasionally caused obstructions of the small bowel, and could result in difficult reoperative situations.

Healing of the intra-abdominal pelvis and APR defects is further rendered more difficult by the radiation therapy (RT) used to further treat low rectal cancers. RT is used to treat patients either before or after the APR procedure. Given pre-operatively before the APR procedure, radiation has been shown to decrease local cancer recurrence rates significantly. It may also reduce the magnitude of the resection required so that LAR becomes an option. However, pre-operative RT increases the local wound complication rate from 1–10% (without radiation) to 10–20% *(3)*. The means by which RT inhibits wound healing is by decreasing the tissue's ability to produce a normal wound-healing response of inflammation, angiogenesis, and deposition of collagen for wound healing. At the time of surgery, the tissues mechanically become stiff and difficult for the surgeon to manipulate, in part also contributing to local wound complications.

In contradistinction to pre-operative RT, post-operative RT has also been used for patients thought to be at high risk for cancer recurrence (e.g., those with positive lymph nodes or extensive invasion of surrounding tissues) and is also associated with reduced rates of local recurrence *(4)*. Post-operative RT is generally not started until the surgical field is healed, and therefore, it generally does not affect immediate post-operative wound healing. However, the small bowel that occupies the pelvic space after APR would be simultaneously radiated at the time of the tumor bed treatment. The bowel, adherent and unmoving in the pelvis because of surgical adhesions, is relatively sensitive to RT, increasing the likelihood of small-bowel radiation enteritis, stricture, and fistula formation. Radiation injury to the small bowel is reduced by limiting the total post-operative dose that is delivered—but this also tends to prevent an optimal treatment of the cancer bed *(5)*.

Placement of vascularized flaps into the perineum at the time of APR directly addresses many of the issues of wound healing and tumor treatment with radiation delineated in this chapter *(6)*. The vascularized tissue of a flap can fill the pelvic dead space created after APR with pliable, non-irradiated soft tissue whose blood vessels can carry in healing wound factors and antibiotics. The flap can also serves to block the small bowel from becoming located within the pelvis. This has the dual purpose of preventing a bowel obstruction and keeping the small bowel out of potential post-operative RT fields.

Historically, the most common flap used to fill the pelvis has been the pedicled greater omentum flap. The greater omentum can be dissected off of the transverse mesocolon and the stomach, elongated by dividing some of the vascular arcades, and passed to the right or the left of the midline to place it into the pelvic dead space. The flap is based on either the left or right gastroepiploic vessels. Unfortunately, the omentum may not be available or usable for reconstruction because of previous surgical adhesions in the upper abdomen, previous surgical removal, or insufficient size.

Myocutaneous flaps taken from the abdominal wall are an ideal alternative to the omentum for pelvic and perineal reconstruction. In essence, a trade-off of extra surgery and potential consequences with the abdominal wall is made for a decrease in wound-healing problems in the intra-abdominal pelvis. Considering the difficulty of treating pelvic abscesses, wounds, adhesions, and fistulae, use of the abdominal wall as a donor site for flaps seems justified. These flaps are typically based on the right deep inferior epigastric artery system. The left-sided vessels nourish the left rectus abdominis muscle, which is typically reserved for placement of the end colostomy required for completion of APR. There are three main types of flap "designs" based on the right rectus abdominis muscle and/or overlying skin. A right rectus abdominis muscle flap includes the muscle from above the costal margin to the vascular pedicle near the symphysis pubis. The anterior (above the arcuate line) and posterior rectus fasciae are still present for closing the abdominal wall. The muscle-only flap can improve initial pelvic/perineal wound healing, can be harvested through the same midline incision used for the laparotomy, and preserves the anterior abdominal wall fascia for closure of the abdominal wall. The problem with this flap is its relatively low volume. The muscle flap alone has limited bulk to obliterate pelvic dead space. Also, the muscle atrophies over time owing to division of the intercostal nerves necessary to transfer the flap into the pelvis, and this atrophy allows the small bowel to slowly descend into the pelvis.

As opposed to muscle-only flaps, myocutaneous flaps carry skin, subcutaneous tissue, and muscle based on the right rectus muscle and the right deep inferior epigastric vessels. Most of the flap volume with these myocutaneous flaps is composed of fat, which unlike muscle does not atrophy over time. Therefore, the small bowel is unlikely to slowly descend into the pelvis over time. When the skin is oriented vertically along the length of the rectus muscle, the flap is termed a vertical rectus abdominis myocutaneous flap (VRAM), whereas an oblique skin paddle based on peri-umbilical perforators is called an oblique rectus abdominis myocutaneous (ORAM) flap. The decision of whether to employ a rectus muscle flap, a VRAM, or an ORAM flap depends on pre-existing abdominal incisions, individualized requirements for soft tissue in the pelvis, and surgeon preference *(7)*. The two myocutaneous flap designs each have the potential to transfer skin into the pelvis, to help recreate the lining of the vagina, or to provide external skin at the level of the anus.

The benefits of filling the pelvic dead space with vascularized tissue must be compared to the risks of the procedure. In general, myocutaneous abdominal flaps are dependable, and partial or total flap loss owing to vascular insufficiency is not common. The reconstructive surgeon may attempt to take overlying skin and fat with less muscle in a desire to reduce morbidity of early wound-healing problems and late hernia formation of the abdominal wall. The VRAM flap generally includes the full width of the rectus muscle from the costal margin to the symphisis pubis. This creates the most vascularized flap, but the abdominal closure requires a moderate amount of medial advancement of fascia and skin. The ORAM flap bases the skin blood flow on perforators found near the umbilicus. Only a strip of muscle containing the right deep inferior epigastric vessel is harvested with an ORAM, leaving more muscle and fascia present for closing of the abdominal wall. However, muscle-sparing flaps may have more unpredictable blood flow and thus an increased risk of partial or even total flap loss.

Collections of fluid can accumulate at the donor sites from which the flap soft tissues were removed. These fluid collections (seromas) may be prevented with drains placed at the time of surgery. Although drains are usually effective, these seromas can cause small wound separations that become apparent 1–2 weeks after surgery. The trade-off of a small wound problem on the anterior surface of the abdomen is generally accepted to decrease the chances of a deep pelvic abscess or wound-healing complication. Another complication with these flaps is late abdominal hernia formation from the harvest of a portion of the rectus abdominis muscle. Because of the contaminated nature of the bowel resection, the use of permanent synthetic meshes are best avoided at the time of surgery to reinforce an area of the abdominal wall weakened by flap harvest. An example of an ORAM flap placed into the abdomen is represented in Figure 13.1.

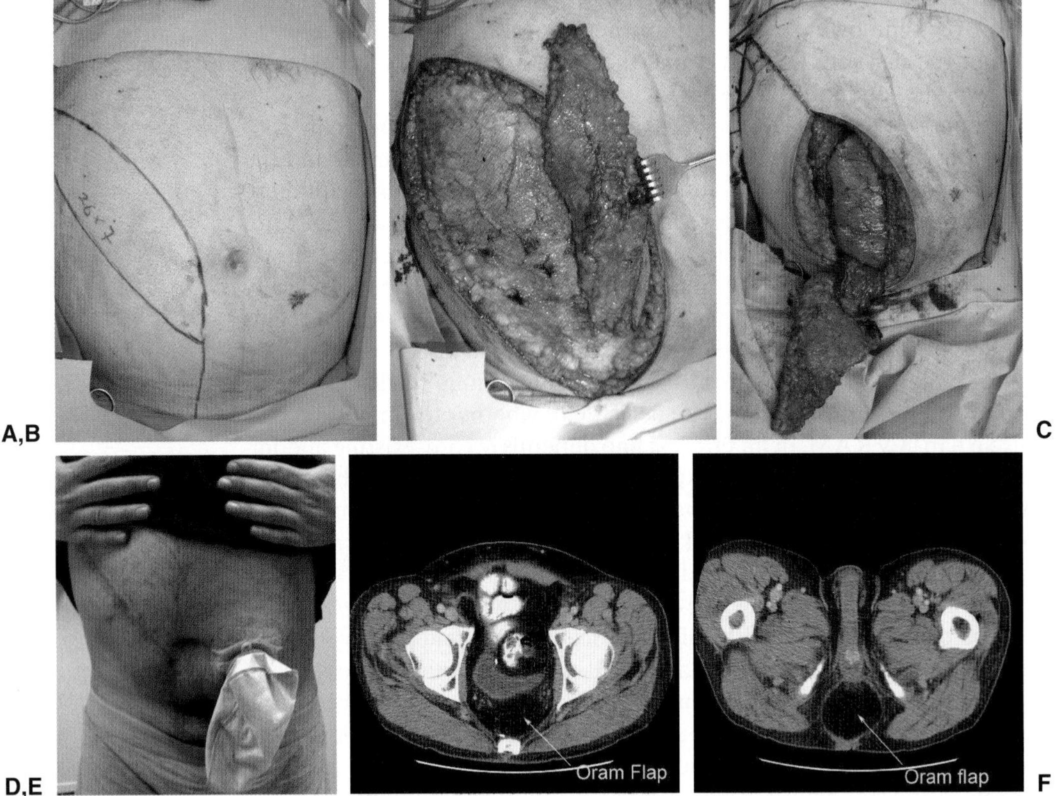

Figure 13.1. An ORAM flap was used to fill an intra-abdominal pelvis defect created after APR. Pre-operative RT had been given to the patient. **(A)** Drawing of the flap design and the pre-operative marking for stoma placement. **(B)** The flap is being elevated. **(C)** Rectus muscle dissection. The lateral border of the rectus muscle is still intact on the abdomen. The upper aspect of the incision is closed. **(D)** Post-operative photograph demonstrating the relationship of the incision to the stoma appliance. **(E)** The CT scan at 2-years follow-up with view of the upper aspect of pelvis showing the flap and bladder. **(F)** The CT scan at 2-years follow-up with view of the lower aspect of intra-abdominal pelvis showing the ORAM flap in place and the small bowel has been excluded from the area.

As described in this chapter, flaps have been used prophylactically in order to prevent a problem of the intra-abdominal pelvis. Flaps can also be useful in the treatment of wounds that develop after pelvic surgery. Pelvic wounds that occur after APR and without a previous flap can be difficult to treat. The wounds are typically in the lower aspect of the bony pelvis, radiated, chronically contaminated with bacteria, and can be painful. The bowel is located just superior to the wound, making debridement of the wound difficult and at risk for the creation for an enterocutaneous fistula. In order to avoid another laparotomy, gracilis flaps can be harvested from the inner thigh and tunneled into the wound. The muscle or myocutaneous gracilis flaps have been used successfully to treat non-healing wounds and sinus tracts of the perineum after APR. The abdominal flaps are generally performed at the time of ablative surgery, to help fill dead space and to help prevent perineal wound complications. The gracilis flap is generally smaller and can often fill only the lowest aspect of the rectal defect. It is less effective for filling the pelvis and preventing the small bowel from descending into the pelvic space. Therefore, the gracilis flap is often reserved for established wounds of the perineum after APR, rather than for their prevention.

Perineal Reconstruction

Vaginal Reconstruction

The vagina can be reconstructed by several methods, and the optimal technique depends on the reason for the vaginal absence. In vaginal atresia, the soft tissues of the perineum are intact, and often a tubed skin graft placed inside-out into a space created between the bladder and rectum can be used to construct a vaginal wall. However, vaginas constructed from skin grafts tend to contract over time, and dilators are generally required to maintain the size of the neovagina.

Tumor resections for cancers of the introitus, vagina, and cervix remove enough tissue that skin grafts generally cannot be reliably used for reconstruction. For low and small defects, local perineal skin flaps can be transposed to reach the remnant of the vaginal cuff. Adducting the patient's legs usually allows the donor site to be closed primarily *(8)*.

The optimal means of reconstruction for larger defects depends on the method of tumor extirpation. Vaginal tumors are often removed without a laparotomy. Reconstruction of the resulting defects is often performed using bilateral gracilis myocutaneous flaps. The skin paddles are sutured together to create a vascularized tube, which is inset into the perineum. The flap requires bilateral inner-thigh donor-site incisions that are usually cosmetically acceptable. One shortcoming of this reconstructive method is that occasionally the skin overlying the gracilis muscle does not remain viable during the flap transfer. The flaps can also be also difficult to sew into place with just a perineal (without a laparotomy) approach. The vascularized tissue is anchored deeply within the bony pelvis, and these stitches are much easier for the surgeon to place when the abdomen is entered at the time of tumor extirpation. These flaps are also more easily inset when there is a larger tissue defect, such as occurs with an APR or pelvic exenteration.

An alternative to bilateral thigh flaps for vaginal defects is a myocutaneous flap taken from the abdomen. When a vaginal tumor is removed during a laparotomy, then the rectus abdominis muscle with overlying skin can be tubed and transferred into the perineum. The skin used for the vaginal reconstruction will come mostly from above the umbilicus, resulting in a visible scar on the patient's upper abdomen. Despite that drawback, this method of reconstruction may be more reliable than bilateral tubed gracilis flaps. An example of reconstruction of the posterior aspect of the vagina, removed with the APR for locally advanced rectal cancer, is shown in Figure 13.2.

Other methods of vaginal reconstruction are less frequently used. Tubed fasciocutaneous flaps can be harvested from various remote locations and transferred into the pelvis using microsurgery. These are technically difficult operations, requiring several hours of surgery for the microvascular reconstruction, and with a chance of failure if the vascular anastomoses were to thrombose. Another alternative for vaginal reconstruction is transfer of a vascularized, defunctionalized segment of bowel into the pelvis, with the superior end sutured closed and the inferior end sutured to the perineal defect. This provides a tubed epithelial structure with its own mucous production for lubrication. Many surgeons avoid this means of vaginal reconstruction, however, because of its technical difficulty, need for bowel anastomoses, and the constant production of mucous, which often requires the patient to always wear a sanitary pad for hygiene.

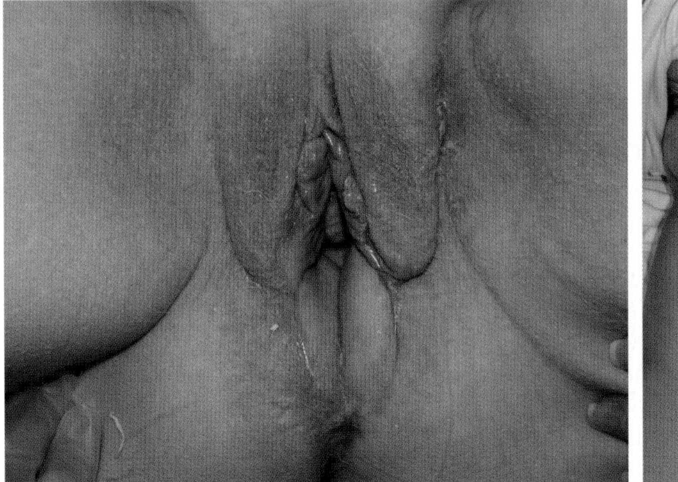

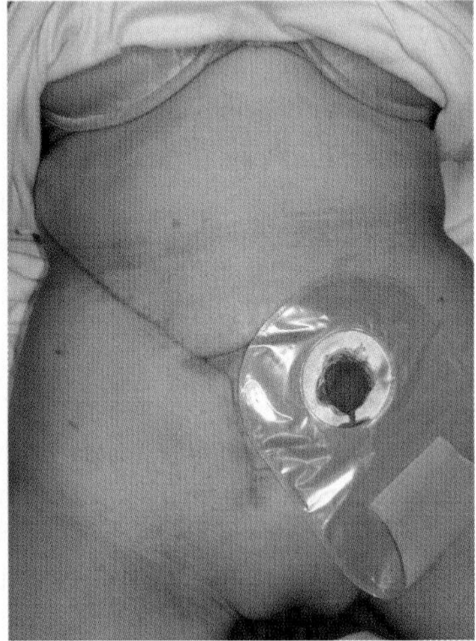

Figure 13.2. **(A)** Post-operative photograph of an ORAM reconstruction of the perineum after APR and partial (posterior) vaginectomy. The posterior vaginal wall and perineal skin were reconstructed with the ORAM flap harvested from right side of abdomen. **(B)** The APR was performed and the same incision used to harvest the right ORAM flap. An end colostomy was created through the left rectus abdominis muscle.

Perineal Skin Reconstruction

Although reconstruction of both the intra-abdominal pelvis and the vagina requires a "three-dimensional" reconstruction of the pelvic cavity and/or creating an internal lining of skin, reconstruction of the perineum typically requires only a two-dimensional reconstruction of the missing perineal skin. However, this skin replacement is often complicated by the need to preserve the exit sites for the vagina and urethra.

Perineal reconstruction may be required after removal of large primary tumors and smaller recurrent tumors of the labia, vagina, cervix, urethra, bladder, and penis. When the tumor involves the superior aspect of the vagina, the anus, and/or the rectum, perineal reconstruction may be required in conjunction with reconstruction of the pelvis and vagina.

Squamous cell cancer of the vulva is one of the most common tumors of the perineum, and the treatment of vulvar cancer is primarily surgical. The primary tumor is excised, and dissection of the inguinal lymph nodes may be performed at the same time, if indicated. Wound closure after resection of a small to moderately sized primary vulvar cancer is typically possible by adducting the patient's legs, flexing the patient at the waist, and advancing the thigh skin medially and the lower abdominal skin inferiorly. Larger primary tumors can be excised and the defect skin grafted if the area has not already received RT.

When vulvar cancers recur, secondary surgery is difficult because the tissues may be tight owing to prior removal of the primary tumor and/or RT. Tumor re-excisions result in large defects of the perineal skin. Thin skin flaps from the thighs or abdominal wall are the optimal coverage of these defects. Skin grafts alone may be insufficient as these areas are typically irradiated, contaminated with bowel flora, and under the stress of chronic movement. Skin flaps used in this area should be thin because even the thinnest skin flap may be more bulky than native tissue and be redundant and bothersome during ambulation. A representative case of a perineal defect repaired with an ORAM flap is demonstrated in Figure 13.3; the urethra and the vagina were inset into an opening created in the center of the skin flap. The underlying fat of skin flaps may be thinned at a delayed setting using liposuction once several months have elapsed since the surgery.

Obese patients have thick skin flaps, rendering the use of an abdominal flap difficult because of the marked difference between the thick layer of fat beneath the thin perineal skin. An alternative to the use of a skin flap for obese patients is a skin-grafted muscle flap. Both the gracilis muscle and the rectus abdominis muscle will reach the perineum, and can provide excellent interfaces between the irradiated bed and the skin graft to improve the "take" of the graft and to achieve wound healing. However, it is more difficult for the surgeon to create "exit sites" for the urethra, vagina, and anus when using a skin-grafted muscle flap in comparison to a skin flap, and consequently skin-grafted muscle flaps are not generally the first choice of reconstructive surgeons for perineal defects.

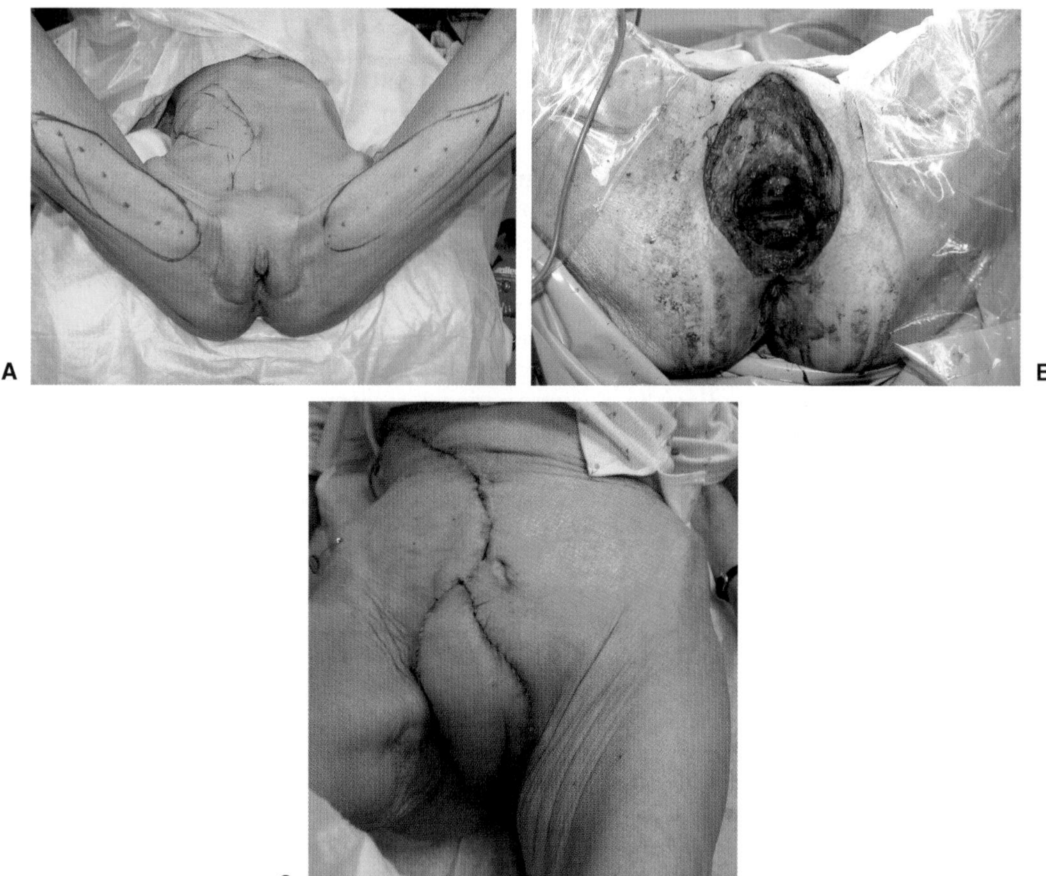

Figure 13.3. A 75-year-old woman with recurrent squamous cell carcinoma of the vaginal introitus was treated initially with RT and surgery. **(A)** The design of bilateral gracilis flaps (not used for the reconstruction) and an ORAM flap are marked on the patient. **(B)** Surgical resection with grossly negative margins. **(C)** Photograph at 3 weeks after a pedicled ORAM flap. An opening in the center of the flap was created for the exit of the vagina and urethra.

Anal/Buttock Skin Reconstruction

Squamous cell cancers of the anus, very low rectal cancers, and other tumors of the buttock skin, including melanoma, can involve the skin of the anus and buttocks. Anal cancer is different from other cancers described in this chapter, in that non-surgical treatment involving chemotherapy and RT alone is effective in preserving the anus in up to 85% of patients *(9)*. Failures of treatment can still be salvaged with an APR, though the radiation used for initial treatment becomes problematic in achieving wound healing. An ORAM or VRAM flap can be transferred to reach the anus and to facilitate incisional healing. Such a flap is performed at the time of APR, when the abdomen is completely open. The

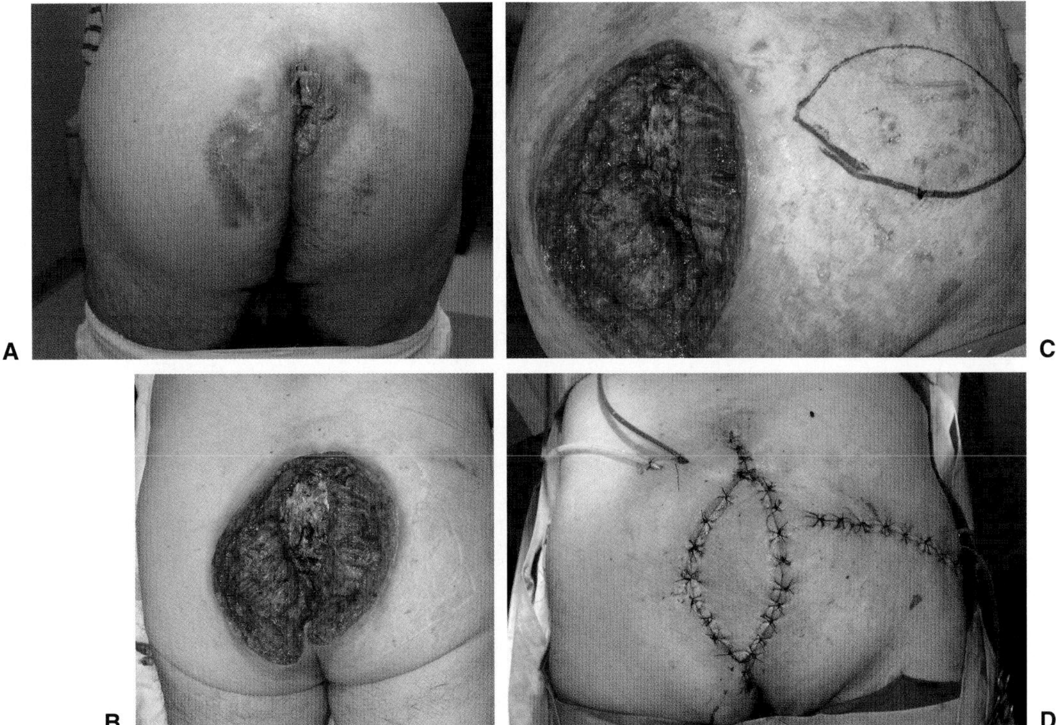

Figure 13.4. **(A)** A 64-year-old man with squamous cell carcinoma (Marjolin's ulcer) arising from a chronic pilonidal cyst. **(B)** Surgical resection with grossly negative margins. **(C)** The design of a superior gluteal artery perforator flap is marked on the right buttock. **(D)** Photograph of the reconstruction with donor and recipient sites closed.

flap is tunneled through the intra-abdominal pelvis to reach the buttock skin for wound closure.

Squamous cell carcinoma (Marjolin's ulcer) can develop in chronic perineal wounds present for prolonged periods of time. Figure 13.4 represents an unusual case of a large squamous cell carcinoma arising out of a chronic pilonidal cyst that had been present for 30 years. An important surgical consideration is that attention must be paid to diminishing the potential injury of the donor site for an ambulatory patient, particularly gluteal muscle function. Rather than creating a myocutaneous buttock flap for wound closure, a large gluteal perforator flap was harvested, leaving the entire gluteus maximus muscle in place while transposing the buttock skin to achieve wound closure. Another important consideration is the prevention of pressure on the incision during the early post-operative period. Pressure relief sand mattresses are employed for 7–10 days so that the patient can lie directly on the flap to decrease the chances of breakdown at the incision line and to prevent pressure on the vascular pedicle.

Conclusion

Successful tumor excisions of the intra-abdominal pelvis, perineum, vagina, and buttocks require not only a plan of how best to remove the tumor, but also a detailed plan as to how best to reconstruct the patient. Well-vascularized flaps are employed to fill dead spaces, prevent migration of the bowel into tight pelvic recesses, provide epithelized tissue for reconstruction of the vagina, and to achieve wound closures of the perineum and buttocks. The role of the reconstructive surgeon is to use the most reliable flap with the smallest long-term side-effects to the patient to achieve the desired goals.

References

1. Del Pino A, Abcarian H. The difficult perineal wound. Surg Clin North Am 1997;77:155–174.
2. Silen W, Glotzer DJ. The prevention and treatment of the persistent perineal sinus. Surgery 1974;75:535–542.
3. Stockholm colorectal cancer group. Randomized study on preoperative radiotherapy in rectal carcinoma. Ann Surg Oncol 1996;3:423–430.
4. Ota DM. Preoperative radiotherapy for rectal cancer: benefits and controversies. Ann Surg Oncol 1996;3:419–420.
5. Saclarides TJ. Radiation injuries of the gastrointestinal tract. Surg Clin North Am 1997;77:261–268.
6. Kroll SS, Pollock R, Jessup JM, et al. Transpelvic rectus abdominis flap reconstruction of defects following abdominal-perineal resection. Am Surg 1989;55:632.
7. Lee MJ, Dumanian GA.The oblique rectus abdominis musculocutaneous flap. Revisited clinical applications. Plast Reconstr Surg 2004;114:367–373.
8. Dumanian GA, Donahoe PK. Bilateral rotated buttock flaps for vaginal atresia in severely masculinized females with adrenogenital syndrome. Plast Reconstr Surg 1992;90:487–491.
9. Grabenbauer GG, Kessler H, Matzel KE, et al. Tumor site predicts outcome after radiochemotherapy in squamous-cell carcinoma of the anal region: long-term results of 101 patients. Dis Colon Rectum 2005;48:1742–1751.

14

Management of Chemotherapeutic Agent Extravasation and Radiation Therapy Adverse Effects

Ida K. Fox and Howard N. Langstein

Introduction

Although chemotherapy and radiation therapy are very effective modalities against cancer, both of these powerful therapies can have significant adverse effects on oncology patients. Chemotherapeutic agents can extravasate from veins, damaging nearby tissues, whereas therapeutic irradiation also can cause extensive tissue damage. Each member of the healthcare team should recognize and help to prevent these complications among oncology patients. Furthermore, cancer reconstructive surgeons may be called upon to repair tissues that become damaged.

This chapter outlines the biologic effects of these two treatment modalities as well as pathophysiological mechanisms that lead to adverse effects among oncology patients. First-line and more advanced reconstructive interventions, specific clinical scenarios, and ongoing research to repair such damages will also be discussed.

Chemotherapy Extravasation Injury

Incidence and Agents Associated with Extravasation Injury

Extravasation is defined as the leakage of any injected fluid from a blood vessel into the interstitial space. A number of agents including anti-tumor agents, hyperalimentation, potassium chloride solution, vasoactive medications, and various antibiotics can cause deleterious effects once extravasated. Treating extravasation injury is far from straightforward, and the medical literature is replete with reports of different drug and surgical regimens for controlling local tissue ulceration *(1)*.

The incidence of oncologic chemotherapeutic agent extravasation is estimated as 0.1–7.0% in adult populations *(2–5)*. In a 26-month Australian hospital study involving 3258 vesicant chemotherapeutic administrations, the extravasation rate was only 0.01% *(2)*. However, rates reflect differences among patient populations and among specific chemotherapeutic agents being used. For example, the extravasation rate was 11%

among pediatric patients *(1)*. Extravasation rates specifically related to doxorubicin appear to be 0.1% *(6)*.

Chemotherapeutic agents are classified as being irritants, vesicants, or non-vesicants; however, there can be some overlap. On the other hand, biologic agents such as interferons, interleukins, and monoclonal antibodies generally do not cause extravasation injury problems and in some cases, such as for interleukin-2 are even routinely administered subcutaneously *(7)*.

In general, although irritants may cause pain and inflammation if extravasated, they generally do not cause tissue necrosis. However, if an extremely large amount of a concentrated irritant is extravasated, it can cause ulceration *(4)*. Examples of the more commonly agreed upon irritants include carmustine, dacarbazine (may on occasion have vesicant potential *(4,7–9)*, melphalan, thiotepa, streptozocin, and cyclophosphamide. Some consider the topoisomerase II inhibitors, teniposide and etoposide, to be irritants *(2,10–12)*, but others consider them to be low-potential vesicants *(4,7)*. In the platinum analogs, carboplatin acts as an irritant *(4,5,11)* whereas cisplatin *(2,4,7,9,12,13)* and oxaliplatin *(4,14)* are usually irritants but occasionally vesicants. These agents are also sometimes classified as irritants: bleomycin, plicamycin, mitoxantrone, pentostatin, topotecan, and irinotecan *(4,12)*.

Vesicants cause local tissue damage such as blistering and tissue necrosis when extravasated. Agents that are clearly classified as such include: anthracyclines (doxorubicin, daunorubicin, epirubicin and idarubicin), vinca alkaloids (vinblastine, vincristine, vinorelbine and vindesine), alkylating agents (mechlorethamine/nitrogen mustard and amsacrine), and anti-tumor antibiotics (mitomycin, dactinomycin/actinomycin-D and mitoxantrone) *(2,4,5,7,9,11–13,15)*. The taxanes, paclitaxel (versus usual irritant *[12]*) and docetaxel, are generally considered vesicants as well *(4,5,7,11,13,15,16)*. Liposomal doxorubicin was originally reported as a pure irritant *(11,17)* but, in large amounts, it appears to have vesicant level effects *(4,7,18)*. Vesicants may also be classified on the basis of being DNA-binding, the alkylating agents, anthracyclines, and anti-tumor antibiotics; and non-binding, vinca alkaloids and taxanes.

Several related compounds are called non-vesicants because they do not cause tissue damage when extravasated. They include aldesleukin, asaparaginase, cladribine, cytarabine, liposomal daunorubicin, floxuridin, 5-fluorouracil, gemcitabine, and irinotecan *(2,11)*.

Pathophysiology

Agent factors

Any of a number of seemingly innocuous agents can cause adverse local effects if extravasated *(19)*. For instance, hyperalimentation, hypertonic glucose, IV contrast agents, and some antibiotics lead to cell death through osmotic imbalances across cell membranes. Vasopressors, such as norepinephrine and dopamine, and cationic agents, such as potassium and calcium solutions, cause local vasoconstriction and tissue ischemia. Meanwhile, most oncologic chemotherapeutic agents cause direct cellular toxicities. For all these agents, simple mechanical compression caused by the volume-related increase in interstitial pressure can lead to venous congestion and arterial compromise. Subsequent localized bacterial infections can also lead to further complications *(20)*.

Specific damage often varies with drug type. Typically, irritants cause pain, edema, and phlebitis whereas vesicants cause cytotoxicity with blistering and tissue necrosis. Non-vesicants rarely cause tissue necrosis. Other factors such as drug concentrations, amount extravasated, pH, osmolarity, and diluent or vehicle may play an important role *(7)*.

Subsequent metabolism, whether it entails inactivation or prolonged activity of a drug once it is extravasated, has important implications. For example, some DNA-binding vesicants can cause cyclical effects if they remain active and are released by dead cells. If taken up by adjacent healthy cells, they may lead to progressive tissue necrosis *(1,7,13)*.

Administration of therapy factors

The caretakers who administer chemotherapy agents play an important role in recognizing drug extravasation and determining tissue damage *(10)*. Only experienced personnel should insert IVs used for chemotherapy, but all caretakers should know which drugs are being administered and be able to recognize the signs and symptoms of extravasation.

Patient factors

Patients with a history of vascular disease are at higher risk of extravasation. Fragile and small vessels often are seen in patients with diabetes, collagen vascular disease, and in areas that have undergone radiation treatment. Previous venous thrombosis, phlebitis, and a depleted nutritional state also can make patients more susceptible to extravasation. Patients who cannot localize pain because of neurological diseases such as stroke, paraplegia, or diabetic neuropathy, or who cannot describe pain such as the very young or others with diminished capacity, are at risk for having larger volume extravasations because of delayed diagnosis *(19)*.

When chemotherapeutic agents are administered into the venous system via central venous access devices, the risk of extravasation diminishes but is not eliminated *(10,21)*. Central venous access device extravasation can occur due to incomplete placement of needle into port reservoir, dislodging of needle, blockage at catheter tip owing to thrombus or fibrin sheath formation, catheter/port separation, break in catheter or port, vein perforation or dislodging from vessel by the catheter tip, and catheter fracture. Also, the thickness of the port septum varies and a thicker septum port, for example, 11.5 mm in Port-A-Cath may have fewer problems than that seen in thinner septum products such as the Mediport (7 mm) and Infus-a-Port (3 mm) *(22)*.

Site of access factors

The site where extravasation occurs has important implications in defining subsequent injury. Extravasation and subsequent ulceration in areas where there is little soft tissue, such as the hand, may lead to damage of tendons, bones, and other vital structures. Extravasation in the antecubital fossa can cause joint contracture, leading to functional defects. Extravasation also can occur near superficial sensory nerves leading to chronic pain or complex regional pain syndrome (formerly referred to as reflex sympathetic dystrophy) *(23)*.

When chemotherapy agents extravasate from central venous access devices into surrounding breast tissue or into the chest cavity, they can cause significant soft tissue changes *(16)* or may lead to mediastinitis *(24–26)*. This type of extravasation typically occurs when needles dislodge, catheters thrombose, or when the catheters separate from the access port.

Recognizing Extravasation and Record Keeping

Recognizing the injury

In cases of extravasation, patients often will note that the treatment feels different from previous treatments and may note sensations such as pain, burning, and tingling *(13,27)*. There may be a decreased rate of flow of agent through the venous access device, localized edema and erythema, and when attempts are made to withdraw the catheter, often there is resistance and no flashback of blood *(13)*. Symptoms may be more subtle with use of implanted devices because extravasation injury may be confined to the chest cavity (if catheter tip perforates the superior vena cava) or deep in subcutaneous tissue (if port and catheter become dislodged). Vigilance in assessing patient symptoms, such as chest pain, as well as making sure of continuous easy flow of therapy forward and aspiration of blood backward are vital *(21)*.

Continued extravasation can, depending on the agent, lead to discoloration of the skin, induration, and desquamation or blistering, then ulceration, and, ultimately, tissue necrosis. Damage of skin can extend into subcutaneous tissue and underlying structures, and local vessels may thrombose. Severe large-volume extravasation can lead to nerve compression, vascular compromise, and limb loss. Immunosuppressed patients may develop supra-infection at the site of an extravasation injury because the local microvasculature becomes severely compromised.

Keeping track of the injury

Essential facts related to extravasation should be collected with a detailed chronology in the patient record. Memorial Sloan Kettering Cancer Center in New York designed a flow sheet to document extravasation injuries that can be duplicated for non-commercial use *(3)*. It includes the nurse and physician involved in administering the treatment, agent, amounts administered and estimates of how much was extravasated, IV site, needle type and gauge, and number of attempts to place that line. Patient symptoms and appearance of the site should be described along with a drawing or diagram to show the exact anatomic site; photographs can aid in following injury progression. Outlining the area of erythema or color change on the patient's skin can also be useful. Further, include all applications of cooling agents, antidotes, and wound dressings or other follow-up treatments *(2,4,7)*.

Healthcare providers need to be aggressive in following these patients either by direct contact or by phone. There is a need to evaluate localized skin integrity, temperature, edema, mobility, color, and pain. Specific signs, such as pain, erythema, and lymphangitic streaking, as well as systemic symptoms such as fever can mean supra-infection. Follow-up entails observation every other day for the first week, then weekly until symptoms resolve spontaneously or through surgery.

Medical Treatment Options

Immediate interventions

Immediate treatment primarily involves limiting volumes of extravasated agents. The infusion should be stopped and the indwelling device aspirated to remove residual medication site. However, aspiration may be painful and may not be that effective in removing the agent *(2)*. Although some reports recommend removing the peripheral IV, others prefer first to administer any agent-specific antidote through the line before removing it *(4,7)*. If a central venous access device is being used, make sure the needle is in the port by aspiration of blood; if catheter-to-port detachment or leakage is suspected, a radiology study may be warranted.

The affected extremity should be elevated for 48–72 hours, but pressure to the site should be avoided. For most agents, especially anthracycline extravasation, ice packs should be used immediately *(4,13,28–30)*, then for 20-minute intervals four times per day for 72 hours *(7)*. For vinca alkaloids, however, warm compresses should be used *(4,5,7,13,30)*. Several reports recommend leaving extravasation sites open to air at first. But with development of ulcers or supra-infection, specific, individualized wound-care treatment may be indicated.

Subsequent interventions

For more severe injuries, splints and physical therapy to maintain range of motion and prevent stiffness may be helpful. Pain management should be an integral part of the treatment regimen. For open ulcerations or necrotic areas, silver sulfadiazine topical treatment has been recommended *(4)*. In the case of non-healing ulcers, persistently painful areas, or necrotic or supra-infected wounds, surgical consultation is recommended.

Antidote treatment

There is a broad movement away from use of specific antidotes for treating extravasation. Historically, although topical corticosteroids were used to reduce inflammation, the consensus is that they are not effective and, in the case of doxorubicin and vinca alkaloids, can be detrimental *(4,7,10)*. Another agent, sodium bicarbonate, was used to change the local pH in an effort to induce cellular uptake of extravasated medications. However, it too was believed to be more harmful than beneficial because it can act as a vesicant if extravasated *(2,4,7,10)*.

Use of hyaluronidase to degrade hyaluronic acid and allow faster absorption of extravasated agents remains controversial. Hyaluronidase has been used for treating extravasated vinca alkaloids *(4,5,10,28)*, epipodophyllotoxin, and paclitaxel but not for anthracyclines and not in infected areas *(4)*. It can be reconstituted with normal saline to 150U/mL, injected directly via the extravasation IV line or subcutaneously, and administered as 1mL of the hyaluronidase solution for every 1mL of extravasated agent. A repeat dose may be given 3–4 hours later *(4)*.

Sodium thiosulfate has been used for the treatment of mechlorethamine *(4,5,7,10,28,31)* and large amounts of cisplatin extravasation injuries *(4)*. The sodium thiosulfate serves as a surrogate target for the extravasated agent, instead of cellular elements. The thioester byproducts that are created are non-toxic and undergo renal excretion. A 0.17mol/L solution can be injected directly into site of extravasation (use 4mL of 10% weight per volume sodium thiosulfate with 5mL sterile water). Approximately 2mL of the sodium thiosulfate should be administered for each 1mg of mechlorethamine or each 100mg of cisplatin extravasated via the extravasation IV line, then an additional 1mL may be injected subcutaneously and this subcutaneous dose should be repeated several times over the next 3–4 hours *(4,7)*.

Di-methyl sulfoxide (DMSO) is a solvent, free-radical scavenger and antioxidant, which may hasten absorption of extravasated agents by increasing skin permeability. It has been used for extravasated anthracyclines and mitomycin *(4,5,7,10,32)*. In clinical trials, it was used topically as 99% DMSO, four drops per 10 cm^2 of body surface area affected, every 6–8 hours for 7–14 days *(4,5,7,33)*. Treatment areas should be exposed to air because bandaging may lead to blistering *(32,34)*. Adverse effects include halatosis and a burning sensation.

Dexrazoxane, a derivative of ethylenediamine tetra-acetic acid (EDTA), is an intracellular chelating agent that blocks free-radical formation *(35)*. Used to minimize the cardiac toxicity of doxorubicin and other anthracyclines, it has been proposed as a treatment for extravasation of these agents *(5,16,35,36)*. There are case reports of success with use of dexrazoxane administered for treatment of epirubicin *(35)* and doxorubicin *(16,36)* extravasation. It can be administered intravenously at a dose of 1000mg per patient body surface area in m^2 immediately, then repeated 24 and 36 hours later *(35)*.

Both granulocyte colony stimulating factor (G-CSF) *(5)* and granulocyte-macrophage colony stimulating factor (GM-CSF) *(36)* have recently been proposed for use in treating anthracycline extravasation by promoting proliferation of various blood cell precursors to hasten wound healing. One group reported success with treatment of chronic doxorubicin extravasation ulcers by local subcutaneous injection of small amounts of 30mg/L GM-CSF solution three times a week for 2 weeks *(36)*.

Surgical Treatment Options

There are two major surgical strategies for dealing with extravasation. One entails aggressive early surgery to limit the extent of such injury, and the second delayed approach aims to excise non-healing ulcers to achieve durable wound closure.

For example, because anthracycline vesicants can significantly injure tissues, some reports advocate wide excision within 24 hours to 1 week to prevent the cyclic effects attributable to dead cells releasing the agent, which is then taken up and damages neighboring cells *(23,27)*. Excision is followed by frequent dressing changes and delayed skin grafting. Some advocate use of fluorescence microscopy and frozen section to precisely determine the margin of resection *(37)*.

However, most recommend conservative care initially in these often debilitated patients. The plastic surgery service can help to determine whether patients will benefit from surgical intervention. In some cases, local wound care allows healing, whereas in others serial debridement, skin graft, or flap closure may be required.

Delayed excision may be performed for patients who continue to have persistent pain at the site of ulceration or large areas of necrosis after many weeks *(4,10)*. Also extravasation injuries that involve large volumes of the agent or anthracyclines are more likely to require surgery *(7,10)*. In these cases of delayed treatment, some advocate magnetic resonance imaging (MRI) to help delineate extent of tissue damage prior to resection *(38)*.

Prevention of Extravasation Injury

All members of the medical team, but especially those who directly administer therapy, should actively help to prevent chemotherapy-related extravasation. Safe and appropriate use of venous access devices is paramount. For instance, plastic cannula peripheral intravenous devices should be inserted into patients at sites with adequate soft-tissue padding, and sites with any vessel thrombosis, lymphedema, or irradiation damage should be avoided. Although central venous access devices reduce the risk of extravasation, they should be inspected periodically for any evidence of port leak or detachment. Among some patient populations, particularly among the obese, it is preferable to use a tunneled central access device rather than one that must be accessed percutaneously by needle.

Prior to and intermittently during infusion of chemotherapeutic agents, the healthcare provider should draw back and flush the insertion site with saline to assess for patency. Clear plastic dressings should be used to ensure that catheters remain visible throughout the treatment. Whenever possible, drugs should be diluted before being administered and vesicants, which can injure vessels, should be administered before other, less-toxic agents. Pressure bags and infusion pumps should be avoided when possible *(2,7,28,30)*.

Clinical and Pre-Clinical Research

Because there are few if any case-control studies of extravasation injury, the literature on this subject is limited mainly to case reports involving patients treated in large oncologic centers. For example, the M.D. Anderson Cancer Center reported two case series involving oncology patients, with one series from 1979–1982 *(29)* and another from 1994–2000 *(12)*.

In both series, fewer than 20% of patients who received chemotherapy and were managed conservatively needed surgical intervention to treat extravasation-related injuries. Of those patients who required surgery, excision followed by primary closure or skin graft was most common; requirement for flap closure was relatively rare.

Other institutions report more invasive acute interventions to prevent extravasation-related injuries, including diluting the extravasated agent through subcutaneous injection, clysis, with hyaluronidase *(1,19)*, or saline alone *(1,9,19)*. Others attempt removal of the agent by saline flush-out or liposuction techniques *(39)*. Few institutions resort to early aggressive wide local excision.

Pre-clinical research in animal models has been used to compare putative agents for local subcutaneous therapy such as vitamin C *(40)*, N-aceytylcysteine *(41)*, and dapsone *(33)* but have not been translational. More recent pre-clinical work to study the use of systemic dexrazoxane for treatment of anthracycline has been helpful, and extrapolation of this work to clinical use has been reported as successful *(42)*.

Radiation Therapy Adverse Effects

Introduction

Like chemotherapy, radiation is an important cancer treatment modality that may be used following surgery or by itself. Radiation therapy regimens are empirically derived, balancing effective treatment against the "maximum tolerated dose" *(43)*. Despite extensive use, the biologic effects and unique pathophysiologic mechanism of injury attributable to radiation are not fully understood. Changes and effects vary among individual patients with similar treatment regimens, and these effects sometimes take years to develop. The unique effects of radiotherapy are described as "dysregulation of an integrated wound healing process" *(44)*.

Both acute and chronic effects occur in tissues exposed to radiotherapy, and both can lead to non-healing wounds that profoundly affect reconstruction efforts, with the most obvious examples being for patients with breast or head and neck cancer. In this part of the chapter we will review the adverse effects associated with therapeutic radiation treatment as well as grading systems to classify these effects, the pathophysiology behind them, common clinical scenarios, and how cancer reconstructive surgeons play a role in addressing these issues. Specific patterns of injury associated with non-healing radiation therapy-associated wounds and with breast and head and neck cancer reconstruction will be discussed.

Recognizing the Problems and Classifying Injuries

Radiation can cause highly visible, easily recognized acute effects, whereas longer-term effects are part of a "silent epidemic" that has proved difficult to define *(45)*. This obscurity has helped mislead some into believing that the adverse effects of radiotherapy are routinely so minor that cure is achieved with minimal intervention and surgery can be avoided. To overcome this misconception, surgeons, radiation oncologists, and others who deal with cancer patients need to recognize these adverse effects to help patients make well-informed choices *(45)*.

Recent attention to the injury patterns associated with radiotherapy led to development of two systems for classifying acute and long-term effects. Both systems can help to codify injury patterns, identify appropriate management strategies, and provoke interest in developing innovative treatment plans. The Common Toxicity Criteria (CTC) grading system, developed at the National Cancer Institute, is used to describe acute effects from radiation therapy as well as chemotherapy *(46)*. The late effects normal tissue (LENT) system grades tissue responses using "SOMA" categories, namely S, for subjective effects, including pain and numbness; O, for objective effects, including changes seen on physical exam, through imaging studies, and laboratory tests; M, for management, including topical medications and surgical interventions; and A, for analytic, which includes results from additional imaging or other specific tests *(44)*.

Clinical Manifestations

Although the CTC and LENT systems can be useful, radiotherapy-related tissue injuries typically prove more fluid and thus are more commonly classified as acute, consequential effects, and late effects *(47)*.

Acute effects

Acute effects, seen immediately or during the first few weeks after radiation therapy is administered, are attributed to the effects of radiation on cell populations, such as those in the mucosa and hematopoetic system, with rapid turnover. Radiation ionizes molecules within cells, inducing free radical formation and damaging DNA. Some cells, including lymphocytes, spermatocytes, salivary gland, and intestinal crypt cells, with damaged DNA undergo apoptosis. Fibroblasts, on the other hand, differentiate and produce more collagen than usual, leading to fibrosis. There is also a generalized cytokine-mediated increase in inflammation, coagulation, and fibrosis. Other acute effects include erythema of the skin in the area of irradiation, edema of the spinal cord, mucosal slough and diarrhea, and pneumonitis *(47)*.

Consequential effects

The incidence of consequential effects is increasing because of more aggressive radiotherapy, as well as regimens that combine radiotherapy with chemotherapy *(48)*. Consequential effects (also called consequential late effects) include those acute effects that fail to resolve after radiotherapy courses are completed. They may involve the gastrointestinal, genitourinary, and dermatologic systems through loss of epithelia, exposing the underlying connective tissue to stress, including mechanical and chemical forces against which it is ordinarily shielded. Because the severity of consequential effects is directly related to the severity of the acute effects of radiation therapy, minimizing acute toxicities significantly limits the subsequent effects *(47)*.

Late effects

Late effects are those that occur months or even years after radiation is completed. The mechanism of injury is not known and clinical manifestations vary significantly, ranging from vascular injury, fibrosis, necrosis, and atrophy, to the development of secondary malignancies. Such late effects may develop in complex waves of increased vascular permeability, cytokine production, fibrosis, cell death, atrophy, and tissue necrosis. These changes, unlike more acute effects, also affect cells with slower rates of turnover, including those in soft tissue, muscle, brain, kidney, and liver *(47)*.

Factors Affecting Radiation Injuries

Agent factors

Several factors directly affect adverse reactions associated with radiation treatment: the volume and type of tissue being treated, the total as well as the dose per treatment being administered, and the treatment schedule and intervals between treatments. Overall, administering radiation in multiple smaller doses imparts less acute injury compared to administering a single large dose for the same total dose. However, simply prolonging the time period over which radiotherapy is administered does not eliminate late reactions *(49)*. Another important factor is the rate of dose accumulation. Administering relatively small doses in a short period (dose-intense radiotherapy) suppresses natural repair processes that are normally induced after each treatment *(50)*.

The type of radiation used for therapy helps to determine tissue-related effects and damage. For example, external beam, or tele-, radiation has more diffuse effects than does brachytherapy, which consists of radioactive implants that exert more localized effects. Moreover, several different types of external beams are now in use, including orthovoltage, which consists of low-energy X-rays that cannot penetrate deeper tissues and is generally restricted to treatment of skin tumors. Meanwhile, the more extensively used megavoltage, external beam, high-energy radiation has a skin-sparing effect because its maximal dose is achieved deep within target tissues *(49)*. Radiation therapy may also vary by radiation energy source, but the impact of these differences has not been fully assessed *(47,49,51)*.

Although most radiation-induced secondary malignancies are carcinomas, sarcomas do occur but typically only after a large dose of radiation is delivered to a specific anatomic site *(52)*.

Patient factors

Radiation is striking in the wide variation of effects seen from one individual to the next. Some of these differences reflect surgical procedures or other medical conditions affecting the treatment site such as diabetes or other vascular diseases. Other less-straightforward differences are attributed to genetic variations, such as differences in ability to repair DNA damage. An extreme example is patients with ataxia telangiectasia, who may develop tissue necrosis or secondary malignancies *(52)* after standard radiation therapy dosing.

Another specific patient population for whom radiotherapy may be contraindicated is those with collagen vascular disease. Patients with rheumatoid arthritis may tolerate radiation therapy, but other patients with active collagen vascular disease often cannot. However, the small numbers of such patients makes it difficult to know what is normal variation and what is attributable specifically to the collagen vascular disease *(53)*. Variations observed among individuals with BRCA 1 and 2 mutations, who may have increased radiosensitivity along with an increased risk for breast and other malignancies, are also unpredictable *(52)*.

Pathophysiology and Mechanism of Radiation-Induced Damage

Introduction

Radiation therapy kills not only rapidly dividing cancer cells but also other non-malignant cell populations. Historically, such cell death was attributed simply to radiation-induced DNA damage. However, this view is changing to account for the complex changes on the cellular and systemic levels that occur but which are still not fully understood *(43)*. Developing a better understanding of radiation-induced effects could also lead to development of agents to prevent or treat them *(44)*.

Molecular and cellular response to radiation

Basic trauma to cells, through radiotherapy or other means, leads to responses, including cell death, tissue hypoxia, fibrosis, and angiogenesis, that are regulated by cytokines, growth factors, cell adhesion molecules, and the extracellular matrix *(44)*. In radiation injury, fibrogenesis and angiogenesis tend to counterbalance one another; increased fibrosis is, however, paradoxically greater in those sites with decreased wound healing *(50)*.

Radiation, even in small doses, produces free radicals that damage DNA and other molecules such as proteins, lipids, and carbohydrates. Higher doses administered at a rapid rate exacerbate this damage, and cell signaling systems play a role in this re-injury pattern *(50)*. For example, transforming growth factor beta (TGFβ) may be a marker or the responsible agent for such damage. When TGFβ is elevated at baseline, which occurs for some cancer subtypes, radiation-induced fibrosis often is exacerbated *(44)*. An imbalance of matrix metalloproteinases, which become active in tissues that are remodeling, is also associated with radiation-induced damage. The renin-angiotensin system may play a role, especially in patients who have had whole-body radiation, in the development of renal and pulmonary complications *(44)*.

Vascular effects

Radiation affects vessels of all sizes. Capillaries may thrombose, dilate, (leading to telangiectasias), and rupture. Irradiated arterioles and small arteries often have fibrosis along the vessel wall and a media filled with hyaline. Medium-sized arteries also undergo fibrosis and have partial obstruction of the lumen through plaque formation and the presence of lipid-laden foam cells. Although these effects affect tissue inflow, whether tissue ischemia is wholly a result of vascular changes is not known *(50)*. It is also unclear whether radiation-damaged tissues can fully revascularize. In any case, patients with pre-existing vascular disease processes tend to rapidly develop tissue ischemia-related problems following radiation therapy. If vascular disease develops post-radiation, patients may not develop complications until a critical point is reached as part of that secondary disease process *(50)*.

Recognizing Radiation-Induced Effects

Early skin effects

Radiation-induced effects in skin are often seen within days but may last for weeks as acute erythema and desquamation, attributable to protease release, increased vascular permeability, and local inflammation. Dry desquamation is caused by patchy epithelial cell death often seen with intermediate doses of radiotherapy (less than 30 Gy) and manifests as scaling, pruritic skin. Wet desquamation, which refers to exudates of serous fluid from the exposed dermal layer, comes with higher doses of radiotherapy (greater than 40 Gy) and is caused by the death of epidermal cells. Although healing occurs with re-epithelialization from skin-associated adnexal elements or the periphery, such damaged areas tend to remain fragile, with bullous characteristics and a thin epidermis *(49,51,54)*.

Late skin effects

Subsequently, skin pigmentation may increase or, owing to melanocyte death, decrease. The skin may become fibrotic with abnormal eccrine and sebaceous gland functions. In some cases, the skin becomes nearly translucent, fragile, and painful. Permanent hair loss indicates that radiation injury damaged hair follicles, which are normally the skin adnexal agents that allow re-epithelialization after desquamation. Skin necrosis or ischemic ulcers often signal underlying abnormal vasculature *(49,51,54)*.

Effects on wound healing

Wound healing in irradiated areas typically is diminished *(54,55)*. Basal layer keratinocytes of the skin normally re-epithelialize open areas, but these rapidly dividing cells are particularly susceptible to radiation. Fibroblasts are also injured by radiation and this leads to formation of wounds with a diminished tensile strength. These effects are compounded by hypoxia owing to abnormal vascularity. These processes are irreversible and can grow worse, even years after treatment *(55)*.

Treatment of Radiation Damage

Treatment for acute effects

Avoid trauma to the affected skin, including shaving, sun and wind exposure, or scratching. If areas require dressing, minimize the use of adhesive tape. Cleanse skin gently with mild soaps and rinse thoroughly. Iodine may be used if disinfection is required *(56)*. Topical lubricants, Eucerine (Beiersdorf Inc., Wilton, CT) and Lubriderm (Pfizer Inc., Morris Plains, NJ), and protective ointments, such as A and D ointment (Schering-Plough HealthCare Products Inc., Kenilworth, NJ), may be applied to dry areas. For pruritis, cornstarch or Aveeno products (Johnson and Johnson Inc., New Brunswick, NJ) are acceptable except in damp areas, where their use may encourage fungal infection. Steroids (1% hydrocortisone) may be used sparingly in severe cases of pruritis, but not if there is suspicion of infection. Avoid topical alcohol, menthol, or heavy metals such as zinc and aluminum, which are found in deodorants *(49,51)*.

Wet desquamation requires regular cleansing with normal saline, water, or half-strength hydrogen peroxide *(51)*, and gentle debridement. For denuded areas, topical agents such as silver sulfadiazine or antibiotic ointment may be useful. Hydrocolloid, Duoderm (Bristol-Myers Squibb Co., New York, NY), or clear adhesive, Tegaderm (3M, St. Paul, MN) or Opsite (Smith and Nephew PLC, London, England), dressings can be used to absorb drainage, prevent drying out, or simply to protect the affected site *(49)*.

Subsequent treatment

Irradiated skin must be protected from the sun and observed carefully for secondary malignancy formation *(49)*. Wash affected areas only with mild soaps with a pH of less than 7.5, such as Dove (Unilever, Englewood Cliffs, NJ) or Basis (Beiersdorf Inc., Wilton, CT). The skin can also be protected with lubricants such as petroleum, mineral oil, Lubriderm (Pfizer), Nivea (Beiersdorf), or Aquaphor (Beiersdorf) *(49)*.

Treatment specifics

There are two approaches to developing agents to mitigate radiotherapy damage. One involves radiosensitizers to make tumors more susceptible to radiation. The other involves radioprotectants that make bystander cells more resistant to radiation damage. There are few options for protecting cells against direct radiation damage to DNA. However, radioprotectants might be developed to limit free radical-mediated effects of radiation. For example, amifostine is approved for use to decrease xerostomia in patients with head and neck cancer. Although this option appears promising, the deployment of radioprotectants will requires careful balancing so as not to jeopardize the efficacy of radiation treatment *(57)*.

Hyperbaric oxygen treatment

Hyperbaric oxygen (HBO) therapy involves treatment with 100% oxygen at greater than normal atmospheric pressure and is typically administered daily for 90–120 minutes in specially designed chambers.

HBO is often used for treating radiotherapy-induced tissue damage. During treatment, increased tissue oxygenation promotes angiogenesis, fibroblast activity, and other processes that accelerate wound healing *(59)*. For example, HBO has been used successfully to treat hemorrhagic cystitis *(60)*, proctitis *(61)* after pelvic radiation, and osteoradionecrosis after radiation for head and neck cancers *(62,63)*. HBO has also been used for treating pediatric patients for a variety of radiation-induced effects *(64)*. Ongoing studies will better define the indications, utility, and cost-benefit ratio of HBO for treatment of radiation adverse effects *(59)*.

Surgical treatment

Irradiated tissue does not respond like normal tissue to surgical interventions. In cases where surgery must be done in a radiation-treated area, it is better to complete radiation at least 3–6 weeks before surgery *(49)*. However, for non-healing radiation-induced ulcers that demand immediate surgical intervention, there are a number of empirical recommendations for improving outcomes.

Initially, radiation wounds should be serially debrided back to bleeding tissue prior to closure. A viable edge to which a transposed flap can be attached is necessary. In general, flaps of non-irradiated muscle are recommended for treating wounds in irradiated areas. In one clinical study, patients with non-irradiated muscle brought in for wound coverage had far fewer complications than did those whose flaps were taken from within the radiated site. Even though local radiated muscle flaps may look viable at transfer, they subsequently developed necrosis or became infected *(65)*.

Another group looked at surgical treatment of radiation-induced wounds in the breast, axilla, and mediastinum. They also recommend closure with well-vascularized muscle flaps after wide debridement of the affected area. They further suggest that outcomes will be improved if vessels supplying the affected tissue are outside the radiation field *(66)*, although large pedicle vessels within the field are probably safe.

Specific flaps may be helpful for covering irradiated wounds. For example, for anterior chest wounds, pectoralis major and latissimus dorsi muscle flaps can provide coverage with healthy muscle supplied by vasculature that is well outside the radiation field. In comparison, rectus abdominis muscle, with inflow through the superior epigastric pedicle, may be less reliable. For large, central, and inferior chest wall defects, omentum, with its robust intra-abdominal blood supply, may be a better option *(67)*.

Site-Specific Effects of Radiation Treatment

Breast cancer

There is a continuing trend toward the greater use of adjuvant radiation therapy for patients following mastectomy, with the goal of improving survival *(68,69)*. Thus, the number of women receiving radiation and surgical therapy who present for reconstruction will likely increase. Radiotherapy-induced fibrosis of the breast and axilla can develop years after the initial treatment and may be severe *(70,71)*. Breast reconstruction in these patients is both complicated and somewhat controversial. Overall, higher complication rates are seen among all irradiated patients who undergo immediate breast reconstruction regardless of type when compared to patients who do not receive irradiation *(72)*.

One question that deserves special attention is the impact of immediate reconstructive surgery on subsequent radiation therapy. Thus, patients who immediately undergo reconstruction may compromise the efficacy of subsequent radiation therapy because changes in breast geometry may impair the delivering of radiation. However, there are no conclusive data to indicate whether early reconstructive surgery changes recurrence or survival rates *(73)*.

Reconstruction using breast implants in the context of previous or subsequent radiation therapy can be problematic. In one study, unplanned reoperation for implant removal or exchange is required in 18.5% of such patients *(74)*. Among patients who had bilateral mastectomies and implant reconstruction but unilateral post-operative radiation therapy, there were higher rates of capsular contracture on the radiated side. However, overall symmetry, aesthetic outcomes, and patient satisfaction were graded as good. This study included only 12 patients and had a relatively short follow-up period (23.5 months) *(75)*.

Autologous tissue reconstructions may tolerate radiotherapy better than implants. There is continuing disagreement regarding the acceptability of outcomes in irradiated pedicled flap reconstructions *(76,77)*. Initially, there was some hope that the superior vascularity of free tissue transfer would improve results after radiotherapy. Thus, even in patients who would receive radiation, immediate reconstruction with preservation of the mastectomy flap skin envelope would be possible *(72,76)*. However, results after radiotherapy still remain difficult to predict. One proposal is to perform "delayed-immediate" breast reconstruction. The skin envelope is maintained by immediate placement of a saline-filled implant. In patients who do not require radiation, the implant can be removed and reconstruction performed. The implant can be deflated to allow for unhindered radiation or may be left inflated depending on the preferences of the radiotherapist, and reconstruction can be performed once treatment is completed *(78)*. Because no approach is definitive, individual patients and surgeons should consult to develop a plan that best minimizes risk and maximizes benefit on a case-by-case basis.

Head and neck cancer

Radiation of the head and neck area leads to a spectrum of adverse effects that require careful management. Many of the recommended treatment protocols are empirically based and will change as new developments in therapeutic agents and data from clinical trials come forward.

Early and often transient effects seen with radiation to the head and neck include mucositis and taste loss. Mucositis can be prevented by minimizing intra-oral irritation from irregular fillings, dental appliances, spicy or acidic foods, and avoiding alcohol and tobacco. Established mucositis is treated with pain medication, topical anesthetics, and oral barrier suspensions such as sucralfate *(79)*. New modalities, such as GM-CSF may also be useful *(80)*.

Xerostomia, or dry mouth owing to decreased salivation, may occur acutely and then remain a chronic problem that can then lead to the development of radiation caries. Prevention by carefully planning the radiotherapy field to spare some salivary gland tissue is helpful. A more radical means to preserve salivary tissue is by pre-treatment surgical transposition of the submandibular glands outside of the planned radiation field *(47,79,81)*. Pilocarpine and amifostine are medications that may help prevent and treat xerostomia *(79,81)*. To prevent subsequent caries development, fluoride treatment and meticulous oral hygiene are important *(81)*. Trismus, which can be treated by physical therapy and stretching exercises, and dysphagia may also occur *(82)*.

Osteoradionecrosis, exposed irradiated bone that fails to heal, is the most dreaded complication of head and neck radiation treatment. To prevent this, a thorough dental exam should be performed prior to starting radiation treatment. All teeth that have caries, periodontal or periapical disease, partially erupted teeth, and teeth adjacent to the tumor should be removed. This will hopefully obviate the need for any invasive dental procedures during the period of radiation treatment. If extraction during treatment is necessary, antibiotics and HBO treatment may be helpful *(79)*.

The grading system for osteoradionecrosis is under development *(83)*, but certain general treatment strategies should be followed. Sequestrum, pieces of devascularized bone, should be removed. Again, HBO may be helpful *(62,63,84)*. Larger diseased areas that do not respond to serial debridement or that are associated with orocutaneous fistulas, pathologic fractures, or full-thickness involvement of the bone may require radical debridement followed by free tissue transfer *(85,86)*. It should be noted that free tissue transfer in this setting may be complicated by the difficulty of finding adequate inflow vessels in an irradiated field *(87)*.

Research

There is much that needs to be learned about the mechanism of radiation-induced effects and the inter-individual variation of genetic susceptibility to those effects. Understanding how wound healing occurs after radiation treatment would also allow a better treatment of wounds that do not heal. Treatment regimens such as amifostine, antioxidants, free-radical scavengers, and other protective agents should be assessed *(47)*.

Cellular signaling pathways such as the renin-angiotensin system may play a role in radiation-mediated damage and angiotensin-converting enzyme inhibitors and angiotensin II receptor blockers (currently used for treatment of hypertension) may be useful *(44)*. Topical TGFβ1 has been shown in animal studies to help prevent or treat acute radiation induced damage to the skin. Paradoxically, TGFβ1 inhibitors may help to prevent the late effect of radiation-induced fibrosis; this demonstrates the importance of balance of TGF-β1 and its effects on connective tissue formation *(51)*. Use of factors such as GM-CSF may also be helpful for treatment of acute skin effects. Unfortunately, topical treatment with vitamin C, non-steroidal anti-inflammatory drugs (NSAIDs), hydrocortisone, and lasers have not proven effective *(44)*. HBO treatment also deserves further bench and clinical investigation.

Conclusion

This chapter provides an overview of adverse effects associated with two common cancer treatment modalities—chemotherapy and radiation—that improve disease-free survival in oncology patients. Because they are so powerful, these therapeutic modalities often inflict significant morbidity on an already vulnerable patient population. Prevention, early recognition, and use of up-to-date, evidence-based treatments for these adverse effects are imperative. Ongoing efforts to improve our understanding of the underlying pathophysiology of these treatment modalities could lead to development of pharmaceutical agents, such as antioxidants or growth factors, that prove effective for treating or preventing some of the damage that they cause.

References

1. Heckler FR. Current thoughts on extravasation injuries. Clin Plast Surg 1989;16(3):557–563.
2. Cox K, Stuart-Harris R, Abdini G, Grygiel J, Raghavan D. The management of cytotoxic-drug extravasation: guide-lines drawn up by a working party for the Clinical Oncological Society of Australia. [erratum appears in Med J Aust 1990;152(3):168]. Med J Aust 1988;148(4):185–189.
3. Davis ME, DeSantis D, Klemm K. A flow sheet for follow-up after chemotherapy extravasation. Oncol Nurs Forum 1995;22(6):979–983.
4. Ener RA, Meglathery SB, Styler M. Extravasation of systemic hemato-oncological therapies. Ann Oncol 2004;15(6):858–862.
5. Schrijvers DL. Extravasation: a dreaded complication of chemotherapy. [see comment]. Ann Oncol 2003;14(3):iii26–30.
6. Larson DL. Alterations in wound healing secondary to infusion injury. Clin Plast Surg 1990;17(3):509–517.
7. Albanell J, Baselga J. Systemic therapy emergencies. Semin Oncol 2000;27(3):347–361.
8. Napoli P, Corradino B, Badalamenti G, et al. Surgical treatment of extravasation injuries. J Surg Oncol 2005;91(4):264–268.
9. Scuderi N, Onesti MG. Antitumor agents: extravasation, management, and surgical treatment. Ann Plast Surg 1994;32(1):39–44.
10. Camp-Sorrell D. Developing extravasation protocols and monitoring outcomes. J Intraven Nurs 1998;21(4):232–239.
11. Goolsby TV, Lombardo FA. Extravasation of chemotherapeutic agents: prevention and treatment. Semin Oncol 2006;33(1):139–143.
12. Langstein HN, Duman H, Seelig D, Butler CE, Evans GR. Retrospective study of the management of chemotherapeutic extravasation injury. Ann Plast Surg 2002;49(4):369–374.
13. Boyle DM, Engelking C. Vesicant extravasation: myths and realities. Oncol Nurs Forum 1995;22(1):57–67.
14. Foo KF, Michael M, Toner G, Zalcberg J. A case report of oxaliplatin extravasation. Ann Oncol 2003;14(6):961–962.
15. Ajani JA, Dodd LG, Daugherty K, Warkentin D, Ilson DH. Taxol-induced soft-tissue injury secondary to extravasation: characterization by histopathology and clinical course. J Natl Cancer Inst 1994;86(1):51–53.
16. El Saghir NS, Otrock ZK. Docetaxel extravasation into the normal breast during breast cancer treatment. Anticancer Drugs 2004;15(4):401–404.
17. Madhavan S, Northfelt DW. Lack of vesicant injury following extravasation of liposomal doxorubicin. J Natl Cancer Inst 1995;87(20):1556–1557.
18. Lokich J. Doxil extravasation injury: a case report. Ann Oncol 1999;10(6): 735–736.
19. Khan MS, Holmes JD. Reducing the morbidity from extravasation injuries. Ann Plast Surg 2002;48(6):628–632.
20. Hansen DL, Mathes SJ. Problem wounds and principles of closure. In: Mathes SJ, (ed.), *Plastic surgery*. Philadelphia: Elsevier; 2006:901–1030.

21. Schulmeister L, Camp-Sorrell D. Chemotherapy extravasation from implanted ports. [see comment]. Oncol Nurs Forum 2000;27(3):531–538.
22. Lokich JJ, Moore C. Drug extravasation in cancer chemotherapy. Ann Intern Med 1986;104(1):124.
23. Heitmann C, Durmus C, Ingianni G. Surgical management after doxorubicin and epirubicin extravasation. [see comment]. J Hand Surg Br 1998;23(5): 666–668.
24. Anderson CM, Walters RS, Hortobagyi GN. Mediastinitis related to probable central vinblastine extravasation in a woman undergoing adjuvant chemotherapy for early breast cancer. Am J Clin Oncol 1996;19(6):566–568.
25. Bach F, Videbaek C, Holst-Christensen J, Boesby S. Cytostatic extravasation. A serious complication of long-term venous access. Cancer 1991;68(3): 538–539.
26. Bozkurt AK, Uzel B, Akman C, Ozguroglu M, Molinas Mandel N. Intrathoracic extravasation of antineoplastic agents: case report and systematic review. Am J Clin Oncol 2003;26(2):121–123.
27. Banerjee A, Brotherston TM, Lamberty BG, Campbell RC. Cancer chemotherapy agent-induced perivenous extravasation injuries. Postgrad Med J 1987;63(735):5–9.
28. Anonymous. Suggestions to prevent and manage chemotherapy extravasation. Oncology 1993;7(9):42.
29. Larson DL. What is the appropriate management of tissue extravasation by antitumor agents? Plast Reconstr Surg 1985;75(3):397–405.
30. Pattison J. Managing cytotoxic extravasation. Nurs Times 2002;98(44): 32–34.
31. Birdsall C, Naliboff AR. How do you manage chemotherapy extravasation? Am J Nurs 1988;88(2):228–230.
32. Bertelli G, Gozza A, Forno GB, et al. Topical dimethylsulfoxide for the prevention of soft tissue injury after extravasation of vesicant cytotoxic drugs: a prospective clinical study. J Clin Oncol 1995;13(11):2851–2855.
33. Sommer NZ, Bayati S, Neumeister M, Brown RE. Dapsone for the treatment of doxorubicin extravasation injury in the rat. Plast Reconstr Surg 2000; 109(6):2000–2005.
34. Olver IN, Aisner J, Hament A, Buchanan L, Bishop JF, Kaplan RS. A prospective study of topical dimethyl sulfoxide for treating anthracycline extravasation. J Clin Oncol 1988;6(11):1732–1735.
35. Bos AM, van der Graaf WT, Willemse PH. A new conservative approach to extravasation of anthracyclines with dimethylsulfoxide and dexrazoxane. Acta Oncol 2001;40(4):541–542.
36. El-Saghir N, Otrock Z, Mufarrij A, et al. Dexrazoxane for anthracycline extravasation and GM-CSF for skin ulceration and wound healing. Lancet Oncol 2004;5(5):320–321.
37. Andersson AP, Dahlstrom KK. Clinical results after doxorubicin extravasation treated with excision guided by fluorescence microscopy. Eur J Cancer 1993;29A:1712–1714.
38. Yama N, Tsuchida Y, Nuka S, et al. Usefulness of magnetic resonance imaging for surgical management of extravasation of an antitumor agent: a case report. Jpn J Clin Oncol 2001;31(3):122–124.
39. Gault DT. Extravasation injuries. Br J Plast Surg 1993;46(2):91–96.
40. Yilmaz M, Demirdover C, Mola F. Treatment options in extravasation injury: an experimental study in rats. Plast Reconstr Surg 2002;109(7):2418–2423.
41. Schwartsmann G, Sander EB, Vinholes J, et al. N-acetylcysteine protects skin lesion induced by local extravasation of doxorubicin in a rat model. Am J Pediatr Hematol Oncol 1992;14(3):280–281.

42. Langer SW, Sehested M, Jensen PB. Treatment of anthracycline extravasation with dexrazoxane. Clin Cancer Res 2000;6(9):3680–3686.
43. Peters LJ. Radiation therapy tolerance limits. For one or for all?—Janeway Lecture. Cancer 1996;77(11):2379–2385.
44. Stone HB, McBride WH, Coleman CN. Modifying normal tissue damage postirradiation. Report of a workshop sponsored by the Radiation Research Program, National Cancer Institute, Bethesda, Maryland, September 6–8, 2000. Radiat Res 2002;157(2):204–223.
45. Fisher JC. Introduction to radiation injury. Another silent epidemic. Clin Plast Surg 1993;20(3):431–433.
46. Trotti A, Byhardt R, Stetz J, et al. Common toxicity criteria: version 2.0. an improved reference for grading the acute effects of cancer treatment: impact on radiotherapy. Int J Radiat Oncol Biol Phys 2000;47(1):13–47.
47. Stone HB, Coleman CN, Anscher MS, McBride WH. Effects of radiation on normal tissue: consequences and mechanisms. Lancet Oncol 2003;4(9): 529–536.
48. Dorr W, Hendry JH. Consequential late effects in normal tissues. Radiother Oncol 2001;61(3):223–231.
49. Bernstein EF, Sullivan FJ, Mitchell JB, Salomon GD, Glatstein E. Biology of chronic radiation effect on tissues and wound healing. Clin Plast Surg 1993;20(3):435–453.
50. Denham JW, Hauer-Jensen M. The radiotherapeutic injury—a complex 'wound'. Radiother Oncol 2002;63(2):129–145.
51. Mendelsohn FA, Divino CM, Reis ED, Kerstein MD. Wound care after radiation therapy. Adv Skin Wound Care 2002;15(5):216–224.
52. Hall EJ. Do no harm—normal tissue effects. Acta Oncol 2001;40(8): 913–916.
53. De Naeyer B, De Meerleer G, Braems S, Vakaet L, Huys J. Collagen vascular diseases and radiation therapy: a critical review. Int J Radiat Oncol Biol Phys 1999;44(5):975–980.
54. Burns JL, Mancoll JS, Phillips LG. Impairments to wound healing. Clin Plast Surg 2003;30(1):47–56.
55. Miller SH, Rudolph R. Healing in the irradiated wound. Clin Plast Surg 1990;17(3):503–508.
56. Porock D, Nikoletti S, Kristjanson L. Management of radiation skin reactions: literature review and clinical application. Plast Surg Nurs 1999;19(4): 185–192.
57. Grdina DJ, Murley JS, Kataoka Y. Radioprotectants: current status and new directions. Oncology 2002;2:2–10.
58. Zamboni WA, Browder LK, Martinez J. Hyperbaric oxygen and wound healing. Clin Plast Surg 2003;30(1):67–75.
59. Mayer R, Hamilton-Farrell MR, van der Kleij AJ, et al. Hyperbaric oxygen and radiotherapy. Strahlenther Onkol 2005;181(2):113–123.
60. Neheman A, Nativ O, Moskovitz B, Melamed Y, Stein A. Hyperbaric oxygen therapy for radiation-induced haemorrhagic cystitis. BJU Int 2005;96(1):107–109.
61. Jones K, Evans AW, Bristow RG, Levin W. Treatment of radiation proctitis with hyperbaric oxygen. Radiother Oncol 2006;78(1):91–94.
62. Curi MM, Dib LL, Kowalski LP. Management of refractory osteoradionecrosis of the jaws with surgery and adjunctive hyperbaric oxygen therapy. Int J Oral Maxillofac Surg 2000;29(6):430–434.
63. Peleg M, Lopez EA. The treatment of osteoradionecrosis of the mandible: the case for hyperbaric oxygen and bone graft reconstruction. J Oral Maxillofac Surg 2006;64(6):956–960.

64. Ashamalla HL, Thom SR, Goldwein JW. Hyperbaric oxygen therapy for the treatment of radiation-induced sequelae in children. The University of Pennsylvania experience. Cancer 1996;77(11):2407–2412.
65. Arnold PG, Lovich SF, Pairolero PC. Muscle flaps in irradiated wounds: an account of 100 consecutive cases. Plast Reconstr Surg 1994;93(2): 324–327.
66. Bostwick J, Stevenson TR, Nahai F, Hester TR, Coleman JJ, Jurkiewicz MJ. Radiation to the breast. Complications amenable to surgical treatment. Ann Surg 1984;200(4):543–553.
67. Arnold PG, Pairolero PC. Chest-wall reconstruction: an account of 500 consecutive patients. Plast Reconstr Surg 1996;98(5):804–810.
68. Gebski V, Lagleva M, Keech A, Simes J, Langlands AO. Survival effects of postmastectomy adjuvant radiation therapy using biologically equivalent doses: a clinical perspective. J Natl Cancer Inst 2006;98(1):26–38.
69. Prosnitz LR, Marks LB. Postmastectomy radiotherapy: quality counts! J Natl Cancer Inst 2006;98(1):3–4.
70. Johansson S, Svensson H, Denekamp J. Timescale of evolution of late radiation injury after postoperative radiotherapy of breast cancer patients. Int J Radiat Oncol Biol Phys 2000;48(3):745–750.
71. Roychoudhuri R, Evans H, Robinson D, Moller H. Radiation-induced malignancies following radiotherapy for breast cancer. Br J Cancer 2004; 91(5):868–872.
72. Kronowitz SJ, Robb GL. Breast reconstruction with postmastectomy radiation therapy: current issues. Plast Reconstr Surg 2004;114(4):950–960.
73. Schechter NR, Strom EA, Perkins GH, et al. Immediate breast reconstruction can impact postmastectomy irradiation. Am J Clin Oncol 2005;28(5): 485–494.
74. Ascherman JA, Hanasono MM, Newman MI, Hughes DB. Implant reconstruction in breast cancer patients treated with radiation therapy. Plast Reconstr Surg 2006;117(2):359–365.
75. McCarthy CM, Pusic AL, Disa JJ, McCormick BL, Montgomery LL, Cordeiro PG. Unilateral postoperative chest wall radiotherapy in bilateral tissue expander/implant reconstruction patients: a prospective outcomes analysis. Plast Reconstr Surg 2005;116(6):1642–1647.
76. Halyard MY, McCombs KE, Wong WW, et al. Acute and chronic results of adjuvant radiotherapy after mastectomy and transverse rectus abdominis myocutaneous (TRAM) flap reconstruction for breast cancer. Am J Clin Oncol 2004;27(4):389–394.
77. Spear SL, Ducic I, Low M, Cuoco F. The effect of radiation on pedicled TRAM flap breast reconstruction: outcomes and implications. Plast Reconstr Surg 2005;115(1):84–95.
78. Kronowitz SJ, Hunt KK, Kuerer HM, et al. Delayed-immediate breast reconstruction. Plast Reconstr Surg 2004;113(6):1617–1628.
79. Vissink A, Burlage FR, Spijkervet FK, Jansma J, Coppes RP. Prevention and treatment of the consequences of head and neck radiotherapy. Crit Rev Oral Biol Med 2003;14(3):213–225.
80. McAleese JJ, Bishop KM, A'Hern R, Henk JM. Randomized phase II study of GM-CSF to reduce mucositis caused by accelerated radiotherapy of laryngeal cancer. Br J Radiol 2006;79(943):608–613.
81. Kahn ST, Johnstone PA. Management of xerostomia related to radiotherapy for head and neck cancer. Oncology (Williston Park) 2005;19(14):1827–1832.
82. Trotti A. Toxicity in head and neck cancer: a review of trends and issues. Int J Radiat Oncol Biol Phys 2000;47(1):1–12.

83. Schwartz HC, Kagan AR. Osteoradionecrosis of the mandible: scientific basis for clinical staging. Am J Clin Oncol 2002;25(2):168–171.
84. Reuther T, Schuster T, Mende U, Kubler A. Osteoradionecrosis of the jaws as a side effect of radiotherapy of head and neck tumour patients—a report of a thirty year retrospective review. Int J Oral Maxillofac Surg 2003;32(3): 289–295.
85. Hao SP, Chen HC, Wei FC, Chen CY, Yeh AR, Su JL. Systematic management of osteoradionecrosis in the head and neck. Laryngoscope 1999;109(8): 1324–1327.
86. Kobayashi W, Kobayashi M, Nakayama K, Hirota W, Kimura H. Free omental transfer for osteoradionecrosis of the mandible. Int J Oral Maxillofac Surg 2000;29(3):201–206.
87. Bengtson BP, Schusterman MA, Baldwin BJ, et al. Influence of prior radiotherapy on the development of postoperative complications and success of free tissue transfers in head and neck cancer reconstruction. Am J Surg 1993;166(4):326–330.

Index

Printed in Germany